BONE

Evolution of Bone-Body Fluid Continuum

The diagram on the following pages illustrates the evolution of the physiologic function of skeletal tissue, the changes in the chemical composition of the fluids of the body, and the mechanisms of calcium homeostasis.

In the cyclostomes, the ancestors of the most primitive marine vertebrates, the concentrations in mg/100 ml of serum calcium are 50 per cent lower than the concentrations of calcium in the marine invertebrates and 50 per cent lower than in sea water; calcium homeostasis is maintained by membrane phenomena and protein binding of metal ions. In the elasmobranchs, the concentrations of calcium in the serum are lower than in the cyclostomes, but calcium homeostasis is maintained not only by membrane phenomena but also by deposits of apatite in calcified cartilage in the endoskeleton. In the teleosts, the concentrations of calcium are 25 per cent of that of sea water, and bone cells and vitamin D function as specialized agencies of calcium homeostasis. In the sturgeon, a chondrostean with very little bone tissue in the endoskeleton, the serum calcium is lower than in any other vertebrate, frequently less than 9 mg/100 ml. In the amphibians and all higher terrestrial vertebrates, parathyroid glands evolved to provide fine regulation; parathyroids operate through a negative feedback mechanism that controls calcium ion concentration in the fluids of the body.

EVOLUTION OF BONE-

CLASS	SKELETON	ION REGULATION	TOTAL SERUM CALCIUM mg/100ml	ION CONCE TRATI mmols/L
Mammalia	bone cells	↑	↑	↑
Aves	bone cells			
Reptilia	bone cells			
Amphibia	bone cells	Parathyroid glands + vitamin D	9	280
Teleostei	acellular & cellular bone	Vitamin D + apatite + membrane phenomena	10	300
Marine Elasmobranchii	calcified cartilage	Apatite + membrane phenomena	20	900
Marine Proto-Vertebrates	cartilage	Membrane phenomena + tissue proteins	24	1200
Marine Invertebrates	connective tissue	Membrane phenomena + tissue proteins	40	1200
Sea Water		Primeval seas	44	1200

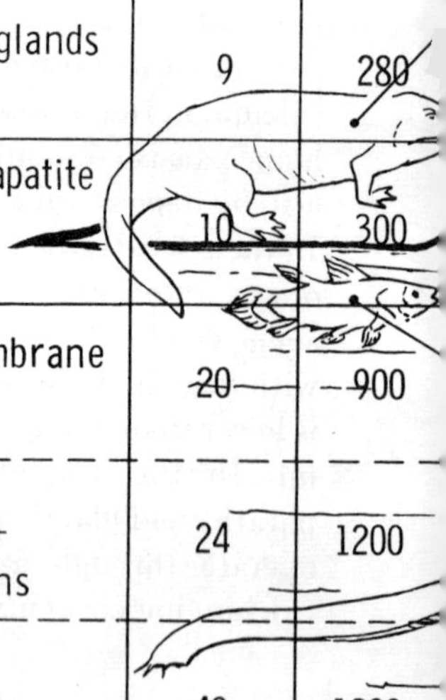

DY FLUID CONTINUUM

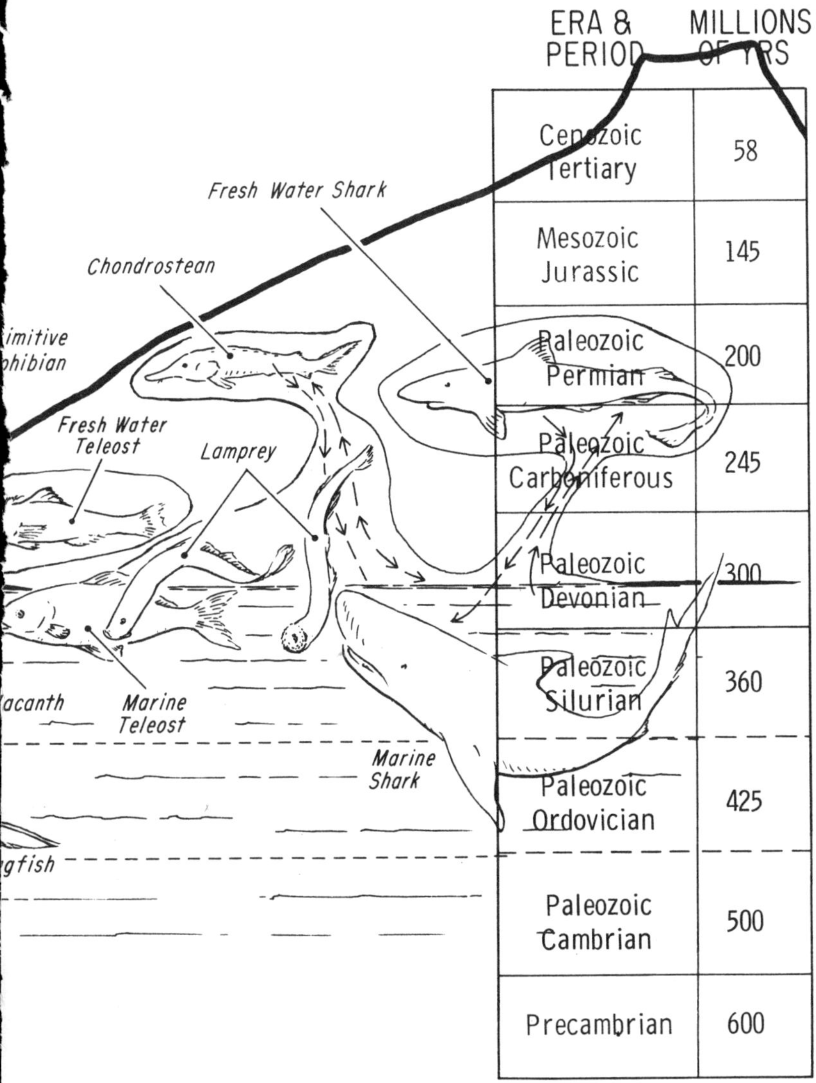

ERA & PERIOD
MILLIONS OF YRS
Cenozoic Tertiary
58
Mesozoic Jurassic
145
Paleozoic Permian
200
Paleozoic Carboniferous
245
Paleozoic Devonian
300
Paleozoic Silurian
360
Paleozoic Ordovician
425
Paleozoic Cambrian
500
Precambrian
600
Fresh Water Shark
Chondrostean
imitive
phibian
Fresh Water Teleost
Lamprey
acanth
Marine Teleost
Marine Shark
gfish

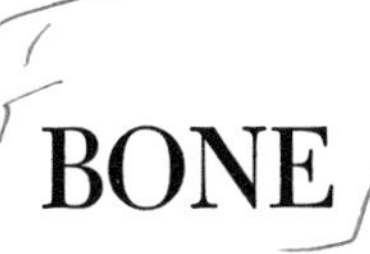

BONE

Fundamentals of the Physiology of Skeletal Tissue

THIRD EDITION
REVISED AND ENLARGED

BY
FRANKLIN C. McLEAN
AND
MARSHALL R. URIST

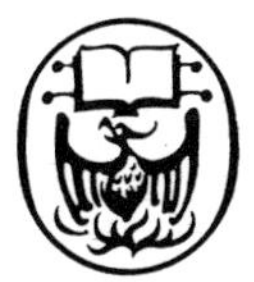

THE UNIVERSITY OF CHICAGO PRESS
CHICAGO & LONDON

THE UNIVERSITY OF CHICAGO PRESS, CHICAGO 60637
The University of Chicago Press, Ltd., London

 Published 1955. Second Edition 1961. Third Edition 1968 Second Impression 1973. Printed in the United States of America

International Standard Book Number: 0–226–56073–2
Library of Congress Catalog Card Number: 68–16703

Foreword

As recorded in the Foreword to the first edition of this book, published in 1955, its origin goes back to our association with A. Baird Hastings and later with William Bloom, beginning about thirty-five years ago. It was largely due to their stimulus and guidance that our interest was directed first to calcium metabolism, and then to all aspects of the physiology of bone.

In the thirteen years since the first edition appeared there has been rapid progress in many aspects of the subject matter of this book, as there has been in most branches of medical science. In reflecting this progress the third edition represents an extensive revision, amounting, for the most part, to a complete rewriting. The previous organization, however, has been retained, and an entirely new, final chapter entitled "Evolution of Bone" has been added. The literature with which the book deals has been much expanded, and this has meant a material increase in the size of the book and in the number of illustrations. The subtitle of the book has been changed to *Fundamentals of the Physiology of Skeletal Tissue*, which is more descriptive of its contents.

Acknowledgment is again made to the Josiah Macy, Jr. Foundation, which supported much of our early work and also influenced its direction through the Macy Foundation Conferences, which were also largely responsible for the establishment and popularity of the Gordon Research Conferences on the Chemistry, Physiology, and Structure of Bones and Teeth, which have been held annually since 1954. In many respects this book reflects the advances reported to the Gordon Research Conferences, of which there exists no other record. We owe much to those who have collaborated with one or both of us, directly or indirectly, over the years. Their names appear frequently in the bibliography, and it is not possible to mention them individually here. It is also impossible to acknowledge our debt to the many who have contributed by their published work, by their stimulus in discussion, and by their aid in formulating the statements of fact and of opinion expressed herein.

Work in our laboratories has been supported from many sources, and specific acknowledgment is made in individual publications. It is appropriate that special mention be made here of the National Institute of Arthritis and Metabolism, and the National Institute of Dental Research, both of the National Institutes of Health of the United States Public Health Service. Other federal agencies that have contributed substantially include the United States Atomic Energy Commission, the United States Army Medical Research and Development Command, and the Office of Naval Research. Non-governmental agencies that have given support include the Ayerst Laboratories, Inc., the Squibb Institute for Medical Research, The Easter Seal Research Foundation of the National Society for Crippled Children and Adults, and the Southern California Chapter of the Arthritis and Rheumatism Foundation.

More than to any other person we owe a debt of gratitude to Dr. Ann Marie Budy, now of the Department of Medicine of the University of Hawaii. She has been associated with us throughout, and has made major contributions to the work in our laboratories, as well as to the planning and actual writing of this book. It is not too much to say that the book appears in print largely because of her help in bringing it through three editions.

FRANKLIN C. MCLEAN
MARSHALL R. URIST

CHICAGO, ILLINOIS
LOS ANGELES, CALIFORNIA

Table of Contents

Illustrations

Tables

CHAPTER I

Introduction

By whatever pathway one comes to the study of bone, one finds oneself in the midst of a complex system of structure and function on the macroscopic, microscopic, and ultramicroscopic levels, with numerous and varied chemical and physiologic interrelations. These furnish the subject matter of the physiology and biochemistry of bone, to which this is directed. The approach is multidisciplinary. Morphology, experimental embryology, histochemistry, enzyme chemistry, crystallography, electron microscopy—to mention only a few—have all been brought to bear on the problems of bone.

This book is concerned with bone as a tissue rather than with its mechanical function in providing the skeletal support of the body or with the shape, adaptation, or development of individual bones. Bone, far from being passive and inert, has a complicated physiology of its own and presents a series of challenges to all the medical sciences. The intent has been to bridge the gaps remaining between the various disciplines and to contribute to the unification of the subject. That this requires the use of the vocabularies of many branches of science is inevitable.

This is not intended as a full-scale monograph on the physiology of bone. Historical treatment is reduced to a minimum; documentation is limited; illustrations are few. On the other hand, the text provides an extended treatment of the current state of the literature. The authors are naturally most familiar with their own work and that of their collaborators, but these contributions have not been overemphasized.

Although there is a logical sequence in the arrangement of the chapters and the material has been developed accordingly, each chapter is intended to stand by itself, to be read and understood independently by those especially interested. To this end there is a minimum of cross-references between chapters; where the need for these is felt, the Table of Contents should serve the purpose. This method of treatment necessarily results in a certain amount of repetition; where the same subject appears in different chapters, the attempt has been to furnish a fresh point of view in each instance.

This book is to complement the many clinical treatises on bone. Few of the pathologic conditions of unknown etiology and none of the tumors of bone are considered here. Disorders of metabolism are treated from the standpoint of pathologic physiology rather than of diagnosis and treatment. The chapter on healing of fractures presents knowledge that can be applied to practical use in clinical work. It is incidental, however, to the results of research on the physiology of bone, a field of endeavor in its own right. This book is written for an audience to include those desiring both a broad acquaintance with the skeletal system and a deep insight into its fundamental problems.

CHAPTER II

Bone as a Tissue

Bone is a highly specialized form of connective tissue, composed of interconnected cells in an intercellular substance and forming the skeleton or framework of the bodies of most vertebrates. Certain characteristics differentiate it from other forms of connective tissue, of which there are many types; the most striking difference is that bone is hard. This hardness results from deposition, within a soft organic matrix, of a complex mineral substance, composed chiefly of calcium, phosphate, carbonate, and citrate. Bone has cells peculiar to it; they are specialized forms derived from cells common to connective tissue.

The interstitial substance, in addition to being calcified, has a fibrillar structure similar to that of connective tissue; the fibers are mainly those of collagen; reticular fibers have also been demonstrated. The ground substance, as in connective tissue, is characterized in bone by its content of mucopolysaccharides. Connective tissue and bone have in common the important function of the support of organs or elements of organs.

Bone is also closely related to cartilage, another specialized form of connective tissue. Most of the embryonic skeleton is laid down first as models of hyaline cartilage, the cells of which hypertrophy and undergo changes in their chemical characteristics immediately prior to their replacement by bone. Part of the cartilage matrix remains, is calcified, and serves as the cores of trabeculae of bone. Following a fracture of a bone that was initially preformed in cartilage, cartilage and fibrocartilage appear in the first attempt at repair—the callus. In certain locations either tendon or calcified cartilage may be incorporated within bone and may undergo direct transformation to bone tissue.

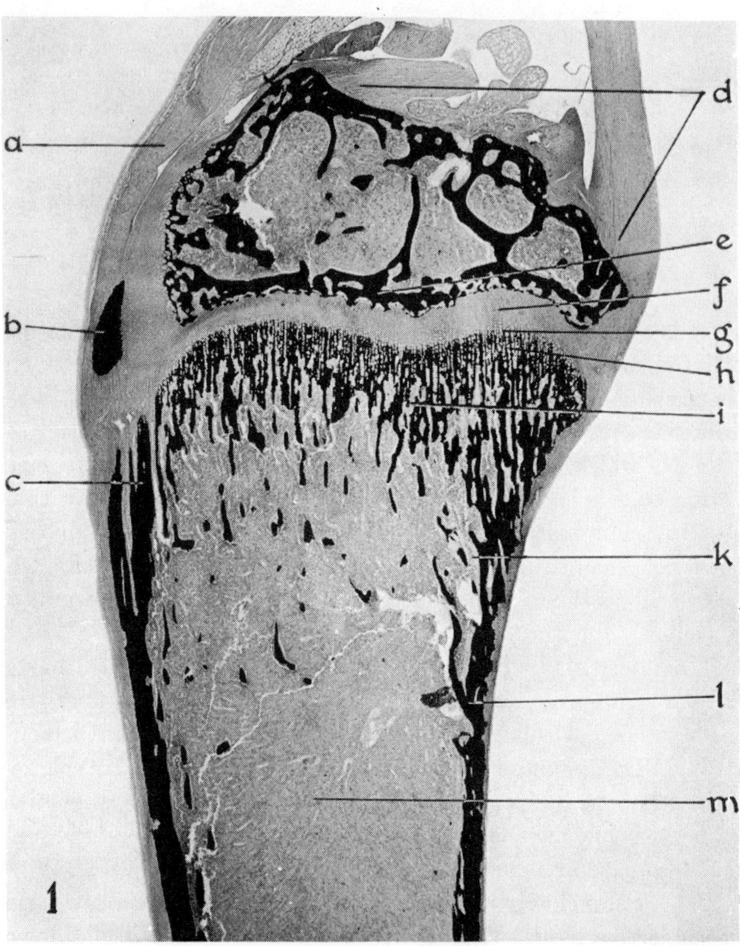

FIG. 1.—Sagittal section of head of tibia of normal rat. Cut, without decalcification, by method of McLean and Bloom and stained with silver nitrate (von Kóssa) to illustrate distribution of calcified tissues. Age 7 weeks, weaned to Bill's diet at 3 weeks. *a*, Patellar tendon; *b*, ossification center of anterior tibial tubercle; *c*, intratendinous ossification in insertion of patellar tendon; *d*, insertions of crucial ligaments; *e*, area in epiphysis where osteoid is frequently seen; *f*, epiphyseal cartilage plate; *g*, zone of hypertrophic cartilage and of provisional calcification; *h*, primary spongiosa; *i*, secondary spongiosa; *k*, area at junction of spongiosa with shaft, where osteoid is frequently seen; *l*, shaft; *m*, bone marrow. Silver nitrate–hematoxylin-eosin. ×10. (From original of Pl. 1, Fig. 1, McLean and Bloom, Anat. Rec. 78:855. Reproduced by courtesy of the publishers.)

Cells of Bone

Three cellular components of bone are associated with specific functions: *osteoblasts* with the formation of bone; *osteocytes* with the maintenance of bone as a living tissue; and *osteoclasts* with the resorption of bone. These three represent one cell type which changes its appearance as it carries out different functions. Such reversible morphologic changes are examples of *modulation,* in contrast with *differentiation,* a term limited to progressive, apparently nonreversible specialization in structure and function. In addition, bone and its membranes include other connective tissue cells with latent potencies for forming the cells of bone under appropriate stimulation. This *osteogenic potency* may become activated during the normal growth of bone; as a result of experimental intervention; or following injury, as in the healing of fractures. When this occurs, the cells assume the forms and functions of the cells characteristic of bone. These *precursors* of the specialized cells of bone, when in a resting state, are present in the inner layer of the periosteum, where they are morphologically indistinguishable from fibroblasts, and in the bone marrow and endosteum as *reticular* or *endosteal cells.* They may also be present as undifferentiated *perivascular connective tissue cells* (fibroblast-like or spindle-shaped).

When such cells, sometimes referred to as *preosteoblasts* or *osteoprogenitor cells,* are changing into osteoblasts, they undergo mitosis and may then be identified by their uptake of tritiated thymidine, as demonstrated by autoradiography; they are also recognizable by their specific morphologic changes as they become osteoblasts, osteocytes, or osteoclasts. The transformation of these cells from one type to another, which occurs spontaneously more frequently in developing bone, can be demonstrated in adult bone under certain conditions. The most striking of such responses are seen during the healing of fractures, in hyperparathyroidism, or in the bird or the mouse under the influence of estrogens.

Osteoblasts. These appear on the surface of a growing or developing bone. During active growth they appear to be in a continuous layer, frequently connected with one another by thin cytoplasmic processes. They are cuboidal in shape, with a breadth of 15–20 microns. The cytoplasm is intensely basophilic, owing to its content of ribonucleic acid (RNA). The typical morphologic characteristics are absent or unrecognizable when the particular structure with which they have been associated is in a resting state. The osteoblasts then become spindle-shaped and resemble fibroblasts or reticular cells.

With histochemical techniques, the presence of granules staining by the Hotchkiss procedure (periodic acid-Schiff reaction; PAS-positive) can be demonstrated in the osteoblast when new bone is forming. These granules disappear when the osteoblast assumes the spindle form. Alkaline phosphatase is present in the cytoplasm of the osteoblast; the amount depends largely upon the state of development and the functional activity of the cell.

Electron microscopy has added new opportunities for exploration of the *cytoplasmic structure* of cells, permitting much higher magnification, with correspondingly improved resolution, than is afforded by the light microscope. Dimensions may now be expressed in terms of angstrom units (A), to supplement microns (μ); electron microscopes with resolving power of 15 A for biologic materials are now readily available. Of special interest in observation of the cells peculiar to bone are the *plasma membrane* (cell membrane); the *endoplasmic reticulum,* a highly characteristic system of canals and saclike structures, especially prominent in cells engaged in the synthesis of proteins; *ribosomes,* which are accumulations of electron-dense granules of ribonucleoprotein (RNP) about 150 μ in diameter, the presence or absence of which, on the surfaces of the endoplasmic reticulum, defines the difference between *granular reticulum* and *agranular reticulum;* the *Golgi complex,* or the electron microscope analog of the juxtanuclear vacuole area, which consists of vacuoles concentrating a secretory product, vesicles, and agranular membranes (i.e., without ribosomes); *lysosomes,* so named because of their content of hydrolytic enzymes; *mitochondria,* the power plants of the cells, with an internal structure characterized by internal lamellae (*cristae*)*;* and a variety of *inclusions,* which may be temporary constituents of the cell associated with the cell products, such as *secretory granules.* All these components of the cytoplasm are formed or surrounded by membranes; the membrane system is a network of cavities that has led to its designation as a *vacuolar system,* including membrane-bound tubules, vesicles, and flat sacs, or *cisternae,* that show frequent intercommunications.

The characteristics of osteoblasts that can be seen under the light microscope have their counterparts in electron micrographs, which also reveal details of ultramicroscopic structure. The basophilic cytoplasm and the Golgi complex are represented respectively by the rough- and smooth-surfaced membranes of the endoplasmic reticulum, denoting the presence or absence of *ribosomes*. Such membranes are striking features of these cells, and are found in greater profusion than in other fibrogenic cells (Fig. 2). The particles of ribosomes that cover the outer aspect of the membranes

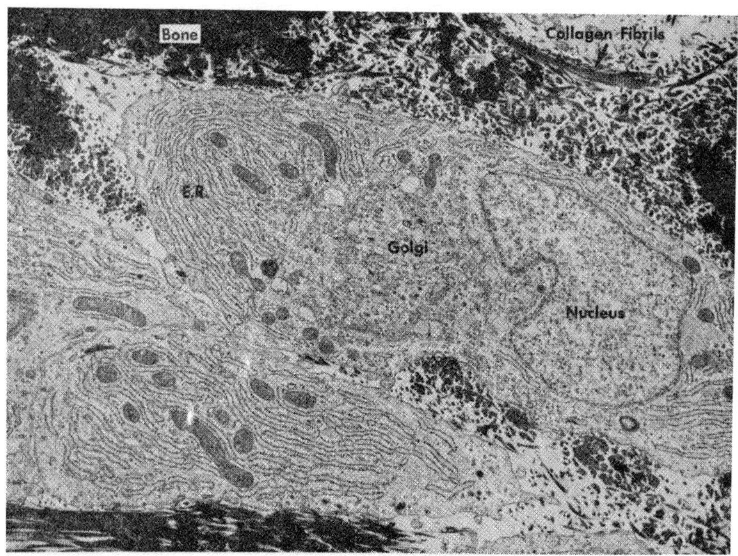

Fig. 2.—Electron micrograph of an osteoblast. Parts of three cells are visible. The central cell nucleus, juxtanuclear vacuole (Golgi apparatus), endoplasmic reticulum, and mitochondria are clearly visible. ×6,560. (Reproduced by courtesy of B. Boothroyd, University of Liverpool.)

are very numerous and appear to be arranged in rows; in sections that run tangentially to the cisternae, the particles are in spirals. Within the cisternae there is material that may have a granular or a fibrillar appearance.

Mitochondria are numerous in the cytoplasm of osteoblasts of actively growing bone. They are usually round or oval in shape, but may be elongated and branched. They have the characteristic double-membrane structure, although the cristae are less regular than those seen in other cells. Lipid droplets and objects that may be lysosomes or secretory granules may be found in small numbers in the cytoplasm. The plasma membrane is continuous, though sometimes indistinct. Small processes extend from the surfaces of the cells and may mingle with those of other osteoblasts; commonly larger processes too extend into the forming matrix.

Osteocytes. The osteocyte is an osteoblast that has been surrounded by calcified interstitial substance. The cells are now enclosed within lacunae, and the cytoplasmic processes extend through apertures of the lacunae into canalicules in the bone. Like the osteoblast, the osteocyte undergoes transformations; it may assume the form of an osteoclast or of a reticular cell. PAS-positive granules have also been demonstrated in osteocytes; those in newly formed bone matrix contain many granules, whereas those in quiescent bone have few. The osteocytes are rich in glycogen; the cytoplasm is faintly basophilic.

In electron micrographs the osteocytes show much the same characteristics as osteoblasts, but the endoplasmic reticulum may not be so profuse. The nuclei are also similar to those of osteoblasts. Osteocytes have processes that extend into the canalicules in the surrounding matrix for some distance. These processes are surrounded by nonmineralized intralacunar matrix. How far these cytoplasmic processes extend into the bone canalicules in adult mammals has not been determined. The osteocyte itself, by its fine structure and relationship with the intralacunar matrix, seems to be engaged not only in the maintenance of the open pathways in bone, but also in the transport mechanism by which transfer of materials from blood to bone and from bone to blood is accomplished (Fig. 3).

There is increasing evidence, beginning with the paper of Heller-Steinberg (1951), that the osteocytes exert an influence on the bone tissue surrounding the lacunae, resulting in increased reactivity of the bone mineral, with *osteolysis*, defined by Bélanger (1965) as an active physiologic phenomenon taking place within the intimacy of the bone under the influence of the osteocytes, whereby bone matrix is modified and bone salt is lost. A current opinion holds that the osteocytes thus play a role in the release of mineral from bone to blood, and hence in the homeostatic regulation of the concentration of calcium in the fluids of the body.

Osteoclasts. The osteoclast is a giant cell with a variable number of nuclei, often as many as fifteen or twenty. The nuclei resemble

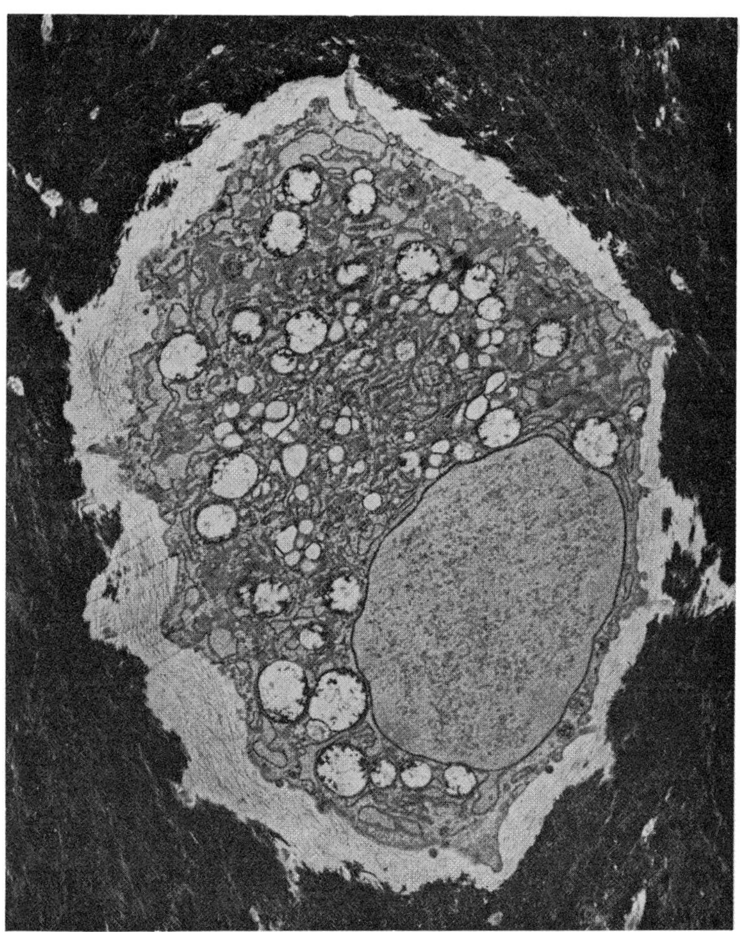

FIG. 3.—Electron micrograph of an osteocyte from a young mouse. Specimen was fixed in permanganate and sectioned without demineralization, stained with lead acetate. An abundance of cytoplasmic organelles is evident. A relatively thick layer of unmineralized intralacunar matrix separates the cell from the mineralized matrix. The interlacunar matrix contains collagen fibrils and an amorphous interfibrillar material. ×2,460. (From original of Fig. 4, Wassermann and Yaeger, Z. Zellforsch. 67:641. Reproduced by courtesy of the publishers.)

those of osteoblasts and osteocytes; the cytoplasm is often foamy; the cell has extensile processes. These cells may arise from precursor cells in the stroma of the bone marrow, or they may represent fused osteoblasts and may also include fused osteocytes liberated from resorbing bone. They are usually found on the surfaces of bone, in close relationship with areas of resorption, and frequently lie in grooves, known as Howship's lacunae. This suggests that the

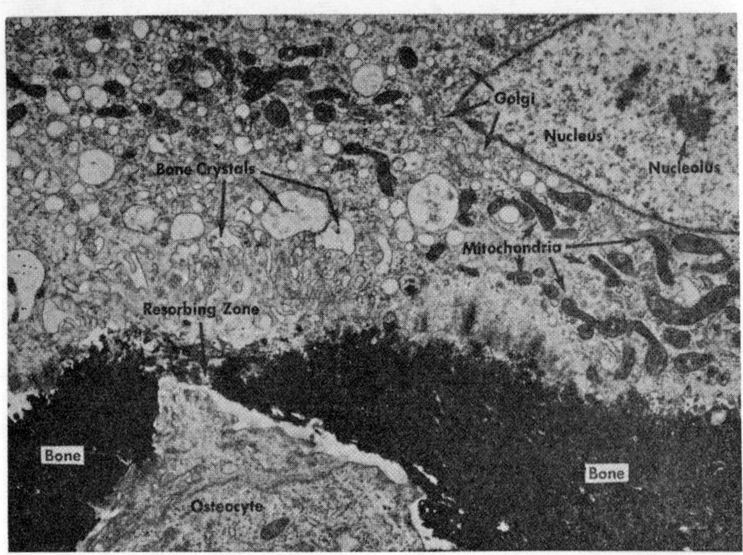

Fig. 4.—Electron micrograph of an osteoclast resorbing bone. Golgi vacuoles are near the nucleus. Bone crystals are in vesicles at the resorbing site. There are no positively identified lysosomes. The cell underneath the resorbing site is an osteocyte. ×6,560. (Reproduced by courtesy of B. Boothroyd, University of Liverpool.)

lacunae were formed by an erosive action of the overlying osteoclasts. For many years the osteoclasts have been considered to play the principal role in the resorption of bone. In the growth and reformation of trabeculae of spongy bone in rapidly growing animals they are commonly seen enveloping the tip of each spicule of bone undergoing resorption.

PAS-positive granules have been demonstrated in osteoclasts and are indistinguishable from those observed in osteoblasts and osteocytes. A brush border, appearing in fixed preparations between the osteoclast and the underlying surface of bone, is now interpreted by some to correspond with a very active ruffled and undulating membrane, seen in time-lapse motion pictures of bone undergoing resorption in tissue culture. Like the osteoblast and osteocyte, the osteoclast can transform into reticular cells.

In electron micrographs the plasma membrane of osteoclasts follows a complicated pattern because of the many projections from the cytoplasm in contact with resorbing bone; this constitutes the brush border. The projections may be finger-like or in folds with the spaces between them extending varying distances into the cytoplasm. Other parts of the plasma membrane, not in contact with bone undergoing resorption, are relatively smooth (Fig. 4).

There are many vacuoles in osteoclasts. The larger ones may be several microns in diameter. There tends to be an array of them close to the brush border. Within some of the vacuoles apatite crystals may be seen; they are believed to be taken up by invagination of fluid through the plasma membrane, by a process designated as *pinocytosis*. Osteoclasts appear to have a greater number of mitochondria in a given volume of cytoplasm than can be seen in osteoblasts; this affords some indication of relative cellular activity. They are spread throughout most of the cytoplasm, and under certain conditions may be packed with an amorphous aggregation of calcium and phosphate.

Interstitial Substance

The intercellular portion of bone is a calcified collagenous substance that makes up the great mass of bone. In ordinary sections this appears to be homogeneous, but with special techniques and staining methods collagenous fibers may be demonstrated. The interstitial substance includes the organic framework or matrix, the inorganic part or the mineral of bone, and water. The organic matrix has two chief components—the collagenous fibers and the ground substance.

Membranes of Bone

Periosteum. Except in certain locations, such as the neck of the femur, the patella, and intracapsular joint surfaces, the connective tissue surrounding bone is a specialized membrane, the periosteum. In the young animal, especially in the regions of rapid growth, this consists of an outer dense layer of collagenous fibers and fibroblasts and an inner looser layer of osteoblasts and their precursor cells. In the quiescent state, in the adult, the periosteum serves for the attachment of tendons and carries blood vessels, lymphatics, and nerves. The inner layer retains its osteogenic potency and in fractures is activated to form osteoblasts and new bone.

Endosteum. The endosteum is a thin layer of reticular cells, lining the walls of the bone marrow cavities and of the haversian canals of compact bone and covering trabeculae of cancellous bone. It is a condensed peripheral layer of the stroma of the bone marrow and has both osteogenic and hemopoietic potencies; like the periosteum, it takes an active part in the healing of fractures.

Bone Marrow

Many of the cellular elements seen in loose connective tissue are absent from bone tissue, but their counterparts are seen in large numbers in the stroma of the bone marrow. The bone marrow, although more commonly thought of in relation to its hemopoietic functions, also participates actively in osteogenesis. The reticular cells of the stroma of the bone marrow can display osteogenic activity and undergo transformation into the cells of bone. Similarly, the cells characteristic of bone, when no longer called upon to perform their specific functions, may disappear into the stroma as reticular cells.

Mast Cells in Bone

Mast cells are normally found in large numbers in bone marrow and in loose connective tissue throughout the body. Their large cytoplasmic granules stain metachromatically with basic aniline dyes. They are associated with storage of heparin, histamine, and hyaluronic acid. Mast cells can be made to accumulate in the bones of rats by feeding a diet deficient in calcium and in vitamin D or by inducing other conditions of stress. These cells gather on the surfaces of, within, or under the endosteum when the animal stops growing (Fig. 5).

Blood Vessels of Bone

The vascular anatomy of the skeleton has a characteristic pattern closely related to the functions of bone. The total blood supply to individual bones, together with the corresponding venous drainage, is readily studied by existing methods; the differences in the descriptions in the literature are largely attributable to species differences, to age, and to variations in the patterns exhibited by different bones in the skeleton of the same animal.

Cancellous bone has arteries entering from all sides that branch until they become oriented to each marrow space formed by the individual trabeculae. The smaller subdivisions thus formed are arterioles with definite muscular walls. The thin-walled capillaries or sinuses are seen about the individual trabeculae, or they abut against them, with nutritive exchange apparently occurring at this level. It is difficult to demonstrate where the sinuses of capillaries end and where venous drainage begins. Intraosseous veins are ex-

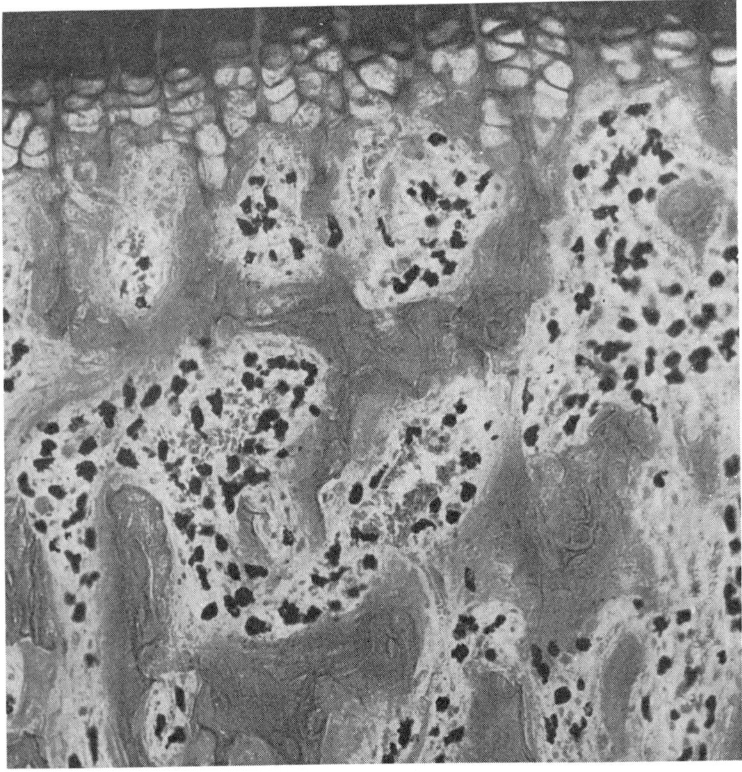

FIG. 5.—Sagittal section of upper end of tibia of a rat, 8 weeks of age, reared on a calcium-deficient diet for four and one-half weeks. Deeply staining mast cells within and upon the endosteal lining of bone trabeculae of spongiosa. Hematoxylin-eosin-azure II. ×160.

tremely thin-walled structures, which enlarge and become spatially arranged, generally parallel to small arteries, and finally exit at the points where the arterial supply enters cancellous bone. On gaining the exterior of the bone, the vein has a thin but discernible wall and is easily differentiated from its accompanying artery.

The blood supply of a long bone comes from three sources: (1) the nutrient artery, (2) the periosteal arteries, and (3) the epiphyseal arteries. The nutrient artery perforates the bone obliquely through the shaft and divides into ascending and descending branches. Each branch arborizes to reach the endosteum, the metaphyses, and the epiphyseal plates.

The periosteum has a rich blood supply, consisting of small arteries and veins, forming a continuous vascular network that ensheaths the bone. The number of periosteal vessels is relatively small in the center of the shaft but adds up to hundreds at the metaphyseal ends of the bone. They are of large caliber and anastomose with the cortical branches of the nutrient artery. The periosteal blood supply is greatly increased when the medullary arterial supply is damaged. The medullary blood supply may increase when the periosteal supply is injured; this represents the collateral route.

The epiphyses are supplied by one to three main epiphyseal arteries, each coursing toward the center and then branching outward to supply a specific area of the spongiosa and articular surface. The epiphyseal plate is supplied by blood vessels from three sources: (1) perforating epiphyseal, (2) perforating metaphyseal, and (3) circumferential epiphyseal arteries.

In compact bone, except for an occasional blind ending, each haversian canal contains one or more blood vessels. Variations in the number from one to four are described, with some disagreement as to whether the number is commonly one, two, or three; again, species differences are not fully taken into account. In the rabbit and in the dog the haversian canal contains a single vessel, which is a simple endothelial tube. In human material the average number is two vessels per haversian canal. In most haversian canals, capillary-like vessels with simple endothelial walls are distinguished. In a few canals of the human tibia an arteriole is seen, with an accompanying venule.

The veins in bone are thin-walled structures; even those that accompany the nutrient artery have walls only two or three cells in thickness. The centrally placed nutrient vein or sinus in the human tibia accompanies the nutrient artery. In the rabbit tibia, there are differences in the venous pattern due to fusion of the tibia and fibula and also to variation in distribution of red marrow. The venous drainage of the epiphysis is by veins that parallel the arterial supply. That of the metaphysis is through a series of longitudinally

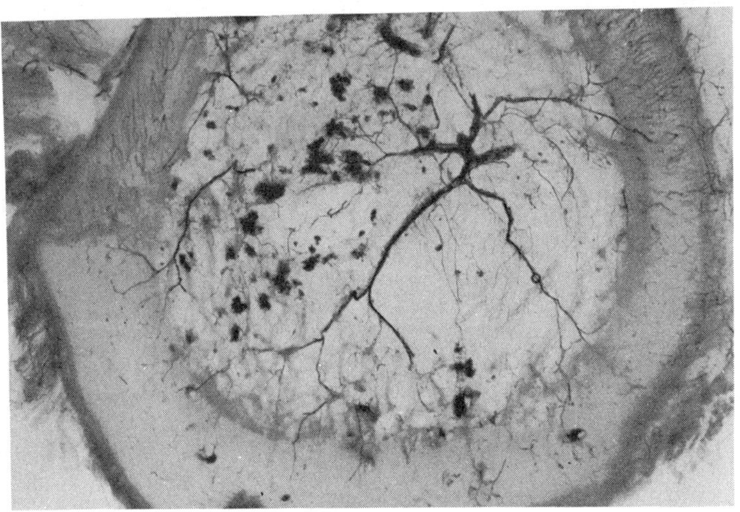

Fig. 6.—Cross-section through the mid-shaft of a human tibia, injected with India ink and cleared by the Spalteholz technique. Radial branches of the nutrient artery ramify in the cortex to supply the vessels of the haversian canals. ×5.25. (From original of Fig. 3-B, Nelson, Kelly, Peterson and Janes, J. Bone Jt. Surg. 42-A:629. Reproduced by courtesy of the publishers.)

arranged sinusoids into which the metaphyseal supply empties after it has coursed into the vessels growing up the columns of degenerating cartilage cells. These vessels drain primarily to the emerging metaphyseal veins.

Nerves of Bone

Combinations of morphologic and physiologic preparations are necessary to demonstrate the nerves of bone. The probability is that there are afferent nerves in the interior of a bone, as well as in the periosteum and endosteum. There is little doubt about the

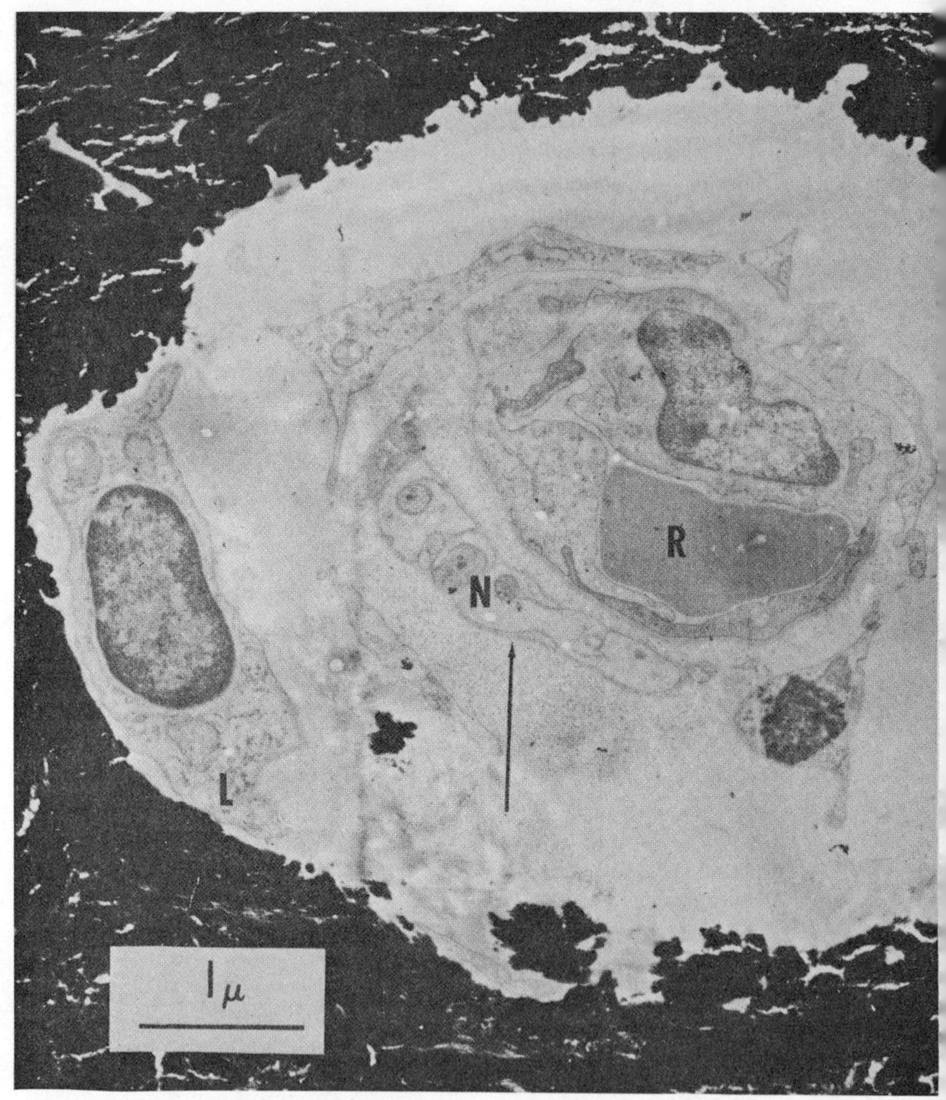

FIG. 7.—Haversian canal in a mature osteon of an adult dog. The lumen of the central capillary contains a portion of a red cell (*R*). An unmyelinated nerve (*N*) is enclosed by its basement membrane (arrow) and surrounded by endoneural collagen fibrils cut in cross-section. One lining cell (*L*) is seen. (From original of Fig. 2, Cooper, Milgram, and Robinson, J. Bone Jt. Surg. 48-A:1243. Reproduced by courtesy of the publishers.)

periosteum; it contains abundant myelinated and nonmyelinated nerve fibers ending in networks on the surfaces of the bone tissue. Some observers also see myelinated and nonmyelinated nerve fibers accompanying the blood vessels in the haversian canals. Myelinated nerves are numerous in the marrow and terminate in the endosteum as delicate fibrils running along the blood vessels.

Lymphatics of Bone

Lymphatic vessels in bone are more difficult to demonstrate by ordinary morphologic techniques than those in any other tissue. Particulate matter may be seen in lymphatic vessels in the periosteum, bone marrow, macrophages, and regional lymph nodes within a few minutes after instillation of India ink or dyes. The lymphatic vessels in the marrow-vascular-cell spaces of compact bone cannot be demonstrated by such means, however. Failure to demonstrate lymphatic vessels in either compact bone or bone marrow has been reported.

CHAPTER III

Histogenesis and Organization of Bone

Bone always arises, both in fetal and in postfetal life, by a transformation of connective tissue. Connective tissue is present throughout the body and assumes many forms. We are concerned with the connective tissue cells that may give rise to the cells of bone and with the interrelations between the cells of connective tissue and those of bone. The requirements for understanding these relationships are: (1) criteria for identification and designation of connective tissue cells, particularly those related to bone and its formation; and (2) a clear and consistent terminology for those cells referred to throughout this book.

Criteria for Designation of Connective Tissue Cells

Morphologic Criteria. Cells found in loose connective tissue—fibroblasts, macrophages, lymphoid wandering cells, mast cells, and plasma cells—are recognizable under the light microscope by their morphology and staining reactions alone. In certain other locations, as in tumors, inflammatory tissue, and perivascular connective tissue, recognition of *fibroblasts* may be difficult; complete characterization of these cells may require criteria other than morphologic. In the absence of definitive criteria, the use of purely descriptive terms, such as *spindle cells*, *spindle-shaped cells*, or *fibroblast-like cells*, is common.

Autoradiographic Criteria. Thymidine is used by the cell in premitosis for the synthesis of deoxyribonucleic acid (DNA). DNA does not undergo subsequent turnover, but when mitosis is complete the newly acquired thymidine is divided between the nuclei of the daughter cells. Tritiated thymidine (^{3}H-thymidine), being specifically incorporated into newly synthesized DNA, affords a label which is retained throughout the life of the cell and through subsequent stages of the cell cycle, and which may be detected by autoradiography. In cells of the bone series, DNA synthesis and mitosis, and consequently ^{3}H-thymidine uptake, are for the most part restricted to rapidly dividing and morphologically unspecialized cells of mesenchymal origin (spindle cells, reticular cells, osteogenic cells). Specialized bone cells (osteoblasts, osteocytes, osteoclasts) are derived from these precursor cells. By means of autoradioggaphy, following administration of ^{3}H-thymidine to the experimental animal, the sequence of the cell cycle is made available for histologic analysis.

Criteria of Location. Many cells, resembling fibroblasts in morphology, may be identified by their locations. Thus the outstretched cells of reticular connective tissue, including the stroma of the bone marrow, are known as *reticular cells.* Among the *perivascular connective tissue cells* are those with mesenchymal potencies, found in close relationship to the small blood vessels; they form the reservoir of *embryonic connective tissue* and preserve embryonic potencies. In the bone marrow, particularly in the zone of cartilage erosion, the perivascular connective tissue cells are reticular cells. Moreover, endosteal cells, associated with bone marrow as well as with bone tissue, represent a condensed layer of reticular cells. *Periosteal cells* form the deeper layer of the periosteum, sometimes called the *cambium layer;* unless participating in osteogenesis and recognizable as osteoblasts, they may be identified only by their location.

Criteria of Origin. All types of connective tissue derive from embryonic mesenchyme. Some *mesenchymal cells* persist in an undifferentiated form in the adult organism, with the capacity of differentiating into new cell types, such as *osteoblasts.* Connective tissue cells may arise in inflammatory processes, such as the reaction to transplants and to injury. The cells may be of local *histogenic* origin, arising from histiocytes (macrophages) or from lymphoid wandering cells; or *hematogenic,* arising from monocytes and also from lymphocytes. Connective tissue cells of inflammatory origin may differentiate into fibroblasts; it is still uncertain whether they may be transformed into the cells of bone.

Criteria of Function. The term *fibroblast* implies that the cell produces connective tissue fibers. Some histologists prefer to reserve the term for cells that have differentiated irreversibly and that, by definition, are not capable of transformation into the cells of bone. Others describe transformation into bone cells, as in ossification of the tendons of the turkey. The issue of the potencies of the fibroblast is frequently avoided by reference to spindle-shaped or fibroblast-like cells. *Reticular cells* are so named because of their intimate relationship with reticular fibers, which they are active in forming. Like the mesenchymal cells of the embryo, they may turn into all types of blood and connective tissue cells; reticular cells of the bone marrow have both hemopoietic and osteogenic potencies.

Criteria of Potencies. A cell with the capacity to transform into an osteoblast and to form bone has *osteogenic potency.* Such a potency is latent; when it manifests itself, either spontaneously or as a result of experimental intervention, the cell exhibits *osteogenic activity.* A reversible change in cellular activity is *modulation;* an irreversible change in potency is either a *differentiation* or *dedifferentiation.* In many instances it is not possible to ascribe specific potencies to cells without having observed the corresponding activities. Connective tissue cells with the capacity to undergo differentiation or modulation and to exhibit osteogenic or other specific activities are called *mesenchymal cells* in embryonic life. In postfetal life their nature is not always clear; some *perivascular connective tissue cells* have these potencies, as do the reticular cells in the bone marrow.

Terminology of Connective Tissue Cells

Precursors of the Cells of Bone. Many connective tissue cells, as identified below, possess osteogenic potency; under appropriate circumstances they are transformed, by differentiation, into the specialized cells of bone; they may therefore be grouped together as the precursors of the cells of bone, either actual or potential. For the most part the cells that will give rise to bone cells (osteoblasts, osteocytes, osteoclasts) are present as cell populations in growing bone, ordinarily in close relationship to osteoblasts in the periosteum, the endosteum, and the growth apparatus, of which the epiphyseal cartilage and the primary spongiosa of growing bone are essential parts. The cells of these populations have in common, in addition to their osteogenic potencies, a relatively rapid rate of proliferation by mitosis, and their identification is aided by the application of autoradiography following administration of ^{3}H-thymidine. Because of the qualities that characterize these cells, they have been designated by various authors as *osteogenic cells*, *preosteoblasts*, or *osteoprogenitor cells*.

Mesenchymal Cell. A *mesenchymal cell* is an embryonic connective tissue cell with an outstanding capacity for proliferation and the capability of further differentiation, as into reticular cells or osteoblasts. When persisting in the adult organism, these cells are usually arranged in loose connective tissue along the small blood vessels and as reticular cells in relation to reticular fibers. They are identified by location as well as by the capacity to differentiate into other cell types, such as into smooth muscle in the formation of new arteries in inflammatory processes, into phagocytes, and into bone.

Reticular Cell. The cell of reticular connective tissue, including the stroma of the bone marrow, where it retains both osteogenic and hemopoietic potencies, is called a *reticular cell*. It is identified by its location, morphology, potencies, and direct origin from mesenchymal cells.

Endosteal Cell. The endosteum is a condensation of the stroma of the bone marrow; its cells are reticular cells, identifiable as *endosteal cells* by their location.

Fibroblast. This is a spindle-shaped cell of the loose and dense connective tissue, with the capacity to form the fibers of these tissues. Opinion differs about the conditions under which it may form bone; we shall not refer to this cell as a precursor of bone cells.

Periosteal Cell. The outer layer of the periosteum is a network of dense connective tissue fibers and fibroblasts. Osteogenic potencies have not been demonstrated for this layer. The inner layer, sometimes called the *cambium layer*, is actively osteogenic during growth; in adult life its cells are identified only by their location and by activation of their osteogenic potencies after an injury.

Connective Tissue Cell. By far the greater number of cells of connective tissue are fibroblasts; these are of doubtful potency with respect to the formation of bone. Where we wish to imply that cells of connective tissue may still possess osteogenic potency, we shall use the general but noncommittal term *connective tissue cell*. When it seems desirable for purposes of clarity, we may further characterize these cells by such terms as *perivascular connective tissue cells*, *undifferentiated connective tissue cells*, or *young connective tissue cells*. At times we may also use the descriptive term *spindle-shaped cells*.

Origin of Bone

Under appropriate conditions, any of the foregoing connective tissue cells may assume the form of osteoblasts and play an active part in osteogenesis. It is useful to think in terms of a pool or population of cells, with osteogenic potencies and in locations where they may contribute to the formation of bone. Such cells may be part of a pool of undifferentiated mesenchymal cells which, depending on their environment, may differentiate in an osteogenic direction, or alternatively in some other direction. One may also conceive of: (1) a pool of mesenchymal cells which are multipotential; and, as a derivative of this pool, (2) a second cellular stage which is committed to osteogenesis and can no longer differentiate in another direction. This second possibility is analogous to the stem cell, or hemocytoblast, committed to the formation of blood cells, and in the case of bone may be thought of as the *stem cell* of the osteogenic cycle.

Once osteoblasts have formed, they produce collagenous fibers and deposit the ground substance of bone. As the interstitial substance surrounds them, they become osteocytes. As resorption occurs, osteoclasts appear in numbers, arising from either osteoblasts or osteocytes or directly from the precursors of the cells of bone. At any stage in these transformations the process may be reversed; the cells characteristic of bone are then no longer recognizable. They may assume the forms of the connective tissue cells from which they are derived, while still retaining their osteogenic potencies. Figure 8 illustrates the relationships of connective tissue cells to bone.

In summary, bone arises in embryonic life by differentiation of mesenchymal cells into osteoblasts; some of the mesenchymal cells may first transform into reticular cells of the bone marrow before becoming osteoblasts. In postfetal life the growth and reconstruction of bone occur mainly by osteogenic activity on the part of the precursors of bone cells, including reticular cells, periosteal cells, endosteal cells, and perivascular connective tissue cells; all of these cells assume the form of osteoblasts while engaged in osteogenesis.

In later chapters the postfetal osteogenesis that occurs in the healing of fractures or following transplants of skeletal tissues will be examined. It will be shown that, when bone is transplanted to a soft tissue, it may lead, by induction, to formation of bone by the connective tissue cells of the host, under the influence of the transplant. Under these conditions the cells that may engage in osteogenesis are the undifferentiated connective tissue cells of the host.

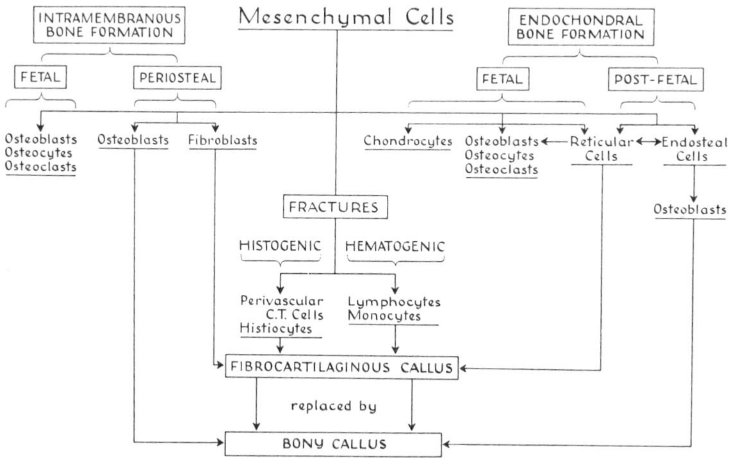

Fig. 8.—Diagram to illustrate origins and transformations of the cells participating in the histogenesis of bone and in the healing of fractures. All these cells are derived from mesenchyme and progress through different pathways in different locations. The repair of fractures depends upon the mobilization of a variety of cells, each contributing to the formation of the provisional fibrocartilaginous callus or to bony union.

In addition, histogenic and hematogenic cells of inflammatory origin may possibly participate in osteogenesis; whether this is the case is not proved. In the healing of a fracture the same reservoirs of connective tissue cells are available; to them are to be added the endosteal and periosteal cells in the fracture area. They are the first to form bone.

Formation of Bone

The formation of bone, particularly in the embryo, may be preceded by the laying-down of a cartilage model, or it may occur by direct transformation of connective tissue. When bone is formed in such a manner as to replace cartilage, either in embryonic or in postfetal life, the process is *endochondral* or *intracartilaginous ossification;* when the transformation is direct, without the presence of cartilage, this is *intramembranous ossification.* It is convenient to describe these two forms of ossification separately.

Bone is characterized by deposition of the bone mineral within an organic matrix. During development and growth this deposition proceeds both in the matrix of the cartilage model in advance of bone formation and in the bone matrix as it is laid down. Calcification will accordingly be described with the histogenesis of bone.

Intramembranous Ossification

Intramembranous formation of bone occurs in every part of the body—in the shafts of the long bones and in the continuous growth, internal reconstruction, and remodeling of every bone. In most vertebrates it is the only form of growth or reconstruction of bone that continues throughout life, after growth in length of the long bones has ceased.

Intramembranous ossification, in its earliest stages and in its least complicated form, is best seen in the formation of the embryonic calvarium. Here, in the places where bone is about to appear, the intercellular substance between the cells of the connective tissue, previously indistinguishable from other connective tissue, increases in amount and density. It assumes a more homogeneous appearance and becomes eosinophilic. Simultaneously, the connective tissue cells increase in size and assume the form of osteoblasts. At about the same time, beginning calcification in the matrix is first demonstrable with the von Kóssa stain. It is then seen as scattered granules of silver, associated with the interstitial tissue. The content of bone mineral of the newly formed matrix rapidly increases as the transformation to bone becomes complete.

Pommer (1885) introduced the concept of *physiological osteoid* as a necessary stage in the formation of bone by apposition. According to this concept, the first step is deposition of a noncalcified *preosseous* or *osteoid tissue;* calcification then follows, and bone is the result. McLean and Bloom (1940), utilizing sections of undecalcified bone stained with silver nitrate (von Kóssa) to demonstrate the bone mineral and observed with the light microscope, concluded that the matrix may be regarded as calcifiable as soon as the tissue is recognizable as bone, and that the delay sometimes observed in the deposit of mineral may be ascribed to a lag in the supply of the necessary materials. Observations with the electron microscope demonstrate that there is always a thin layer, one micron or less, of uncalcified preosseous tissue during the formation of bone, even in animals with an optimum intake of minerals; this layer is no longer

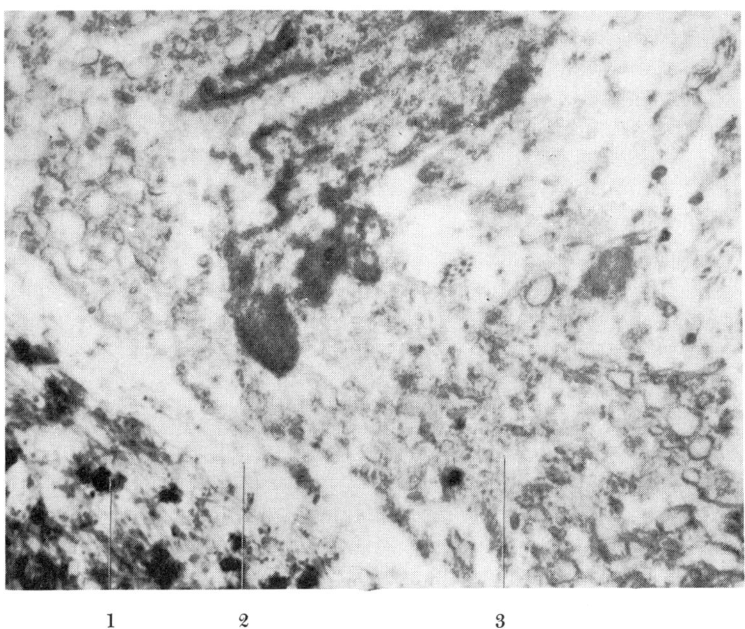

1 2 3

FIG. 9.—Electron micrograph of undecalcified tibia of a rat, fixed with osmic acid. *1*, Zone of calcification; *2*, preosseous tissue; *3*, cross-sections of fibers. (From original of Fig. 9, Knese and Knoop, Z. Zellforsch. 48:465. Reproduced by courtesy of the publishers.)

present after apposition of bone is complete in a given area. Whether this requires a return to the concept of physiologic osteoid, in the sense of Pommer, is a matter of opinion; certainly, the broad osteoid borders observed by him were indicative of a minimal rachitic state rather than of physiologic bone formation (Fig. 9).

INTRACARTILAGINOUS OSSIFICATION

Cartilage models of most of the bones of the skeleton are formed during embryonic life. Initially, these models are made up of hyaline cartilage, relatively free from glycogen, from phosphatase, and from the enzyme systems concerned in glycolysis. At a certain stage of embryonic life, characteristic of each bone in each species, the hyaline cartilage undergoes changes usually described as degenerative, and the cells enlarge. At this time, the hypertrophic cartilage cells accumulate glycogen, and the glycolytic enzymes and alkaline phosphatase appear.

The changes in the cartilage cells occur in certain locations destined to become the ossification centers for the shafts of the bones. As the cells undergo these changes, there is an ingrowth from the periosteum, in one or more places, of vascular mesenchyme. This penetrates the areas of hypertrophic cartilage cells and replaces them with primitive bone marrow, leaving only scattered, short fragments of matrix, upon which osseous tissue is deposited. The entire process of ossification in cartilage models begins in a relatively small number of foci, originating from the mesenchyme forming the perichondrium or periosteum. The mesenchymal cells have both osteogenic and hemopoietic potencies, and from these are formed the ossification centers of the bone and the primitive bone marrow.

From the ossification centers, replacement of cartilage by bone and primitive bone marrow extends centrifugally, until the marrow cavity is free of cartilage cells. Only fragments of cartilage matrix are left; some of the cartilage cells may survive and become osteoblasts. It has been customary to describe this replacement as invasion and erosion, as though the force behind it lies in the mesenchyme, driving it to destroy the cartilage. It is at least equally reasonable to assume that the sequence of events begins with the changes in the cartilage cells themselves and that the ingrowth of the mesenchyme is a response to these changes. In any case, the widespread replacement of cartilage is slowed down only as it approaches the portion of the model destined to form the epiphysis and the epiphyseal cartilage. Here the line of further growth of bone is established, and the replacement of cartilage continues in a more orderly fashion. Formation of the growth apparatus and growth in length of the long bones are thus a direct continuation of the intracartilaginous ossification within the embryonic cartilage model.

At the time that foci of hypertrophic cells are seen in the cartilage models of bone, or shortly thereafter, calcification of the cartilage matrix is demonstrable. In certain bones of the embryonic rat this calcification may begin before penetration by mesenchyme, so that the ingrowth from the periosteum is into an area in which calcification has already begun (Fig. 10). In the bones of larger animals calcification may not occur until penetration is under way, but it proceeds in advance of the invading tissue for at least the space of a few hypertrophied cells. In both cases, replacement of the embryonic cartilage model by bone is guided, just as it is later in the growth of bone, by a network of calcified cartilage matrix.

Also, at about the same time that the cartilage model is being penetrated, a thin layer of calcified subperiosteal bone is formed, encircling the shaft of the model and constituting the *periosteal collar.* Intramembranous formation of bone in this location continues by osteoblastic apposition, and calcification of the osseous tissue follows.

After the line of growth is established and at a time characteristic for each species and each bone, the cartilage forming the epiphyseal ends of the bone is invaded, again by ingrowth of mesenchyme, and replacement of the cartilage by bone follows. The epiphyseal cartilage disk remains oriented toward the marrow cavity of the shaft, its epiphyseal surface commonly being covered by a plate of bone. Within the epiphysis, a framework of spongy bone develops. This gives strength to the ends of the bone and forms the support of the articular cartilage, which is also supported by plates of underlying bone.

Endochondral Growth of Bone

The epiphyseal cartilage is a portion of the embryonic cartilage model that persists through adolescence, proliferates, and participates in the growth in length of the long bones. This occurs by a continuous ingrowth of capillaries into the proliferating epiphyseal cartilage, accompanied by mesenchymal cells with osteogenic potencies; the invaded cartilage is thus replaced by diaphyseal bone. The cartilage disk remains at an approximately constant thickness, being replaced on the diaphyseal front, while new cartilage cells, arranged in rows, arise from the epiphyseal face. The diaphysis increases in length by the amount by which it replaces cartilage. Growth, then, occurs in two places: (1) in cartilage, by division of cells; and (2) in diaphyseal bone, by replacement of

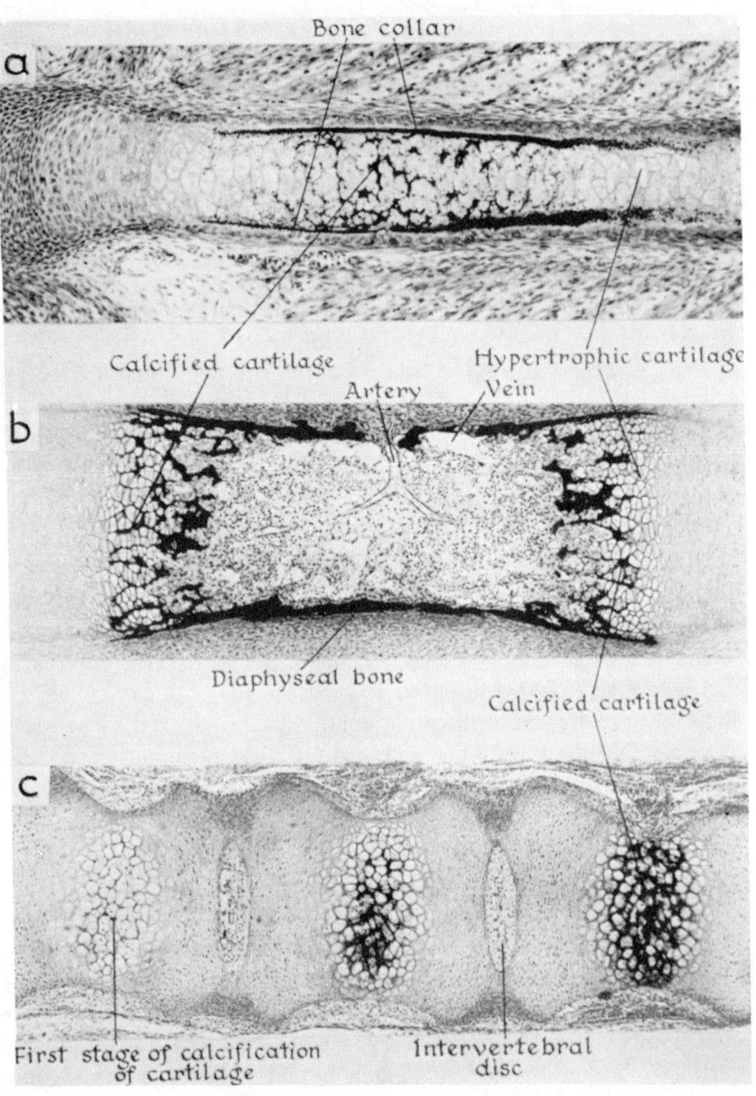

FIG. 10.—Sections to illustrate calcification of bones developing from cartilage models in embryonic and newborn rats. (*a*) Longitudinal section through second rib of 18-day rat embryo. The calcification of the periosteal bone collar is further advanced than that of the cartilage. ×104. (*b*) Section of metatarsal of 4-day-old rat. The matrix of the hypertrophic cartilage is not completely calcified. ×56. (*c*) Section through cartilage models of bodies of three vertebrae of 20-day rat embryo, showing three stages in the calcification of the model. Silver nitrate–hematoxylin-eosin. ×50. (From original of Pl. 5, Figs. 8, 9, 10, Bloom and Bloom, Anat. Rec. 78:523. Reproduced by courtesy of the publishers.)

cartilage. New bone is laid down on a framework of calcified cartilage matrix, which persists when the cartilage is invaded (Fig. 11).

Growth Apparatus

The process by which the long bones continue to grow in length through adolescence is similar to that of the replacement of embryonic cartilage models by bone, with the exception that the epiphyseal cartilage disk and its surrounding structures become organized and oriented to perform a specific function. This requires a complex mechanism, which we have termed the *growth apparatus;* unless this mechanism functions as a whole, growth in length cannot occur or is distorted.

The growth apparatus is based on the epiphyseal cartilage but is not limited to this structure. The epiphyseal face of the disk is made up of cartilage matrix, within which cartilage cells are imbedded. These continue to divide, giving rise to new cells, commonly arranged in rows; for this reason the dividing cells are known as *mother cells,* or *row mother cells;* the rows are separated from one another by cartilage matrix. Replacement of the cartilage cells by bone occurs at the opposite face of the cartilage, i.e., the diaphyseal face or front.

Viewed in sagittal section, the cartilage cells become larger as they near the diaphyseal front and develop vacuoles in their cytoplasm. The nuclei swell and lose most of their chromatin, and the cells degenerate; at this stage they are known as *vesicular* or *hypertrophic* cartilage cells and are ready for penetration by the vascular connective tissue. The *primary spongiosa* is a direct and unreconstructed continuation of the cartilage matrix, the hypertrophic cartilage cells being replaced by vascular connective tissue. Osteoblasts are numerous at the junction of the spongiosa with the cartilage, but, as a rule, little or no new bone is deposited on the matrix of the primary spongiosa.

If the epiphyseal cartilage and the primary spongiosa are viewed in serial cross-section, they resemble a honeycomb in structure, each compartment of which contains a column of cartilage cells growing out from the mother cells and undergoing hypertrophy as they approach the cartilage front. Into each of these columns there grow from the bone marrow one or more minute blood vessels, accompanied by perivascular connective tissue cells. The blood

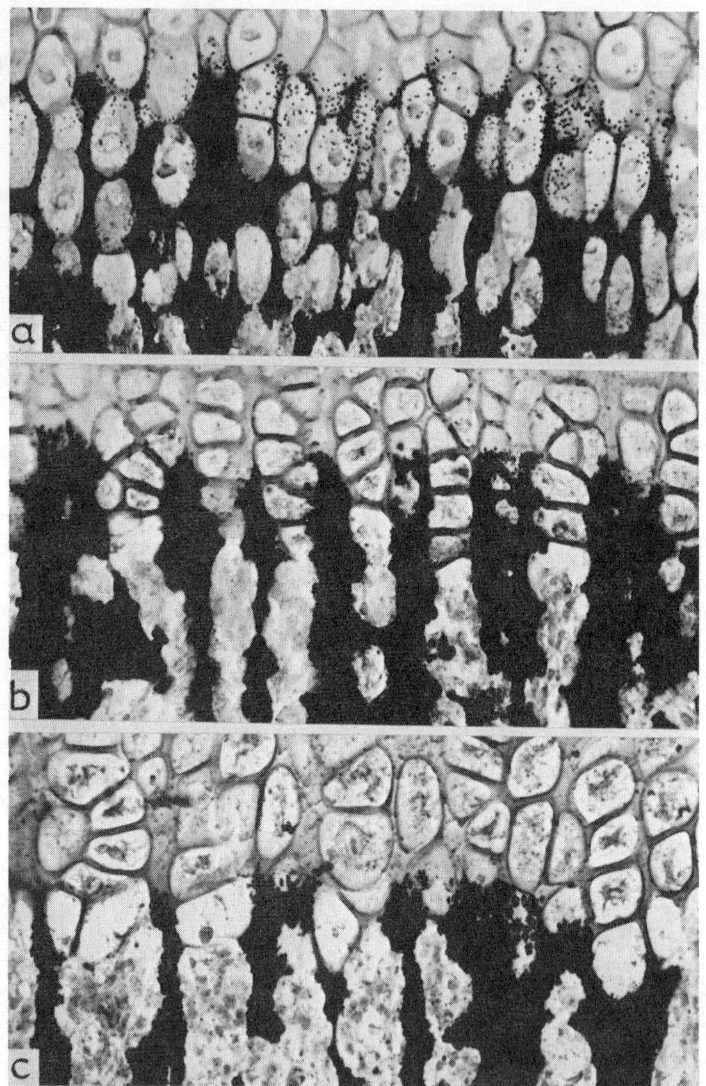

Fig. 11.—Sections through hypertrophic cartilage and zones of provisional calcification in epiphyseal cartilages, to illustrate progress of calcification in the growth in length of the long bones. (*a*) Proximal end of tibia of normal rat, age 28 days. (*b*) Distal end of radius of normal puppy, age 34 days. (*c*) Costochondral junction, same puppy. Note interdigitation of calcified cartilage matrix and cartilage in *a* and *b*, absence of interdigitation in *c*, calcified cross-partitions in *a*, absence of osteoid in primary spongiosa in all. Silver nitrate–hematoxylin-eosin. ×245. (From original of Pl. 2, Figs. 2, 3, 4, McLean and Bloom, Anat. Rec. 78:357. Reproduced by courtesy of the publishers.)

vessels penetrate the hypertrophied cartilage cells, which disappear and are replaced by vascular ingrowth.

In advance of the invading blood vessels, usually to a depth of two to four cells in the cartilage, the matrix making up the walls of the columns becomes calcified. This forms the *zone of provisional calcification,* virtually identical with the *zone of growth,* within which the cartilage cells are displaced by the tissue advancing from the bone marrow. This calcification serves a double purpose: it guides the blood vessels in their progress into the columns of cartilage cells, and it affords structural strength by providing interlocking or interdigitation between the bony diaphysis and the epiphyseal cartilage, bridging the zone of growth. Calcifiability of the cartilage matrix in the region of the hypertrophic cartilage cells is believed to be conferred upon the matrix by some activity of the adjoining cells; this may be the result of degradation of the matrix under the influence of acid hydrolases (proteases) originating from the lysosomes of the cells.

The normal functioning of the growth apparatus has been subjected to mechanical interference in experiments reported by Trueta and Amato (1960). If a plastic membrane is placed in the center of the epiphysis to isolate its marrow from the epiphyseal plate, normal division and row formation of cartilage cells do not occur, owing to the interposition of a barrier to the nourishment of the row mother cells by the blood vessels of the epiphysis. If the membrane is interposed between the metaphysis and the epiphyseal plate, the columns of cartilage cells persist; however, calcification is absent or delayed, and the chondrocytes persist. Here the barrier interferes with the ingrowth of blood vessels from the metaphysis into the growth apparatus.

The barrier that prevents vascular invasion of the columns of cells in the epiphyseal cartilage has a pathologic counterpart in a condition arising from faulty growth of cartilage, usually hereditary and known as *dyschondroplasia* or *Ollier's disease;* the growth apparatus fails to function, and the normal sequence of cartilage degeneration, calcification, and growth is interrupted. A comparable failure of the growth apparatus may be induced by chemical or metabolic interference. If rats are fed a diet deficient in vitamin D and phosphorus, and *rickets* is produced, the hypertrophic cartilage cells persist and accumulate, and the growth sequence fails.

Secondary Spongiosa

The *secondary spongiosa* is a vaulted structure, resting upon the primary spongiosa and transferring the stresses to the shaft. It is a direct continuation of the primary spongiosa, subjected to much more thinning-out and reconstruction, and it is here that deposition of new bone on the cores of calcified cartilage is most prominent. Such bone is ordinarily calcified as it is laid down, with only a thin layer of uncalcified *preosseous tissue* demonstrable by the electron microscope; in well-nourished animals, borders of uncalcified osteoid tissue, visible under the light microscope, are not common. Most of the calcified cartilage matrix disappears during growth and reconstruction. Although cartilage cells at times transform directly into bone cells, this is quantitatively an unimportant part of bone formation or growth in the higher animals. Nothing comparable to the growth apparatus of endochondral ossification is apparent in the growth of bone formed by intramembranous ossification.

Organization of Bone

Bones are organized on two levels: (1) as a tissue, and (2) as organs. Bone as a tissue has a more complex pattern than is apparent in either loose or dense connective tissue. Bones as organs are highly specialized in relation to embryonic development, to growth, to function, and to regeneration following injury.

The organization of bone as a tissue is displayed in the structure of the organic matrix, and in the relation of this matrix to the osteocytes, with their lacunae and interconnecting canalicules. The fibers of compact bone, instead of being arranged in a random fashion, are oriented to the structure of haversian systems.

In primary ossification, beginning in embryonic life, the fibers of bone are interwoven, without a definite structural pattern. Subsequently, after the age of one year in man, all new bone formed in the diaphyses of the long bones is laid down in layers, or lamellae.

The unit of structure of compact bone is the *haversian system*, or *osteon*. This is, when fully formed, an irregularly cylindrical and branching structure, with thick walls and a narrow lumen, the *haversian canal*. The canal carries one or more blood vessels, mainly capillaries and venules. The cylindrical osteons are usually oriented in the long axes of the bones. The walls have a definite lamellar structure, the fibrils of each lamella running spirally to the axis of the canal; the direction of the fibrils changes from layer to layer of the successive lamellae. The haversian system, in addition to being arranged around a central canal, includes large numbers of lacunae, housing the osteocytes and interconnected with each other and with the lumen of the canal by means of branched canalicules (Fig. 12).

Bone, either intramembranous or intracartilaginous, is first formed as trabeculae of spongy bone, with irregular communicating cavities, filled with bone marrow, and with centrally located blood vessels. As the osteoblasts covering the bone produce layer after layer of new lamellae by apposition on the bony surfaces, the marrow spaces are reduced to such an extent that only a small canal remains about a blood vessel. This is, then, a *primitive* or *primary haversian system*, or osteon, with its haversian canal, and it represents the initial state of *compact bone*. In certain small animals, such as the mouse and the rat, organization of bone does not pro-

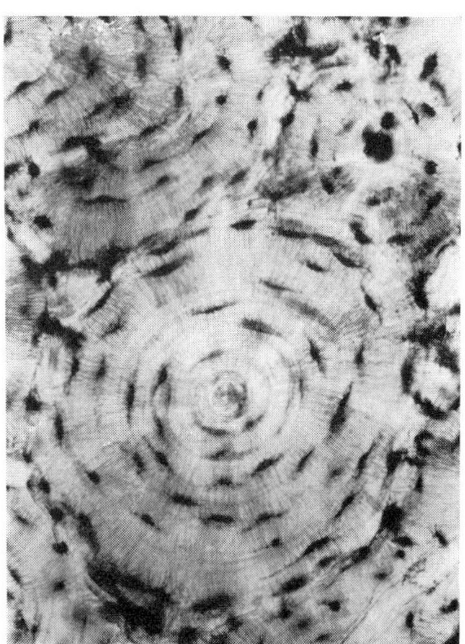

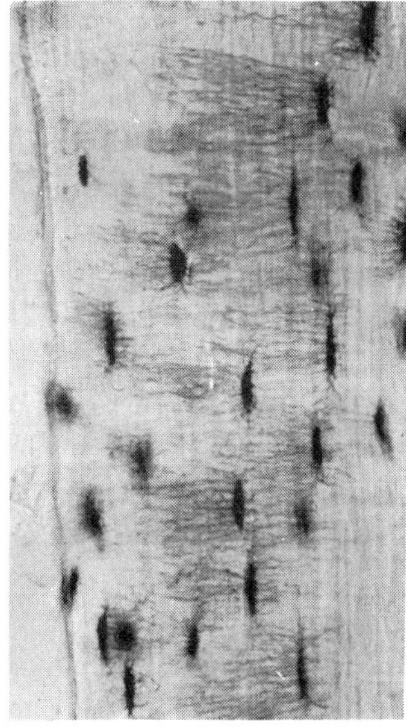

Fig. 12.—Sections through compact human bone, to illustrate haversian systems. *Left:* cross-section, ×180; *right*, longitudinal section, ×215. (From Weinmann and Sicher, Bone and Bones [St. Louis: C. V. Mosby Co., 1947], Figs. 11 and 13, pp. 30 and 32. Reproduced by courtesy of the publishers.)

gress beyond this stage. In larger animals, however, *secondary osteons* are produced by formation of cylindrical *absorption cavities* or tunnels, which are then filled in by deposition of concentric layers or lamellae of bone again, leaving, in each case, a haversian canal. Successive generations of haversian systems are then formed throughout the life of the animal. They cut across the lines of the earlier osteons, leaving irregularly shaped areas of *interstitial lamellae.* Additional circumferential lamellae are formed under the periosteum and endosteum. Compact bone thus consists of lamellar bone, arranged in a variety of ways: in relatively new and regularly shaped osteons; in portions of older osteons, remaining as interstitial lamellae; and in circumferential layers near the surfaces of the structure. All of these lamellae are similar in structure and function; their differences are incidental to the sequences occurring in their formation (Fig. 13).

Internal Reconstruction of Bone

Bones increase in length by the functioning of the growth apparatus and in diameter by apposition of new periosteal bone, while the marrow cavity is being enlarged at the endosteal surface. In addition to the changes in size and shape of the bones as a result of the remodeling incident to growth, there is continuous internal remodeling throughout the life of the individual; this serves an important physiologic function, essential to homeostatic control of the calcium-ion concentration in the blood plasma, and therefore to life itself.

In compact bone there is first the formation of *absorption cavities,* described by Tomes and De Morgan (1853). The appearance of these cavities is associated with the presence of osteoclasts, and the cavities are extended, generally in the long axis of the bone, until they assume the form of tunnels. Regulation of the tunneling process is not understood; it appears to be independent of parathyroid activity, usually associated with osteoclastic activity in other locations. According to Amprino (1965), the regions in which tunnels are formed are determined by the stresses and strains to which the individual bone is exposed; within these regions there is a random distribution of the newly forming absorption cavities or tunnels.

The tunnel, or absorption cavity, as seen in sections, contains blood vessels and connective tissue cells. While resorption is in progress, the cavity is lined with osteoclasts; when resorption comes to an end and rebuilding begins, these are replaced by osteoblasts. The tunnel is then filled in, from its walls toward the center, by apposition of bone in successive layers or lamellae, incorporating the osteocytes, their lacunae, and the canalicules. Wherever the central blood vessel branches, a lateral branch of the osteon is formed to surround it; some of these become the canals of Volkmann (interosteonic canals) and communicate with the marrow cavity of the periosteal surface. The formation of new layers con-

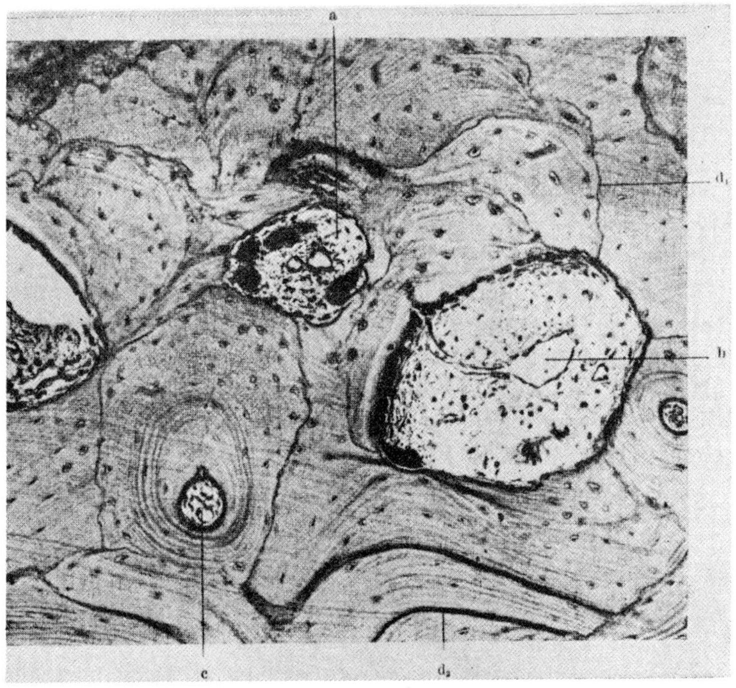

Fig. 13.—Photomicrograph of a ground section of compact bone, from a phalanx of the thumb of a 6-year-old child: *a*, first stage of excavation of a resorption cavity, with osteoclastic activity; *b*, second stage, beginning of formation of lamellar bone by apposition of concentric layers, with osteoblastic activity; *c*, final stage, completed lamellar system, with an excentric haversian canal; *d*, cement lines. ×150. (From Fig. 6, Petersen, Arch. Entwicklungs. Organ. 112:122. Reproduced by courtesy of the publishers.)

tinues until the canal reaches its final diameter, usually approximately 20 microns.

Using lead as a marker, Vincent (1957) has studied the rate of formation and of maturation of new osteons. An average absorption cavity in a dog takes roughly three weeks to form, this being the period required for tunneling or excavation. The building of the new osteon, including partial mineralization of the organic matrix, requires some six to twelve weeks. Primary mineralization of the matrix, to about 70 per cent of the final content, occurs rapidly during and immediately after the deposition of new layers of organic material; completion of secondary mineralization, to maximum density, takes much longer, and has been found to be incomplete for as long as eighteen weeks.

Frost *et al.* (1960), using tetracycline as a marker, found the mean osteon formation time in a fifty-seven-year-old man to be five weeks. The biologic half-life of the osteons was calculated as 2.7 years for the femur and 8.6 years for the tibia. The percentage of the mass of bone turned over, i.e., resorbed and redeposited, per day was 0.036 for the femur and fibula and 0.012 for the tibia.

Throughout the life of the individual, formation of new osteons is begun by the tunneling process referred to, and this stage continues until the absorption cavity is complete, osteoclastic activity ends, and deposition of concentric lamellae of new bone, by osteoblastic activity, begins. This second stage, which includes most of the metabolic activity of bone, has been referred to by Vincent and Haumont (1960) as *metabolic bone;* its completion is marked by the arrival of the haversian canal at its final diameter, and by cessation of apposition of new bone. At this time the osteon assumes its final form and dimensions, and its metabolic activity is at a minimum; it then comes to the resting state of *structural bone*, constituting more than 99 per cent of the total mass of skeletal bone.

Figure 14 illustrates the zones that may be identified in the second stage of formation of a new osteon, during which the changes incident to its formation may be identified as in Table 1.

This figure illustrates a cross-section of a single osteon from the tibial diaphysis of a dog six months of age. *A* represents the section treated with cobalt nitrate; *B* is the microradiograph of the same section. Most prominent in *A* are zones 2 and 3 in Table 1. Zone 2, or the uncalcified preosseous tissue, is radiolucent, and does not

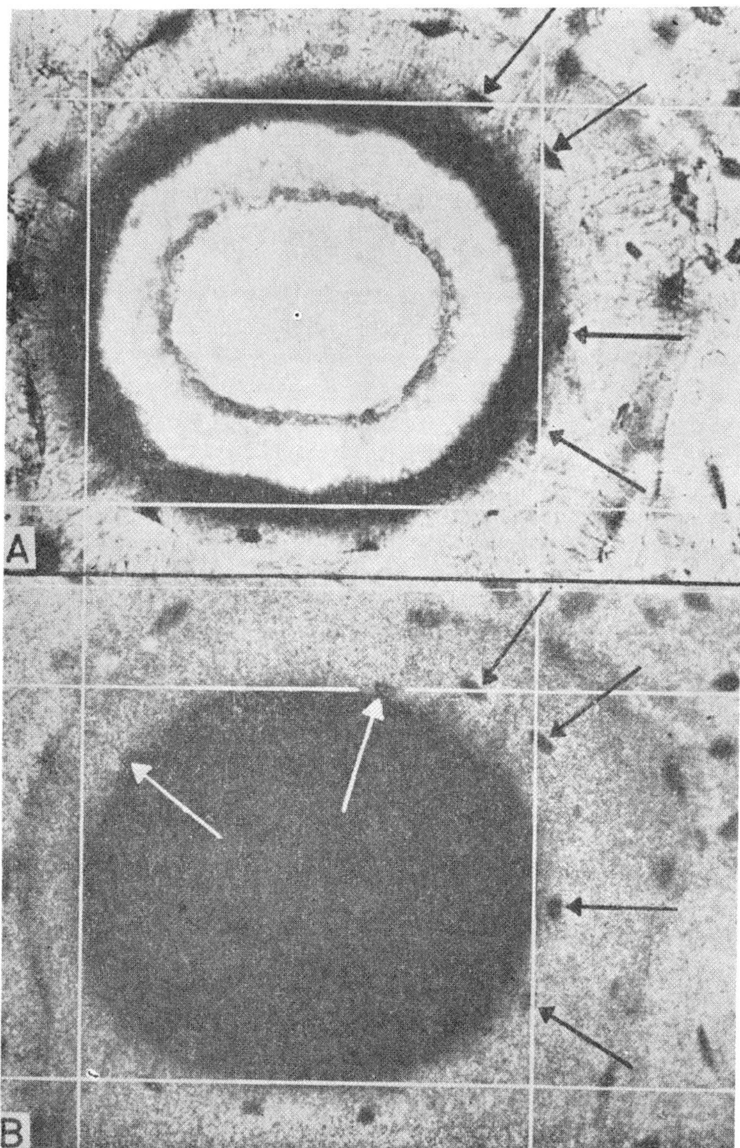

Fig. 14.—Osteon in formation in a cross-section of the tibial diaphysis of a 6-month-old dog. (*A*) Ground section treated with cobalt nitrate. (*B*) Microradiograph. The borders of the canal are indicated by arrows; inside of the points of the arrows there is a preosseous layer which is not calcified and hence does not show in the X ray. ×550. (From Leblond and Lacroix, C.R. Acad. Sci. 249:935. Reproduced by courtesy of the publishers.)

show in the microradiograph. Zone 3 illustrates the reactivity of the calcification line, with beginning calcification sharply demarcated by both the cobalt stain and the microradiograph. The figure illustrates the situation at a particular instant of time; the two zones are, of course, moving toward the center of the canal, and will continue to do so until growth activity ceases and the osteon reaches a resting state.

It is notable that the major activity in a forming osteon is sharply delimited at the border of a completely uncalcified preosseous tissue, which Frost and Villanueva (1960) have estimated as

TABLE 1

CROSS-SECTION OF FORMING OSTEON, FROM CENTER TO PERIPHERY

Zone	Description	Reacts with
1.	Haversian canal, lined with osteoblasts, and housing blood vessels, nerves, lymphatics, and connective tissue	Histologic stains
2.	Uncalcified preosseous tissue, or osteoid seams	Histologic stains, ^{35}S *in vivo*
3.	Calcification line or front	Mineral Component; ^{45}Ca, ^{226}Ra, ^{90}Sr, ^{32}P, Pb, tetracycline, alizarin, etc. Organic Component; ^{65}Zn *in vivo*; Zn also demonstrable in untreated animal Cd (competes *in vivo* with Zn) Co, Sudan Black, and other stains
4.	Partially calcified osteon	^{45}Ca (after *in vivo* or *in vitro* pretreatment with acid)
5.	Cement line (external limit of osteon)	Histologic stains

advancing at the rate of an average of 0.9 microns per day in actively forming haversian systems in adult man; the onset of calcification takes place at a constant distance from the lumen of the canal, this distance being the thickness of the zone of preosseous tissue.

The advance of calcification into the preosseous tissue thus occurs at the same rate at which the uncalcified preosseous tissue advances into the lumen of the haversian canal, and it seems clear that some critical event must occur at the calcification line, moving steadily into the preosseous tissue. The nature of the event that triggers the transformation of the preosseous tissue into a calcified and highly reactive tissue must remain speculative for the present.

The sequence of events in the forming of the osteon suggests that the advance of the calcification line depends upon a catalytic phenomenon. Haumont (1963), working at Lovanium University in the Republic of the Congo, has demonstrated that it is precisely at this line that zinc is demonstrable, and he has found that the zinc is in association with a mucopolysaccharide; it is tempting to postulate a metal-enzyme complex, activated by zinc, which may serve to catalyze calcification. In any event, it is at this line that the continuum between calcium in solution (in the body fluids) and in the solid state (in the bone mineral) is established and maintained during the internal remodeling of compact bone.

It is also noteworthy that zone 3, in which calcification begins, is the zone of maximum reactivity in the newly forming osteon, as indicated by a variety of criteria. It is in this zone that the newly deposited mineral reacts with bone-seeking radioisotopes, and takes up tetracycline, alizarin, and porphyrins. This reactivity of the mineral, leading to deposit of some 70 per cent of the final mineral content of the new osseous tissue, is one of the chief reasons for assuming that the newly deposited mineral is less mature and more reactive than the hydroxyapatite associated with mature bone. Moreover, the organic matrix of the tissue about to undergo calcification is reactive in the sense that it takes up trace metals, e.g., Zn, Cd, and Co, and it is highly reactive with the Sudan Black staining procedure.

Ultrastructure of Bone

While the intimate structure of bone, as observed with the light microscope, has been well described for many years, the exploitation of new biophysical techniques has added information concerning the details of fine structure and has increased knowledge of the relation of structure to function; special emphasis on the interrelations of the chief components of bone is necessary for an understanding of its functions.

The terms *fine structure* and *ultrastructure*, as well as *submicroscopic*, have been used to indicate particles or structures not resolvable by the light microscope. High-resolution electron microscopy refers specifically to dimensions of 30 A or less. At this level, information has been obtained concerning the fibrillar structure of bone and the characteristics of collagen fibers, as well as about the form of the crystals of the bone mineral and their relationship to the collagen fibers and to the ground substance. The potentialities of the electron microscope for elucidating the fine structure of bone, thus permitting further insight into its functions, have by no means been exhausted.

Electron microscopy of bone has been aided by X-ray diffraction, both high-angle and low-angle. High-angle diffraction, particularly

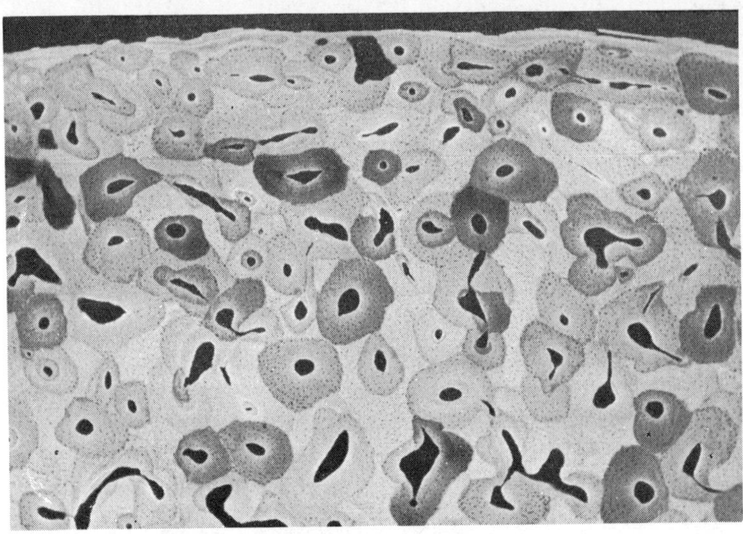

FIG. 15.—Microradiograph of normal human compact bone, from cross-section of a fresh tibia of a woman, age 47. Section, 100 μ thick, cut with high-speed rotary saw without embedding and without further treatment. Radiograph made with 9 kv X rays, on Eastman Kodak 649-0 spectroscopic plate. ×30. (Reproduced by courtesy of R. E. Rowland, Argonne National Laboratory.)

with microdiffraction techniques, has been of assistance in studying the crystallographic properties of bone tissue. Low-angle diffraction has given information about the dimensions of the particles and their orientation.

Microradiography requires the passing of X rays through thin sections and the recording of differences in absorption of the radiation on photographic plates or film, thus permitting enlargement of the image. Whereas ordinary histologic sections of bone do not reveal differences in the density of individual osteons, such differences are clearly demonstrated in microradiograms; the younger osteons are less mineralized and consequently less dense than the older ones (Fig. 15). This has focused attention on the mineralization of osteons, and it is readily demonstrable that the new and less dense osteons take up radioactive calcium, strontium, and phosphorus preferentially.

The results obtained on normal bone tissue by microradiography have been confirmed by microinterferometry. In addition, microinterferometric measurements made on decalcified tissue have shown that the content of organic material varies little from one osteon to another, indicating that the differences seen in microradiograms depend solely upon the content of mineral. The polarizing microscope reveals the arrangement of the molecules in calcified tissue; the close relationship between collagen and the mineral phase of bone was observed by this means as early as 1923. Electron microscopy of the cells of bone has been given consideration in Chapter II.

Relation of Structure to Function

When a radioisotope—for example, strontium 90—has been administered to an animal and undecalcified sections of compact bone have been made, it is possible to prepare photomicrographs, microradiograms, and autoradiograms, all of the same section. These may be enlarged to the same size and compared (Fig. 16). The radioisotope is not only taken up preferentially by the newer and less dense osteons; but far the greater portion of it is taken up by a thin layer of new and only slightly mineralized matrix, which may not be seen at all in the microradiograms, but may be visible in the section under the light microscope. When this layer is absent, no appreciable amount of radioisotope may be taken up by a particular osteon, even though the osteon as a whole is incompletely mineralized, and hence of a density comparable to that of others which do take up the isotope. These combined techniques afford a record of the sequence of events in the growth and mineralization of bone, not seen by any one of the techniques alone.

Such findings as these have given strength to the view, to be treated at length later in this volume, that there is a labile fraction of the bone mineral, located chiefly, if not exclusively, in the newly formed and incompletely mineralized osteons, and more particularly in the newest layer of osseous tissue lining these osteons. This

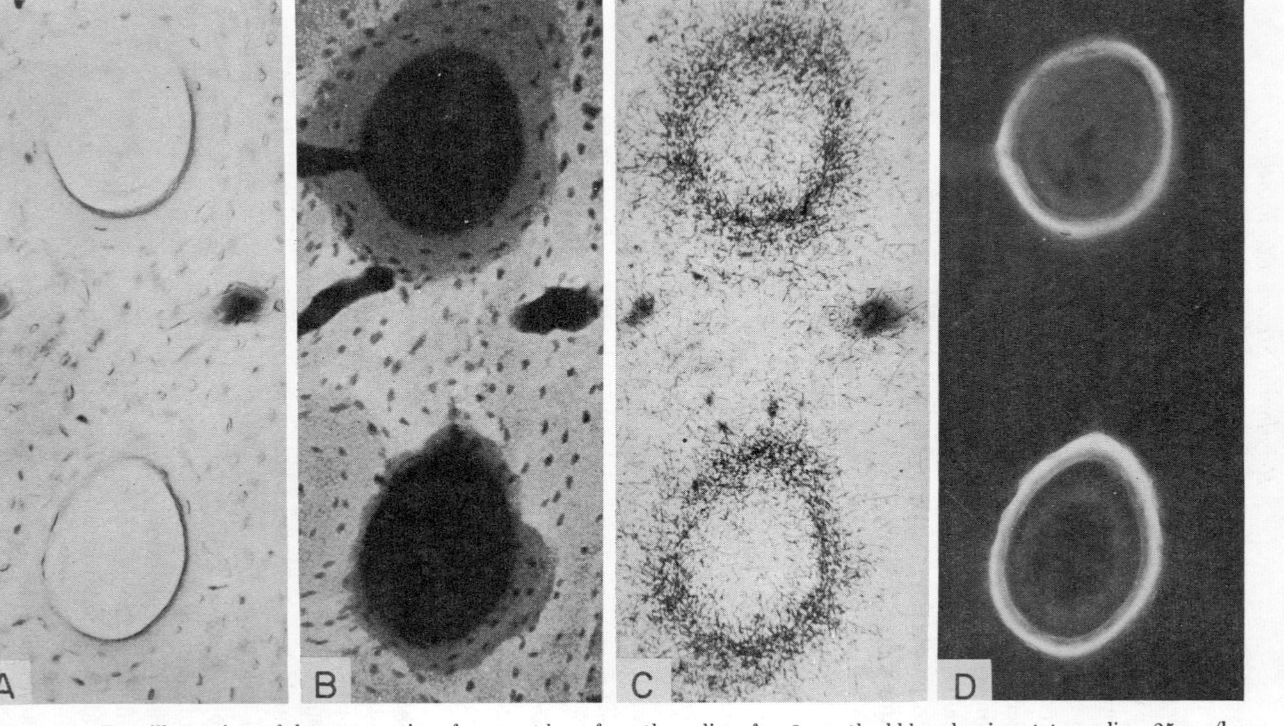

FIG. 16.—Four illustrations of the same section of compact bone from the radius of an 8-month-old beagle, given tetracycline, 25 mg/kg, 4 days and ^{226}Ra, 40 μCi, 2 days before sacrifice—both intravenously. The bone was embedded in methyl methacrylate and the section, 100 μ thick, was cut with a high-speed rotary saw, without further treatment. (*A*) Photomicrograph of unstained section. (*B*) Microradiograph, made with 9 kv X rays on Eastman Kodak 649-0 spectroscopic plate. (*C*) Alpha track autoradiograph, made with stripping film, Kodak Limited AR-10, exposed for 14 days. (*D*) Fluorescent image with UV light, photographed on Kodak Panatomic X film. All ×126. (Reproduced by courtesy of R. E. Rowland, Argonne National Laboratory.)

labile fraction of mineral, associated with bone of maximum reactivity, accounts for the rapid uptake of mineral from the fluids of the body. When the blood plasma is depleted of calcium, there is a rapid movement of this element from the intercellular fluids; this serves to buffer any rapid changes in the Ca^{2+} content of the plasma. The calcium thus transferred from the intercellular fluids is then replenished from the labile fraction of the bone mineral. As a rough guide, it may be said that the transfer of calcium from intercellular fluids to plasma provides for minute-to-minute adjustment; from the labile fraction of bone to the intercellular fluid for hour-to-hour adjustment; and from the stable fraction of the bone to the blood, by hormonal and cellular intervention, for day-to-day adjustment. Taken together, the separate elements of this mechanism provide for the continued life and health of the organism, which without it would be subject to violent fluctuations in the Ca^{2+} concentration in the internal environment.

Bioelectric Effects

The local stimulus that induces osteoblastic activity and bone formation on one side and osteoclastic activity and bone destruction on the other side of a bone trabecula, only a few microns in thickness, is attributed to surface electric currents. Like nearly all material in the solid state and in crystalline form, bone is piezoelectric; that is, it generates an electric current when mechanically deformed. Both the fibrous and the mineral phases of bone tissue are crystalline in form, and therefore capable of generating electric currents. The effect is elicited by deformation of a strip of bone and measured as potential difference equal to as much as 20 millivolts. Opinion differs about the source of the current. Bassett and associates (1964) note that the maximum amount of electricity generated comes when the whole bone, the mineral-collagen-mucopolysaccharide complex is stressed. Shamos and Lavine (1964; 1965) state that the collagen fiber is the main source of stress-induced potentials, whereas Becker and Bachman (1965) maintain that because the system, collagen and apatite, consists of crystals of two different types, it acts as a semiconductor junction of the p-n type. When the crystalline-collagen, covered with many electrons, and the apatite, coated with relatively few, are stressed, the p-n junction could generate an electric current.

A piezoelectric transducer transforms mechanical to electric energy and could incite cellular activity. Bassett (1965) conceives of the process of bone formation as a response to a positive feedback mechanism, and bone resorption to a negative one. When the bone is bent, a negative charge builds up and new bone is deposited on the concave side; when a positive charge builds up on the convex side, old bone is resorbed to straighten it. Diminution of electric current incites osteoclastic activity and bone resorption. Frost (1963) expresses these ideas in the form of laws as follows: compression inhibits osteoclastic and permits osteoblastic activity, while absence of compression inhibits osteoblastic and permits osteoclastic activity. In either event, surface electric signals generated by deformed bone combine to operate as a negative feedback mechanism in which cell activities minimize and correct deformation.

These hypothetical concepts represent an attempt to express those of Julius Wolff in modern terms. Wolff (1892) suggested that bone trabeculae place or displace themselves in the direction of functional pressures. Later Murray (1936) added that genetic factors must determine the gross configuration and that mechanical influences modify and develop the fine detail of bone structure. Mechanical influences upon a bone are the all-inclusive effects of ballistics of cardiovascular action, gravity, muscle tonus, voluntary muscle activities, and impact between skeleton and environment. Assuming that mechanical stimuli from all of these sources are transformed into electric energy on the surfaces of bone cells, Bassett (1965) proposes that generation of electric charge, reversal of charge, space polarization, oxygen saturation, CO_2 tension, and other physical or metabolic environmental factors alter intracellular chemical reactions. In the final analysis, the bioelectrics of bone encompass the fundamental problem of the physical effects of the environment on the cell metabolic machinery, first regulatory genes and eventually even structural genes.

CHAPTER IV

Structure and Chemical Composition of Bone Matrix

The organic fraction of compact bone makes up as much as 35 per cent of the dry, fat-free weight. Only a small part of this is contributed by the cells; the remainder, impregnated with the bone mineral, is the bone matrix. This has been investigated intensively by histologic, chemical, biophysical, and histochemical methods, and numerous electron-microscope studies have been reported.

The organic matrix has two chief components. Of these the most prominent is fibrillar in nature and is chemically a collagen, closely related to the collagens found in other connective tissues. Between the fibers is a ground substance whose best characterized component is a *proteinpolysaccharide,* which is readily degraded, *in vitro,* to a peptide or protein, and to a polysaccharide, *chondroitin sulfate;* small amounts of additional constituents may also be present. The fluid portion of the intercellular elements of the bone matrix, coextensive with the ground substance, is small in amount but is important for the transfer of dissolved substances between the blood and the bone.

The overall composition of bone is best illustrated by a tabulation of its inorganic and organic constituents, in terms of the relations of their amounts in compact bone, expressed as percentages of the dry, fat-free weight of the bone (Table 2). These components are considered separately below.

Collagen

Bone collagen is the substance that yields gelatin or glue when boiled. It makes up 90–96 per cent of the dry, fat-free weight of the organic matter of bone. Most studies on collagen have been made on material from other sources, such as skin and tendon, but increasing attention is now being given to the collagen of bone.

The collagenous fibers in bone are more densely packed than in any other connective tissue of the body. In bone, as in all other connective tissues, collagen is made up of fibrils with double cross-banding at intervals averaging 640 A (Fig. 17). It has a crystalline structure with a characteristic X-ray diffraction pattern. Chemically it is characterized by a low content of aromatic amino acids and a high content of pyrrolidine amino acids and glycine and by its specific hydrolysis by the enzyme *collagenase.* Certain collagens,

TABLE 2

COMPOSITION OF AIR-DRIED COMPACT BONE TISSUE (OX FEMUR DIAPHYSIS)

	Per Cent by Weight
Inorganic matter insoluble in hot water	69.66
(Probably including up to 1 per cent of citrate)	
Inorganic matter soluble in water	1.25
Collagen	18.64
Proteinpolysaccharide	0.24
Resistant protein material	1.02
Fat	0.00
Carbohydrate, other than proteinpolysaccharide	0.00
Water (lost below 105° C)	8.18

From Eastoe and Eastoe, Biochem. J. 57:453, 1954.

such as those from the tendons of the rat's tail and from the swim bladder of fish, are soluble in dilute acid and may be reconstituted as fibrils, with typical cross-banding, by the addition of electrolytes to the solution. The individual fibers, 0.3–0.5 μ in diameter, are often collected into small bundles, 3–5 μ thick.

Knowledge of the chemistry and molecular structure of collagen is growing rapidly. While the collagens from different sources resemble one another, both chemically and morphologically, there are wide variations in solubility.

Collagen is readily digested by pepsin in acid solution, but resists digestion by trypsin in alkaline solution. On hydrolysis, collagen or gelatin yields especially high proportions of *glycine* (25 g/100 g), of *proline* (14.8 g/100 g), and of *hydroxyproline* (14.5 g/100 g). *Hydroxylysine* is found only in hydrolysates of collagen and of gelatin, and in these the content of this amino acid is only about 1 per cent. Alpha amino acids are absent from collagen; aspartic acid, glutamic acid, alanine, and threonine, as well as glycine, are found as terminal residues in various forms of gelatin. Collagen is poor in some of the amino acids essential to protein metabolism. There are species differences, as well as local differences, in the physical and chemical properties of collagen. The life span of the individual fibers is in doubt; the physiologic turnover of collagen in tendons is extremely slow; the same is true for bone.

The collagen molecule has been represented as a rodlike cylinder, 3,000 A long and about 14 A in diameter. Its molecular weight is now generally agreed to be about 300,000. It is a triple-chain coiled coil, twisted to the left, as determined by X-ray diffraction

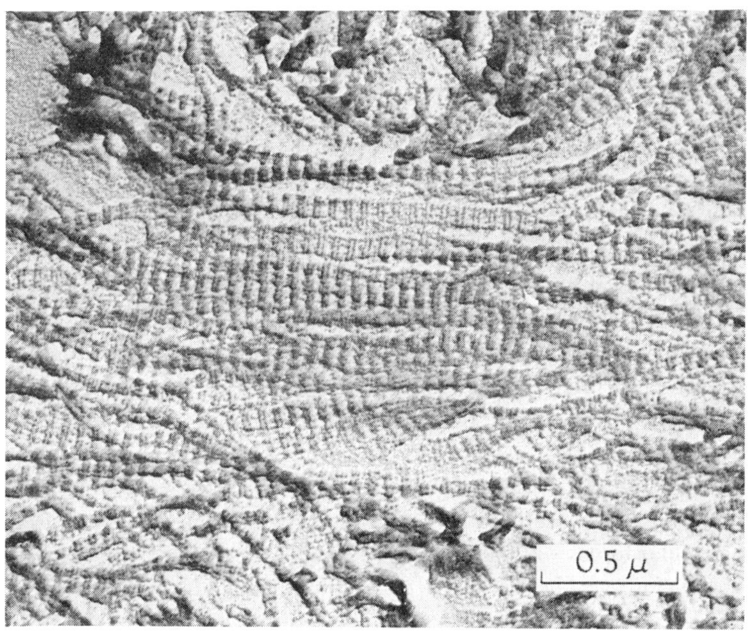

FIG. 17.—Electron micrograph, illustrating collagen fibers in a section of decalcified human femur. Shadowed with uranium at an angle of 5:1. The major doublet bands of the collagen are spaced by 560 A in this area. Incomplete intermediate cross-bands are found in a few places. Continuity of the doublet bands across several fibers at right angles to the fiber direction is observed. Osmium tetraoxide fixation. (From original of Pl. 3, Fig. 4, Robinson and Watson, Anat. Rec. 114:399. Reproduced by courtesy of the publishers.)

measurements, and supertwisted to the right; that is, each polypeptide chain is helical and the three chains are wound around the axis of the molecule, to produce a second helix. Regions with lengths of the order of 10–100 A along the length of the molecule alternate between polar and nonpolar character; this results in the fine band structure seen in electron micrographs of stained fibrils and is related to the positions of polar and nonpolar amino acids along the polypeptide chain. The amino acid composition includes one-third glycine, and sequence data indicate that the glycine residues are in every third position; this is a requirement for the collagen structure.

Seifter *et al.* (1965) summarize the primary structure of the collagen molecule as follows: the periodicity is determined by a specific sequence of nonpolar amino acids in a tripeptide with the general formula Gly-P-X, where Gly represents glycine, P is either proline or hydroxyproline, and X is arginine or another of the less frequent components of the polar polypeptide regions. Gly and P are believed to appear as interbands in electron micrographs; the X component may represent areas of the transition between polar and nonpolar regions of the molecules. In addition, probably included in the peptide backbone are γ-glutamyl peptide bonds.

The lateral association of the chains within the coiled coil is known as cross-linking; the chemistry of the cross-links is not known with certainty. The degree and forms of cross-linking determine how much of the collagen is extractable by ordinary nonhydrolytic procedures. Bone collagen is cross-linked rapidly and extensively while it is being formed, and is difficult to extract and reconstitute. Glimcher and associates (1965) have referred to the weak bonds in the bone collagen molecule as non-covalent intermolecular forces—hydrogen bonds, electrostatic bonds, and van der Waals forces. They succeeded in solubilizing and reconstituting bone collagen first by freezing decalcified tissue at $-70°$ C to expand intermolecular spaces and to decrease net intermolecular forces, and then by thawing the tissue at 2° C in acetic acid. After freezing and thawing, a part of the collagen of bone was dissolved, and could be reconstituted by the addition of salts. The ultrastructural properties of the reconstituted bone collagen indicate that it resembles the native-type fibril and has an axial periodicity of 600–

700 A. The mechanisms responsible for the localization of microcrystals of apatite in skeletal tissues will be considered in detail in Chapter VI.

Ground Substance

Broadly conceived, ground substance may be defined as the extracellular and interfibrillar component of all connective tissues. Formerly described as amorphous, it is now believed to have an organization and ultrastructure of its own, or at least to contribute to the shape and form of connective tissue. The relation of tissue fluid to ground substance is poorly understood. A working concept is that the ground substance varies in consistency and density from that of an interstitial fluid—that is, an ultrafiltrate of plasma—to that of the basement membrane, and that it is coextensive with both; they represent its most fluid and most condensed portions, respectively.

Chemistry of Ground Substance

The ground substance of connective tissue, including bone, is characterized chemically by its content of *proteinpolysaccharides.* Although it is not possible to make a statement that will include all connective tissues, present evidence, derived mainly from cartilage, suggests that there is no free polysaccharide in connective tissue, including bone; all of the polysaccharide is bound to protein. For this reason, the term *mucopolysaccharide* has been largely discarded as representing a constituent of connective tissue, except for such tissues as have been degraded, as by hydrolysis, and the term *proteinpolysaccharide* (PP) has taken its place. A mucopolysaccharide, as such, is an artifact, in that it is not present in the living organism.

In cartilage the polysaccharide bound to protein is mainly chrondroitin sulfate (CS) and keratin sulfate (KS). The proportions differ widely in material from different sources; in bovine nasal cartilage the ratio CS/KS is over 10; in human costal and articular cartilages the ratio is about 1.5. Proteinpolysaccharides may be divided, by centrifugation, into two fractions, heavy (PP-H) and light (PP-L), and these may be further subdivided, by appropriate means.

There are four mucopolysaccharides that possess a very similar structure; these are hyaluronic acid and the three chondroitin sulfates, designated as A, B, and C, which are nonbranched polymers, composed of alternating glucuronic acid and *N*-acetylgalactosamine groups. Little is known of the physiologic specificity of these four compounds; an exception is that hyaluronic acid is a major component of synovial fluid, rather than of the dense connective tissues. Next in the list of mucopolysaccharides is heparin monosulfate, representing a family of compounds chemically related to heparin. A final group is the keratosulfates, which are sulfated polymers of *N*-acetyllactosamine and *N*-acetylglucosamine. Keratin sulfate (KS) is found in cartilage, as already noted, and is also a structural component of the cornea. On hydrolysis, or on digestion with testicular *hyaluronidase*, chondroitin sulfate A yields glucuronic acid, with a repeating unit of chondroitin. Hyaluronic acid yields glucuronic acid with a repeating unit of hyalbiuronic acid.

The amounts of proteinpolysaccharides in bone are small and analytic data are scanty. Dry, fat-free compact bone has been reported to contain 0.1–0.25 per cent of hexosamine (estimated as glucosamine hydrochloride) and 2–4 per cent of total reducing substance (estimated as glucose). Ox shaft bone contains 0.3–0.4 per cent of a sulfated polysaccharide, composed of about equimolar concentrations of hexosamine, uronic acid, and sulfate. Eastoe and Eastoe (1954) reported the isolation of a mucopolysaccharide-protein complex obtained by lime-water extraction of air-dried powder (0.24 per cent by weight). On hydrolysis, they demonstrated both galactosamine, 7.67 per cent, and glucosamine, 1.23 per cent, together with 1.63 per cent sulfate-S. On paper chromatography, they found galactose, mannose, and xylose.

The results from analyses of bone are consistent with the finding of approximately 0.5 per cent of chondroitin sulfate in dentin. Another approach to the estimation of chondroitin sulfate in cartilage and bone is by analysis for total sulfate. The sulfate content of the organic matter of bone is about 15 per cent of that of cartilage. A similar contrast between cartilage and bone is revealed by autoradiographs following administration of ^{35}S to suckling rats. The highly polymerized molecules of chondroitin sulfate do not ordinarily move with the tissue fluid into the blood plasma, but have been reported to be so mobilized under the influence of the parathyroid hormone.

The plant proteases—papain, bromelin, and ficin—have been useful for the study of ground substance. When crude or inactivated papain is injected into a young rabbit, the ear cartilages collapse; within a few days resynthesis and redeposition occur, and the rabbit's ears again become erect. During the phenomenon of collapse there occurs an uncoupling of chondroitin sulfate from the protein to which it is bound in cartilage and connective tissue. This results in complete loss of metachromasia from the cartilage; the metachromatic material accumulates in the adjacent connective tissue, is picked up by the lymphatics, and then appears in the blood and urine. Cortisone prevents the reconstitution of the chondroitin sulfate–protein complex. Similar depletion of basophilia, owing to removal of chondroitin sulfate from growing cartilage or new bone, occurs *in vitro* when vitamin A is added to culture media containing chick-embryo limb buds.

Lathyrism, a syndrome induced in man by diets containing large amounts of peas of the genus *Lathyrus* and characterized by spastic paraplegia, pain, hypesthesia, and paresthesia, has been recognized in man for centuries. It occurs sporadically, especially in times of famine, in India, North Africa, and southern Europe. No skeletal lesions have been observed. A skeletal form of lathyrism produced in rats by diets containing sweet peas (*Lathyrus odoratus*) has been studied intensively; the condition as it occurs in man and that produced in animals appear to be two completely different diseases, caused by different species of *Lathyrus* peas. The disease in rats has been designated as *odoratism,* to differentiate it from human lathyrism.

Odoratism is caused by *aminonitriles.* A number of such compounds have been found in several varieties of sweet peas; these compounds are absent from the legumes of common consumption as well as from the peas that cause human lathyrism. Odoratism in rats is characterized by kyphoscoliosis, exostoses, hernias, and lameness of the hind legs, with other skeletal deformities. The aminonitriles are tissue specific, affecting mesodermal tissues, and appear to have a special affinity for the ground substance. Actively growing epiphyseal plates and certain tendon and muscle insertions are markedly affected by these compounds.

The ground substance of bone, as well as of other connective tissues, is responsible for certain staining reactions—*metachromasia* and a positive *periodic acid-Schiff reaction* (PAS). Metachromasia is the phenomenon, described by Ehrlich, of the staining of certain tissue components in a color different from that of the dye solution itself. Thus, when cartilage is stained with toluidine blue, part of the tissue displays a reddish color. As chondrocytes mature and hypertrophy, the large β-metachromatic (purple-staining) granules differentiate into small γ-metachromatic (pink-staining) granules. Metachromasia is believed to be due to the presence of free electronegative surface charges. The change in type of metachromasia of the granules reflects an increase in the number of free sulfate or carboxyl groups on the mucopolysaccharides, with possibly also a rearrangement of these groups. The ground substance of bone stains metachromatically, but only after decalcification; this reaction is associated with the mucopolysaccharide components, and more particularly with the state in which they are present. When depolymerization of chondroitin sulfate is brought about by the action of hyaluronidase, metachromasia is lost.

The *Hotchkiss procedure*, resulting in the PAS reaction, consists in treatment by periodic acid, followed by staining with fuchsin sulfite (leucofuchsin). The periodic acid oxidizes to aldehyde groups, with cleavage, adjacent hydroxyl or hydroxyl-amino groups in carbohydrate molecules. The colorless leucofuchsin then forms a polysubstituted dye compound with the aldehyde group, pale pink to purple-red in color. The intensity of the color depends on the number of reacting aldehyde groups formed by periodic acid oxidation. Free aldehydes do not contribute to the staining reaction; simple sugars, being water-soluble, also do not affect the color of the sections. The staining reactions of the ground substance are referrable to (1) the content of insoluble polysaccharides and (2) a change in their state. Ground substance containing highly polymerized mucopolysaccharides stains a pale pink color; this is interpreted to mean that it has relatively few reactive groups available for visualization. Depolymerization leads to an increase in color, owing to the release of a greater number of reactive groups.

When these criteria, in part based on assumptions, are applied to the study of bone, it is concluded that the ground substance of fully formed bone, being barely stainable by the PAS reaction, contains only highly polymerized mucopolysaccharides. When bone is being deposited or resorbed rapidly, the stain becomes more intense; this indicates a lesser degree of polymerization. In the epiphyseal cartilage disk of growing bones of rats, the matrix of hyaline cartilage stains a pale pink color. As the zone of provisional calcification is approached, the matrix takes on more color; where the cartilage cells are markedly hypertrophied, the matrix is stained a brilliant purple-red, which persists when the cartilage is incorporated in the spicules of spongy bone.

Reticulin

The composition of reticular fibers, present in small quantities in the organic matrix of bone, occupies a position intermediate between collagen and the mucopolysaccharides of the ground substance. Quantitative data are lacking, but reticulin is believed to be a glycoprotein; that is, a polysaccharide in combination with protein containing fucose, mannose, and galactose, and possibly hexosamine. The relationship between reticular and collagenous fibers is imperfectly understood. The fibers in the skin of newborn rats have an affinity for silver and are, by definition, reticular fibers. Electron microscopy of these fibers reveals the periodic cross-banding characteristic of collagen. With increase in age there is a decrease in the proportion of argyrophilic fibers, without any demonstrable difference in structure. Similar observations on reticulin from the organic matrix of bone have not been reported.

Water of Bone

The water content of bone varies with the species of the animal, with age, with the nutritional state of the individual, and with the nature of the bone tissue under observation. As a representative standard for the compact bone of an adult dog, Robinson and Elliot (1957) have selected a figure of 3.68 per cent of water *by weight*, with 72.17 per cent of mineral and 24.15 per cent of organic matter. Owing to the differences in density, the corresponding figures, in terms of the *volume* of the sample of bone, are 8.2 per cent for water, 53.62 per cent for mineral, and 38.18 per cent for organic matter. Of the water present, some 10–15 per cent of the total volume is in the spaces in the bone occupied by canalicules, haversian canals, and osteocytes; 85–90 per cent is in the organic matrix, including the collagen fibers and ground substance, and in the hydration shells of the crystals of bone mineral. Drying at 100° C removes the water of constitution of the collagen and of other organic matter, but not the water of the bone crystals. The water of compact bone is so firmly bound that little or none can be removed from the finely powdered cortical bone by enormous centrifugal forces—forces sufficient to strip all mechanically held water from the crystals.

Perhaps the most important concept concerning the water of bone is that while the organic matter of normal compact bone remains relatively constant in relation to volume, calcification of new haversian systems occurs by replacement of water by crystals of bone mineral. The space available for mineral is thus the greater part of that occupied by water; crystallization proceeds until there is no space left for further expansion. As crystals form and grow in a fixed volume, by displacement of water, the spaces between the crystals become smaller and smaller; eventually a state of maximal diffusion-locked mineralization is achieved, with inadequate space for the diffusion of new ions.

In spite of the reduction in the ability of ions to diffuse in bone as a result of maximal mineralization, it has been found that when deuterium is administered in the form of heavy water, D_2O, it is able to permeate all areas of bone, and to exchange freely, though slowly, with the hydrogen ion of water. There is thus restricted diffusion of even the deuterium ion. The slow movement of ^{45}Ca into the stable portion of bone, which characterizes long-term exchange, must take place in part by diffusion, where there is sufficient space for the ions to move between crystals, and in part by intracrystalline exchange. The packing of the water spaces with crystals differentiates calcified from soft tissues and is doubtless responsible for the relative inaccessibility of the bone mineral to ion exchange.

Fluorescence in Bone

Bone mineral produces a light-blue fluorescence in ultraviolet light. This physical property can be used to detect calcium salts in new bone in microscopic quantities. Owing to a complex interaction in newly formed bone, it is possible to change the fluorescence from blue to red, yellow, and other colors. In this way, new bone can be differentiated from older deposits of bone. John Belchier (1736*a*, *b*) reported that madder stained the new bone in the skeletons of birds and pigs that had been fed bran and madder; the color depends on ruberythric acid, which yields alizarin on hydrolysis. Synthetic alizarin is 1,2-dihydroxyanthraquinone; fluorescent solutions indicate the presence of unchanged 2-anthraquinone sodium sulfonate. Alizarin, as well as tetracycline, chlortetracycline, and oxytetracycline, has been found to fluoresce brightly in the new bone of animals and man examined under ultraviolet light. Alizarin Red S fluoresces deep red; chlortetracycline, orange; and tetracycline, light yellow. Quercetin, a flavine derivative, fluoresces an intense gold yellow. Other substances—porphyrins, carotenoids, lipofuchsins, and oxidized cytochrome—also produce a red or orange fluorescence, but appear in soft tissue as well and are not useful for experimental work on bone.

CHAPTER V

Crystal Structure and Chemical Composition of Bone Mineral

The hardness of bone, its outstanding characteristic, is the result of the unique properties of a two-phase system in which a mineral is enmeshed in a fibrous organic matrix. The bone mineral and the organic matrix, together with their associated water, make up the interstitial substance of bone. The mineral consists mainly of Ca^{2+}, PO_4^{3-}, OH^-, CO_3^{2-}, and citrate, with an inclusion of small amounts of other ions, especially Na^+, Mg^{2+}, and F^-. The crystal structure and chemical composition of the bone mineral have been under investigation for more than one hundred years, and they remain a subject of intensive study.

Certain statements may be made about the bone mineral, as a guide to its composition, structure, and behavior: (1) the crystals are ultramicroscopic in size, extremely minute, and of hardly more than colloidal dimensions; (2) the bone mineral is not a single, homogeneous chemical individual; (3) it includes an amorphous calcium phosphate with a range of Ca/P molar ratios from 1.45 to 1.55; (4) the basic atomic structure of the crystalline fraction is well known, chiefly from X-ray diffraction patterns, and is that of an apatite mineral, prototypes of which are common in nature; (5) the Ca/P molar ratio of the mineral that is present in calcifying cartilage of growing animals is less than 1.6, while that in bone is 1.6 or more; (6) the chemical composition is not so accurately known, partly because of its variability and partly because of the difficulty of differentiating between (*a*) the constituents of the basic structure, (*b*) the ions having only a surface relationship to the crystals, and (*c*) those possibly admixed with the apatite crystals, in a separate phase; (7) the structure and composition of the mineral correspond most closely to those of hydroxyapatite in all vertebrates studied, although the mineral component includes carbonate and citrate in substantial amounts; (8) various substitutions and exchanges of ions occur in the crystal structure; (9) dissolution and recrystallization may occur; (10) the minute crystals and the voids and discontinuities in the mineral expose large surfaces to the fluids of the body; (11) the ions held by adsorption or by substitution at these surfaces, as well as those incorporated within surface unit cells, with unshared sides, have a considerable influence upon the total composition of the mineral; (12) the surface ions are subject to rapid exchange with the fluids bathing the crystals; and (13) the reactivity of the mineral varies with its age and with its immediate environment.

Crystals of Bone Mineral

The crystals of the mineral of bone have long been known to be extremely minute—too small to be seen with the light microscope. While it was first shown by X-ray scatter patterns that the crystals are of the order of a few hundred A in size, current knowledge of the size and shape of the individual crystals is dependent mainly on electron microscopy. This method has its limitations, but the resolving power of the electron microscope has been increased, and the crystal of bone mineral is within the limits of its resolution.

Early reports of direct observation of crystal size and shape, by means of the electron microscope, described the crystals as minute tablets of a few hundred A in length and breadth, and a thickness of only 20–50 A; later reports tell of rodlets or hexagonal prisms. These descriptions were supported by low-angle X-ray scatter patterns, from which measurements of approximately 200 A in length and 75 A in diameter were calculated. Current estimates are in good agreement, to the effect that the diameters of rodlike crystals range from 25 to 75 A, with an average of 50 A. The rodlike crystals frequently extend over several major periods of the collagen fibrils; some have been traced up to a length of 3,000–4,000 A; all exhibit subunits of about 50 A (Fig. 18).

Internal Structure of Crystals

Much of the present knowledge of the internal structure of the microcrystals of the bone mineral stems from interpretation of the X-ray diffraction pattern of the crystals of bone, as compared with patterns of relatively pure samples of synthetic or naturally occurring crystals of minerals of known composition. When a monochromatic X-ray beam is passed through a regular array of atoms, such as a crystal, a diffraction pattern is produced, related to the atoms in the material, and more especially to their spatial arrangement. With a film near the irradiated sample it is possible to measure the angles between the incoming X-ray beam and the outgoing

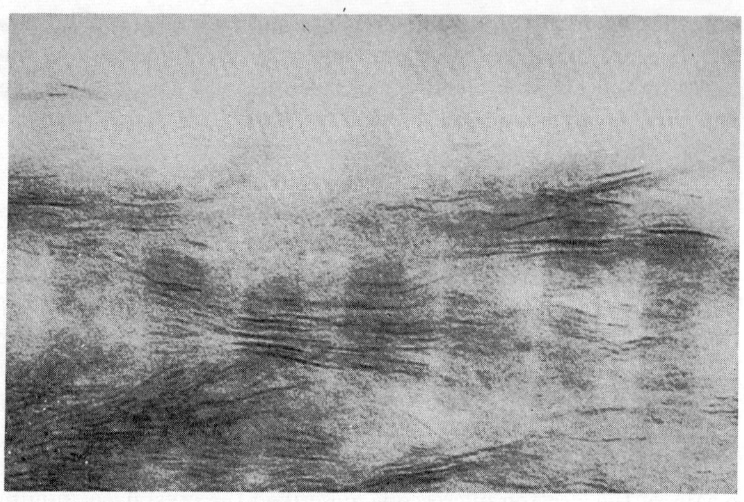

FIG. 18.—Electron micrograph of a section of undecalcified bone, in the long axis of the fibers. Needle-shaped crystals in the same axis appear in relation to the cross-bands. In some instances they extend over the intervals between the cross-bands. ×200,000. (Reproduced by courtesy of M. J. Glimcher, A. Hodge and F. O. Schmitt.)

diffracted beams. Data may thus be obtained concerning the arrangement of atoms within the crystal, including the distances between the atoms, and also concerning the orientation of the crystals.

It is firmly established that the mineral constitution of bone consists chiefly of crystals of a compound of calcium and phosphate with the structure of an apatite. The apatite series contains a number of compounds with their constituent ions arranged similarly in a three-dimensional symmetry pattern. The apatites usually have: (*a*) divalent cations (Ca^{2+}, Pb^{2+}, Sr^{2+}), (*b*) tetrahedral anionic radicals (PO_4^{3-}, SiO_4^{3-}), and (*c*) electronegative anions (OH^-, F^-), all in a hexagonal symmetry array characteristic of this isomorphous series. Certain ions can be substituted one for the other, e.g., Pb^{2+} for Ca^{2+}, F^- for OH^-, without disturbing the symmetry of the structure, although the distance between ions may change, owing to the differences in ionic size. X-ray diffraction techniques can easily detect changes of the order of 0.5 per cent in interatomic differences resulting from isomorphous substitution.

The basic structure of bone mineral is in the form of hydroxyapatite, of which the prototype is:

$$Ca_{10}(PO_4)_6(OH)_2 \text{ (hydroxyapatite).}$$

It is therefore possible to treat the internal structure characteristics of the bone mineral with some degree of certainty; the uncertainties in the exact chemical composition will be treated in later sections.

Unit Cell

The internal structure of the hydroxyapatite crystal is best understood in terms of the *unit cell.* This is a conceptual configuration having no independent existence. It is the smallest expression of the ions found in the same ratios and in the same spatial relationships in which they are present throughout the entire crystal. Imaginary lines connecting the ions, drawn in an arbitrary but regular way, outline the unit cell; when extended through the crystal structure they result in a three-dimensional lattice—the *crystal lattice.*

The crystal structure of hydroxyapatite may be represented in two different ways. In a cross-section of the crystal, perpendicular to the long axis, it may be represented as a series of contiguous hexagons (Fig. 19). At each intersection there is a Ca^{2+} ion, shared between three hexagons, and surrounded by PO_4^{3-} ions, arranged in a complex pattern. At the center of the hexagon there is an OH^- ion, shared by three Ca^{2+} ions. The two OH^- ions of hydroxyapatite are superimposed on each other; three of the six Ca^{2+} ions forming the hexagon share one OH^- ion; the other three share the next.

The second method represents the unit cells. The points corresponding to the OH^- ions in a cross-section of the crystal may be connected in a two-dimensional diagram as a series of rhombi with angles of 120° and 60° at the intersections. When extended in a third dimension, this forms a parallelepiped, or a six-sided right prism, four of whose faces are rectangles, with two faces as rhombi.

Each of these geometric figures is, by convention, a unit cell of the crystal lattice. The rhombi of a unit cell of hydroxyapatite have four equal sides, measuring approximately 9.43 A in length, representing the *a* axes of the cells (Fig. 19). The third dimension, or *c* axis, measures approximately 6.88 A.

The *c* axes of the unit cells are oriented in the long dimension of the crystal of hydroxyapatite. When a diagram of the lattice of an ideal crystal is viewed parallel to the *c* axis, there are continuous columns of calcium and oxygen arranged at the intersections of the hexagons and columns of OH^- ions at the intersections of the rhombi representing the unit cells. From this point of view there is

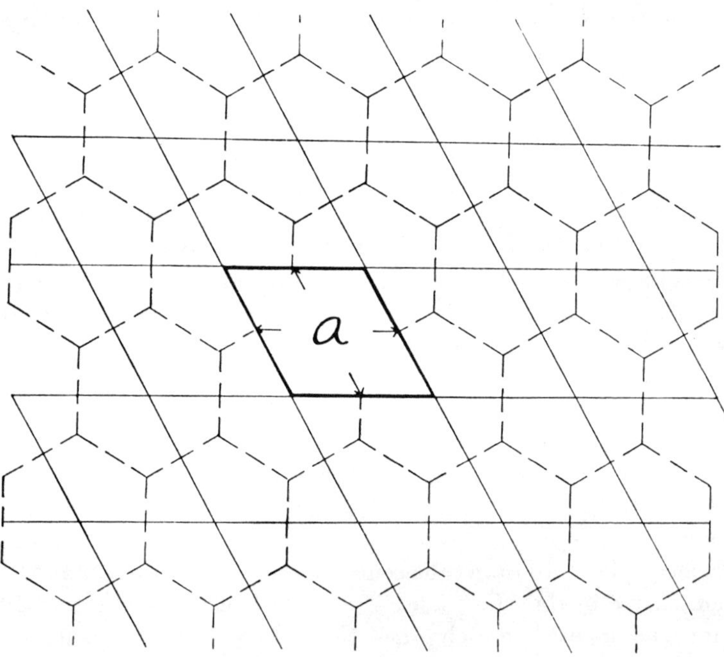

Fig. 19.—Diagram of a cross-section of a crystal of bone mineral, to illustrate internal structure. The parallelograms represent the unit cells of the crystal; these are conceptual, rather than structural, units, since they illustrate only the arrangement of constituent ions in space. The hexagons represent a honeycomb-like arrangement of ions, oriented with the long axis of the crystal. At each intersection of the hexagons is a Ca^{2+} ion. The tunnels are lined with Ca^{2+} ions and packed with PO_4^{3-} ions, with a column of OH^- ions in the center. Scale ×20,000,000 (2 mm = 1 A). The parallel sides of the unit cells (*a* axes) are approximately 9.43 A in length.

a honeycomb arrangement, oriented in the long axes of the crystals. The columns of calcium and oxygen at the intersections of the hexagons give the form to the honeycomb; these columns are surrounded by phosphate, with a column of OH^- ions in the center of each hexagon. In addition, there is a screw axis, running spirally around the columns of OH^- ions; Ca^{2+} ions, in addition to those at the intersections of the hexagons, are symmetrically arranged with respect to this axis, and are also accompanied by phosphate ions.

Variability in Structure

The descriptions just given refer to perfect or ideal crystals of hydroxyapatite. The real crystals, as they occur in bone, are neither perfect nor ideal. Many discontinuities are formed within the structure of a single crystal as it grows, and others form with time. At the surfaces of the discontinuities, which are irregular and occur at random, impurities may exist; in fact, if such impurities are of sufficient magnitude, they may be the cause of the discontinuity. Moreover, substitutions occur in the unit cells; not all unit cells are identical in composition or even in structure.

The crystals of the bone mineral are only a few unit cells thick. The surface is therefore large in proportion to the mass, and 1 gram of the mineral is reported to have a surface area in excess of 100 square meters. Calculations from these figures lead to the rather startling conclusion that the total surface area of the bone crystals in the skeleton of a man weighing 70 kilograms exceeds 100 acres! The implications of the fact that such a large area is bathed by a few liters of body fluid are many.

Because of the small size and the thinness of the crystals, one-half to two-thirds of the unit cells are located in the surface, possess one or more unshared sides, and are subject to special surface conditions. These conditions have created difficulties in characterizing the bone mineral and are as yet not fully understood. When they are taken into account, it is seen that the nature and structure of the bone mineral and the dynamics of its behavior are largely problems in surface chemistry.

Discontinuities in the bone mineral are not limited to the interior of the crystals; the crystals themselves are discrete; the spaces between them are filled with organic matrix, water, and the solid constituents not included in the crystal structure. If one considers bone from which the organic matter and water have been removed, it is as though the bone mineral itself were built up of bricks and mortar rather than as a continuous mass of a homogeneous substance. It thus resembles a brick wall, rather than a monolith, with a pattern peculiar to itself. The bricks are the crystals of apatite; the mortar consists chiefly of citrate and carbonate, with an admixture of other ions. In the living animal the structure is plastic rather than rigid; the organic matrix and the intercellular fluid are also in the spaces between the crystals; the collagen fibers act as reinforcing strands in the loosely assembled intercrystalline portion of the structure. From studies made with the electron microscope it is reported that the crystals lie in the ground substance, forming a ringlike periodic pattern around the collagen fibers. The intervals between the rings are about 640 A, corresponding to the intervals between the cross-banding of the fibers; the crystals have a definite relationship to the cross-banding (Fig. 20). Some of the mineral is deposited *within* the collagen fibers; in this location it may be in a noncrystalline state.

It is convenient to consider the structure of the bone mineral as being made up of a large number of similar, but not identical, complexes. These complexes are not solely the crystals of apatite, although much effort has been expended in attempting to understand the mineral in these terms. Instead, each structural complex may be regarded as including interior unit cells wholly within the crystals; surface unit cells, sharing some of their sides with interior cells; ions bound by surface forces; and a surface hydration shell, containing ions in equilibrium both with the surrounding medium and with the surfaces.

Chemical Nature of Bone Mineral

It has already been noted that the bone mineral is not a single, homogeneous chemical individual; that the chemical composition is not accurately known; that various substitutions and exchanges of ions occur in the structure; that dissolution and recrystallization may occur; and that there are voids and discontinuities in the crystals. All of these factors make for an unsatisfactory situation with respect to the chemical characterization of the initial form of the bone mineral, even though the structure of the mature form, corresponding closely to that of hydroxyapatite, is well established.

Elementary Analysis

Armstrong and Singer (1965) have furnished a summary of their analyses of a single sample of dry, fat-free bovine cortical bone. The standard deviations represent the variations in the analyses, and do not refer to variations of composition between various samples of bone (Table 3).

The most important single value in this tabulation, for our purposes, is the molar Ca/P ratio of 1.656; this corresponds very closely to the theoretical ratio for hydroxyapatite, 1.667. Values for another single sample of bone as found by Bogert and Hastings (1931) differed with the previous treatment of a sample, but were in the range of 1.70–1.80 for untreated bone and bone extracted with water or alcohol. After more vigorous treatment to remove the

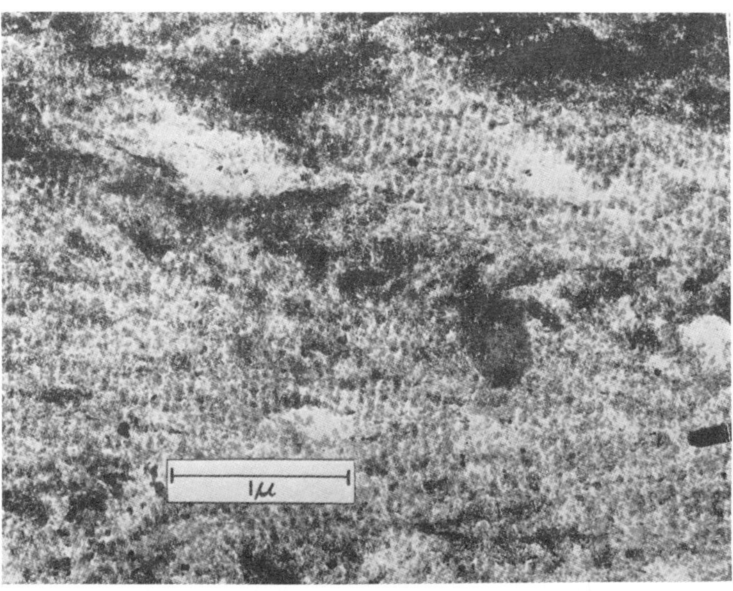

Fig. 20.—Electron micrograph of a section of an undecalcified human rib, to illustrate pattern of arrangement of crystals of bone mineral in relation to collagen fibers. The underlying collagen is barely visible, but the crystals are easily seen in the regularly arranged bands corresponding to the main collagen striation. The longitudinal direction of the fibers is horizontal. (From Fig. 1, Neuman and Neuman, Chem. Rev. 53:4 [courtesy of R. A. Robinson and M. L. Watson]. Reproduced by courtesy of the publishers.)

organic matter, including ashing at such temperatures as to cause little or no loss of carbonate, the range was consistently between 1.57 and 1.61. If allowance is made for the Ca^{2+} required to neutralize the anionic constituents of the mineral, chiefly carbonate, as Bogert and Hastings (1931) and Neuman and Neuman (1958) have done, the residual molar Ca/P ratio is then approximately 1.5, or considerably less than the theoretical value of 1.67. The bone

TABLE 3

COMPOSITION OF DRY, FAT-FREE, AND EXTRACTED BOVINE CORTICAL BONE

	Per Cent ± S.D.	mEq/g
CATIONS		
Calcium	26.70 ±0.015	13.32
Magnesium	0.436 ±0.009	0.358
Sodium	0.731 ±0.015	0.318
Potassium	0.055 ±0.0009	0.014
Strontium	0.035	......
Total	....	14.01
ANIONS		
Phosphorus	12.47 ±0.013	......
as PO_4^{3-}	....	12.06
Carbon dioxide	3.48 ±0.022	......
as CO_3^{2-}	....	1.58
Citric acid	0.863 ±0.004	......
as Cit^{3-}	....	0.138
Chloride	0.077 ±0.004	0.022
Fluoride	0.072 ±0.003	0.038
Total	....	13.84
$\frac{\text{mEq. cations}}{\text{mEq. anions}}$	....	1.01
$\frac{\text{mmoles Ca}}{\text{mmoles P}}$	....	1.656
Nitrogen (per cent)	4.92 ±0.05	......

Adapted from Armstrong and Singer, Clin. Orthop. 38:179–90, 1965.

mineral has been compared with similar apatites, synthetically prepared, and deficient in divalent cations. The calculations of the residual Ca/P ratio in bone mineral do not take into account the cations other than Ca^{2+} that are available for neutralization of the anionic constituents; their inclusion in the calculations would tend to raise the Ca/P ratio toward the theoretical value of 1.67.

There is no doubt about the ability of certain other cations to substitute for calcium in the structure of the bone mineral; this occurs by isomorphous substitution and has been demonstrated in living animals, as well as in synthetic hydroxyapatites, for strontium and for lead; radium also substitutes for calcium. Sodium substitutes for calcium, as does the hydronium ion, H_3O^+. There is no evidence that potassium substitutes for calcium in the bone mineral, and the position of the divalent magnesium ion, Mg^{2+}, is doubtful; it has been suggested that the magnesium found in analysis of the mineral constituents of bone may be in the form of the complex ion $MgOH^+$. As to anions, the most common substitution is that of F^- for OH^-. Fluorapatites occur in nature; the occurrence of F^- in the bone mineral represents a contamination. There has been no suggestion that citrate, found in the mineral of bone in substantial amounts, can be a structural constituent of the apatite crystal; the dimensions of the citrate ion, $C_6H_5O_7^{3-}$, are too large for isomorphous substitution. Citrate is regarded as a separate phase, with a special relationship to the surfaces of crystals.

Noncrystalline Calcium Phosphate

X-ray diffraction patterns reveal only the bone mineral that is in crystalline form, and do not account for any additional component that is poorly crystallized or amorphous. Termine (1966), employing X-ray diffraction, electron spin resonance, and infrared spectroscopy, has found amorphous or noncrystalline calcium phosphate to be a second major phase of bone mineral, separate and distinct from bone apatite. From his work, and from the work of Eanes, Gillessen, and Posner (1965), it appears that the first mineral formed in bone is noncrystalline, and that the amorphous calcium phosphate content of rat femur decreases with age, as its crystalline apatite increases. In the rat, the crystallinity value for the femur levels off at 65 per cent when the rat reaches maturity. This poor crystallinity accounts for the low intensity of the X-ray diffraction patterns obtained with samples of bone mineral. In young growing rats, 8 to 38 days of age, minerals with Ca/P molar ratios ranging from 1.41 to 1.59 have been found, with amounts of noncrystalline calcium phosphate equal to from 36 to 69 per cent of the total inorganic mineral. The evidence produced is stated to be quite conclusive proof that the two-phase nature of bone mineral is universal, and the presence of amorphous calcium phosphate in bone is not an artifact of species specificity. As indicated in Table 4, there is no direct transformation of amorphous calcium phosphate to the crystalline mineral; the amorphous form must be dissolved, and its constituent ions are then redeposited in crystalline form. The physiologic significance of the change in phase from the amorphous to the crystalline form of the bone mineral has as yet to be clarified.

Initial Deposits of Crystalline Mineral in Cartilage and Bone

Urist and Dowell (1967) note that the chemical composition of the earliest deposits of crystalline mineral is different in the zone of provisional calcification from that in the new diaphyseal bone. The Ca/P molar ratio is low in cartilage, the uptake of tetracycline

TABLE 4

Model of Maturation of Bone Mineral

Compound	Symbol	Formula	Ca/P Ratio Molar	Ca/P Ratio Weight
Amorphous calcium phosphate...........	......	....	1.45–1.55	....
Octacalcium phosphate.	OCP	$Ca_8H_2(PO_4)_6 \cdot 5H_2O$	8/6 (1.33)	1.72
Hydrated tricalcium phosphate...........	TCPH	$Ca_9H(PO_4)_6(OH)$	9/6 (1.50)	1.94
Hydroxyapatite........	HA	$Ca_{10}(PO_4)_6(OH)_2$	10/6 (1.67)	2.15

is high, and the yield of pyrophosphate on ignition is high. Urist and Dowell correlate the low Ca/P ratio in diaphyseal bone with the amount of cartilage in the matrix. This could explain why chemical analyses of marrow-free cortical bone by Armstrong and Singer (1965), microchemical analyses by Strandh *et al.* (1965), and electron probe analyses by Mellors (1964) result in values for the Ca/P ratio that is always 1.67, while chemical analyses of fetal or newborn cartilaginous bones by other investigators always give a value near 1.5. The nature of the mineral responsible for the low Ca/P ratio in calcified cartilage is not known, but it is suggested in Table 4 that it is either octacalcium phosphate or another precursor of hydroxyapatite of similar composition and structure.

Carbonate of Bone

Carbonate is universally present as a constituent of the mineral of normal bones and teeth. A carbonate-containing apatite, dahllite, exists in nature and is described as a carbonate hydroxyapatite. Similarly, francolite has been characterized as a carbonate fluorapatite. These have attracted attention because of possible analogies between their composition and crystal structure and those of bones and teeth. Prior to 1937 it was believed that CO_3^{2-} could substitute for 2 F^- or 2 OH^-, thus forming a true carbonate apatite, but this is no longer accepted. Instead, there is now the proposal, advanced and strongly supported by McConnell (1965), that CO_3^{2-} substitutes isomorphically for PO_4^{3-} in the minerals francolite and dahllite. McConnell concludes that dental enamel is composed of a single mineral, carbonate hydroxyapatite (dahllite), and states that there is no valid reason for supposing that the crystal structure or crystal chemistry of bone is significantly different. Against this is the view that CO_3^{2-} is present in the mineral of bone and teeth only in surface positions, where it substitutes for PO_4^{3-}; the evidence is summarized by Neuman and Neuman (1958). Neuman and Mulryan (1967) have demonstrated with exchange studies with $^{14}CO_2$ that 60 per cent of the CO_2, presumably as CO_3^{2-}, resided within the crystal lattice, and 40 per cent, presumably as HCO_3^-, remained in the hydration shells of the crystals. The exchangeable carbonate is lost on drying and in the bone of very young animals amounts to a fraction as high as 47 per cent of the total carbonate in bone mineral. Thus the bone mineral is to be regarded as a substituted hydroxyapatite, with the structural characteristics of the latter.

Without attempting to resolve the differences of opinion concerning the location of carbonate in relation to the structure of hydroxyapatite, it may be said that, in common with certain other minerals, a carbonate hydroxyapatite does not lend itself to stoichiometric formulation, since CO_3^{2-} does not substitute for PO_4^{3-} in any fixed proportions or in any special pattern. Instead, McConnell has supplied the following as a type of formula used to represent minerals with constituents in varying proportions:

$$Ca_{10-x}O_{2+x}H_{2+3x}(PO_4)_{6-3x}(CO_3)_{4x} \quad \text{(carbonate hydroxyapatite)},$$

which reduces to conventional hydroxyapatite when $x = 0$, and to the following when $x = 1$:

$$Ca_9O_3H_5(PO_4)_3(CO_3)_4 \quad \text{(carbonate hydroxyapatite).}$$

However, there is no evidence that natural substances ever have x as great as 1.

There has been little evidence to show that random substitution of CO_3^{2-} for PO_4^{3-}, either within the apatite crystal or on the surface, is of physiologic importance; this question would assume much significance if it could be shown that the presence of CO_3^{2-} is essential for the mineralization of bone. Hydroxyapatite has been produced in essentially pure form without carbon dioxide. Sobel and Hanok (1948) have shown that the carbonate content of the bone mineral depends upon the Ca/P ratio of the serum, as influenced by dietary Ca/P ratios and levels. Neuman and Mulryan (1967) propose that the exchangeable bicarbonate in the hydration phase of bone is the one compartment capable of serving as a useful alkaline reserve in times of acidotic stress.

Maturation of Bone Mineral

There is evidence that: (1) the mineral of bone is initially deposited as an amorphous calcium phosphate, with a Ca/P molar ratio of 1.45–1.55; (2) part of this is redissolved and redeposited as a reactive crystalline precipitate, similar to or identical with octacalcium phosphate; (3) this is transformed, mainly by the addition of Ca^{2+}, through a stage corresponding to Dallemagne's hydrated tricalcium phosphate (1952), or to Posner and Perloff's calcium-deficient hydroxyapatite (1957); and (4) the crystalline portion of the mineral finally matures to the relatively unreactive and stable form of hydroxyapatite. Efforts to describe the mineral in terms of a single chemical individual, corresponding to any of the transition forms, have not been successful. For our purposes it will be more profitable to consider the mineral as a heterogeneous system which, following its initial crystallization, should be regarded as a continuum, rather than as a mixture of transition forms.

It seems now to be well established that the bone mineral undergoes maturation, leading eventually to its stable and best characterized form, approximating hydroxyapatite. In so doing, and in contrast to its earth-mineral prototypes, it is severely limited both with respect to time and to temperature. While the minerals found in the earth have had virtually limitless time for their evolution into their present forms, and in many instances, at least, have been exposed to wide ranges of temperature, the bone mineral must reach its final state during the lifetime of the organism in which it is formed, and must do so at body temperature. When these limitations are taken into account, it is not surprising that the crystallinity of the bone mineral is poor and that its chemical composition and crystal structure are variable.

Table 4 represents an attempt to describe an arbitrary model for the evolution of the stable mineral from its precursors. According to this concept, calcium ions are regarded as missing randomly throughout the crystal structure of the mineral, electroneutrality being maintained by hydrogen bonds between oxygens of adjacent orthophosphate groups. Maturation occurs by an increase in the proportion of calcium in the mineral, as a result of the replacement of hydrogen bonds or of the filling of voids by calcium ions.

This scheme does not insist on a rigid chemical definition of any stage of the formation or maturation of the mineral; it represents rather a model of the continuum referred to above. The general formula for the system, taken from Winand and Dallemagne (1962) may be written as follows:

$$Ca_{10-x}H_x\,(PO_4)_6\,(OH)_{2-x} \quad \text{(apatitic calcium phosphate series).}$$

The case for individual crystalline compounds existing as such is outlined below. Table 4 is intended to illustrate the concept of initial crystallization, following precipitation of an amorphous calcium phosphate, and leading to the evolution of a continuum that eventually stabilizes with an approximation of the hydroxyapatite structure and chemical composition. It illustrates amorphous calcium phosphate as the precursor of the crystalline system, but not included in the continuum as such.

This table, illustrating the maturation of the bone mineral, ignores ions known to be present in bone, such as carbonate and citrate, but not essential to the concept of maturation of the mineral.

Hydrated Tricalcium Phosphate

The formulation of hydroxyapatite calls for a molar Ca/P ratio of 1.667, as already noted. By mixing phosphoric acid and calcium hydroxide in varying proportions one may obtain calcium phosphates with Ca/P ratios as low as 1.5; all of these phosphates give the X-ray diffraction pattern of apatite. Bone mineral with a Ca/P ratio of 1.5 has been described, and referred to as hydrated tricalcium phosphate or as alpha tricalcium phosphate. It was originally given the formula:

$$Ca_9(PO_4)_6 \cdot H_2(OH)_2 \text{ (alpha tricalcium phosphate; original formulation).}$$

Posner and Perloff (1957) modified this view, and indicated that the concept of alpha tricalcium phosphate is a special case of a calcium-deficient hydroxyapatite. They proposed that hydrogen bonding is responsible for maintaining neutrality in low-calcium hydroxyapatites, since hydrogen bonds are present in a series of such compounds in proportion to the missing calcium ions.

Hydrogen bonding in these compounds has been further demonstrated by Winand and Dallemagne (1962), who proposed the following formula for the calcium-deficient apatite containing 9 Ca^{2+} ions for 6 PO_4^{3-} groups:

$$Ca_9(PO_4)_4(OH)(O_3PO\text{-}H \rightarrow OPO_3) \text{ (hydrated tricalcium phosphate; hydrogen bonding).}$$

This formation has been accepted by Termine (1966) for small-sized, calcium-deficient, synthetic apatite crystals, and he also suggests that such defect apatites must be considered as possible intermediates in the formation of mature bone apatite crystals. Defect apatites are no longer considered to be major constituents of the mature bone mineral.

An important characteristic of low-calcium apatite is that, like bone mineral, it has the capacity to yield calcium pyrophosphate following ignition and dehydration. The reaction is:

$$2\ Ca_9(PO_4)_4(OH)(O_3PO_4\text{—}H\text{—}OPO_9) \text{ (hydrated tricalcium phosphate)}$$

$$\downarrow \ 500^\circ \text{ C (synthetic apatite crystals)}; \ 325^\circ \text{ C (bone)}$$

$$Ca_9(PO_4)_5(OH)(P_2O_7)OH(PO_4)_5Ca_9 \text{ (calcium pyrophosphate).}$$

When the Ca/P ratio of a mineral is 1.5, it yields pyrophosphate on heating to the extent of 16.6 per cent of the total phosphorus; when it is 1.3, it yields 33 per cent pyrophosphate. Low-calcium apatites also absorb infrared to produce bands characteristic of numbers of hydrogen bonds and amounts of water; they have a higher reactivity than hydroxyapatite in systems containing fluoride ions or other bone-seeking substances. It is now very much an open question whether there is a specific single mineral that characterizes the initial deposit of bone mineral.

Octacalcium Phosphate

When samples of bone mineral are obtained from the ends of a rapidly growing bone of a young animal, the Ca/P ratio may be as low as 1.3–1.4. If one calcium atom were missing from the crystal lattice, the Ca/P ratio would be 1.5 and the mineral would be comparable to a synthetic low-calcium apatite. If two were missing, the Ca/P ratio would be 1.3, and there would be another possibility for serious consideration. Brown (1962; 1966) proposed that octacalcium phosphate, also called tetracalcium hydrogen triphosphate, $2\ Ca_4H(PO_4)_3 \cdot 2.5\ H_2O$, having a Ca/P ratio of 1.3, may be present in the formative stages of the bone mineral as an intercrystalline lamellar mixture with hydroxyapatite. Their evidence is that: (1) octacalcium phosphate (OCP) produces epitaxial growth of hydroxyapatite (HA); (2) the X-ray diffraction pattern of HA obscures the presence of OCP; (3) bone mineral of young individuals has a higher solubility and higher rate of dissolution and recrystallization, more like OCP than HA; (4) HA has a needle form while OCP has a platy crystal habit closer to that of bone mineral; (5) young calf bone has a Ca/P molar ratio of 8.13/6, reflecting the presence of a large amount of a mineral such as OCP; and (6) a large amount and higher solubility of OCP in growing bone would explain the higher level of serum phosphorus of young animals. However, despite the evidence, the case for OCP as the initial step in formation of the bone mineral is not complete.

Summary

It is generally accepted that the basic crystal structure and chemical composition of the mature mineral of bone is that of hydroxyapatite, $Ca_{10}(PO_4)_6(OH)_2$, with an admixture of variable amounts of carbonate and of citrate, as well as of adventitious ions, both in the crystal lattice and in the crystal surface. A second phase, amorphous or noncrystalline calcium phosphate, has been described, and in this chapter the concept of maturation of the bone mineral has been advanced, leading to the formation of the stable mineral of which hydroxyapatite is the prototype.

CHAPTER VI

Dynamics of Bone Mineral

The preceding chapter has dealt with the crystal structure and chemical composition of the bone mineral, largely in static terms. This chapter will be concerned with its dynamics, including such topics as nucleation, crystal formation, crystal growth, solubility, and reactivity. Study of the dynamics of the bone mineral has been mainly concerned with calcification, including nucleation and crystal growth. In recent years, much attention has also been given to matrix formation, the reactivity of the mineral, and more especially the transfer of ions between bone and blood.

Solubility Relationships

That the bone mineral is difficultly soluble is of far-reaching physiologic significance. This property not only determines the deposition of the bone mineral; it preserves the structure and the rigidity of the bones. Moreover, it is of first importance in maintaining the balance of minerals between the skeleton and the fluids of the body.

The adult organism as a whole is normally in approximate calcium balance; that is, the output of calcium is equal to the intake. There is a constant turnover of the bone mineral; and since the bones account for by far the greater part of the body's store of calcium, an overall calcium balance means that the rates of deposition and of solution of the bone mineral are also in balance. This is true even though deposition and solution of the mineral may occur at different rates in different parts of the skeleton at the same time.

It is desirable to review here the concept of the solubility product constant. An *ion product* is the product of the molar concentrations of ions in solution, relevant to the salt under consideration. The *law of mass action* requires that when an ion is present in the formula of a molecule in numbers greater than one, its molar concentration in the ion product must be raised to the power corresponding to the number of ions in the formula. The ion product of $CaHPO_4$ is $[Ca^{2+}] \times [HPO_4^{2-}]$, while the ion product of $Ca_3(PO_4)_2$ is $[Ca^{2+}]^3 \times [PO_4^{3-}]^2$. In these expressions the brackets are used to indicate *concentrations* in moles per liter. Application of the Debye-Hückel theory of interionic attraction would require that these concentrations be corrected by *activity coefficients;* the physicochemical activity of ions is decreased as the *ionic strength* of the solution is increased. The development of the subject of ion products without these corrections is admittedly an oversimplification; since activity coefficients remain constant at constant ionic strength, it is justifiable to omit them for purposes of comparison when body fluids of approximately constant ionic strength are under consideration.

A *solubility product constant* is the ion product at concentrations of the ions at which the rates of solution and of precipitation of the salt are equal. The solubility product constant thus defines the conditions present at equilibrium; these are identical with those in a saturated solution containing the ions of a difficultly soluble salt.

Numerous attempts have been made to define the solubility of the bone mineral in simple physicochemical terms; that is, by the determination of a solubility product constant. These have not been successful, for several reasons. First, the concept of solubility product constant is meaningless without reference to a known and homogeneous solid phase. The bone mineral does not meet this requirement. Second, equilibrium between the solid and liquid phases of hydroxyapatite is attained *in vitro* only very slowly and with great difficulty. Moreover, the results of equilibration may differ, according to whether the state of saturation is approached from supersaturation or from undersaturation. A part of this difficulty stems from the fact that the solid phase of the mineral may adsorb ions from solution. Third, the solid phase may undergo changes in composition during equilibration. Fourth, the relations between the bone mineral and the fluids bathing it are influenced by certain biologic factors, such as the state of activity of the parathyroid glands.

Levinskas (1953) has made a careful and detailed study of the solubility of a synthetic hydroxyapatite, under widely varying conditions. The reproducibility of the results and the agreement of findings, when undersaturated and supersaturated solutions were employed initially, support the belief that equilibrium was attained. Even under the rigorously controlled conditions of the experiments, however, the constant, well-characterized solid phase employed did not permit determination of a solubility product constant. It was concluded that it is impossible to determine a $K_{s.p.}$ for such examples of the apatite lattice in aqueous systems. The factors entering into this situation are reviewed in detail by Neuman and Neuman (1958), who conclude that the blood serum is supersaturated with respect to bone mineral, but below the point of spontaneous precipitation.

Earlier, Logan and Taylor (1937) brought bone powder to equilibrium with solutions containing calcium and phosphate, and they expressed the conditions at equilibrium as an ion product which they regarded as a solubility product constant, as follows:

$$[Ca^{2+}]^3 \times [PO_4^{3-}]^2 = K_{s.p\,Ca_3(PO_4)_2}$$

$$-\log K = pK_{s.p.Ca_3(PO_4)_2} = 23.1 \pm 0.4 \,.$$

Although, for reasons stated above, their formulation cannot be accepted as defining the solubility of the bone salt, it is still of interest and empirical value. They approached equilibrium from both supersaturation and undersaturation; moreover, they reduced the quantity of the solid phase to the vanishing point, thus minimizing adsorption. We are retaining their values for comparison with results obtained with a biologic end point.

More recently, MacGregor and Nordin (1960) have carried out equilibration studies with human bone powder, comparable to those of Logan and Taylor, but using different methods. In the pH range of 6.58–7.8 they obtained a relatively constant ion product $[Ca^{2+}]^3 \times [PO_4^{3-}]^2$ whether equilibrium was approached from supersaturation or undersaturation. The arithmetic mean product observed was 4.1×10^{-27}, corresponding, in the terms of Logan and Taylor, to pK = 26.39. This figure approximates that obtained by Logan and Taylor when they used a high solid/solution ratio, and was reduced by them to 23.1 when they eliminated the influence of adsorption by using very small quantities of the solid phase. Since the figure obtained by MacGregor and Nordin corresponds to the ion product in normal tissue fluids at pH 6.8, they suggest that this may be the pH at the surface of the bone mineral. This subject is given further consideration in connection with the surface chemistry of the mineral.

Biologic Solubility

Much of the difficulty in expressing the conditions for crystallization of the bone mineral in physicochemical terms has been due to the requirement of attaining equilibrium between the liquid and the solid phases and of determining when this end point has been reached. To avoid the necessity of equilibrium, the concept of *biologic solubility*, with the use of a biologic end point, was introduced some years ago. Such an end point, to be meaningful, may be described in terms of an ion product. It therefore has the characteristics of a solubility product constant, with the exception that the criterion for arriving at the constant is the phenomenon of calcification itself. The limit of biologic solubility is the minimum ion product at which calcification will occur.

If young growing rats are fed diets deficient in phosphate and in vitamin D, the bones continue to grow, but calcification ceases. There follows an overgrowth of cartilage, accompanied by the appearance of uncalcified bone matrix—the osteoid tissue. This condition, characterized by a failure of calcification to keep pace with growth, is *rickets*. If the deficiencies in the diet are corrected, calcification begins again, both in the cartilage matrix and in the osteoid tissue. This occurs also in cartilage matrix *in vitro* when slices of rachitic cartilage are incubated under favorable conditions, and both the locus of calcification and the product obtained are comparable to those observed in the living animal. Most of our information concerning the dynamics of calcification is based on *in vitro* studies, but enough observations have been made *in vivo*, both in rachitic children and in experimental animals, to make it appear that the results obtained *in vitro* are applicable to the living organism. Calcification of the cartilage matrix *in vitro* has been used as the end point for biologic solubility.

Calcification: Humoral Conditions

Calcification, in the systems with which this book is concerned, is essentially the deposition within a soft organic matrix of a difficultly soluble compound of calcium, resembling the hydroxyapatite described in the foregoing chapter. For calcification to occur, certain fundamental conditions must be present. These divide themselves naturally into (1) humoral and (2) local conditions. The *humoral conditions* embrace the supply and transport of the minerals necessary for calcification and their delivery to the locus of calcification in the concentrations required. The local conditions include whatever it is that differentiates a *calcifiable* from a noncalcifiable tissue. This is at times referred to as the *local factor*. Since, however, several interrelated factors, enzymatic and nonenzymatic, appear to be involved, it will be convenient to refer to these collectively as the *local mechanism*. In considering the humoral conditions for calcification, it is apparent that in spite of the difficulties in defining the solubility relationships of the bone mineral, its deposition and its maintenance in the solid state depend primarily upon its solubility.

Howland and Kramer (1921), in the absence of any method for determining either calcium or phosphate ion concentrations in the plasma, introduced a simple empirical product, Total Calcium *times* Total Phosphate, and found that the presence or absence of rickets in infants could be correlated with this product. Further refinement of this formulation has since been possible, and it has now a sound, although incomplete, basis.

Of the 1–2 mmoles per liter of phosphorus in the plasma, as inorganic phosphate, approximately 85 per cent is in the form of the divalent ion HPO_4^{2-}, while 15 per cent is $H_2PO_4^-$ and only 0.0035 per cent is present as PO_4^{3-}. The ions Ca^{2+} and HPO_4^{2-} may combine in a one-to-one ratio, and both are present in the fluids of the body in appreciable concentrations. For these reasons it should not occasion surprise that since the publications of Howland and his associates the findings have been more consistently related to the ion product $[Ca^{2+}] \times [HPO_4^{2-}]$ than to any other combination.

In view of these considerations, the concept of biologic solubility has been used in an attempt to determine whether the ion product of $CaHPO_4$ or that of $Ca_3(PO_4)_2$ is critical for calcification. The results are presented, with the reservation that the theoretical significance of the ion product $[Ca^{2+}]^3 \times [PO_4^{3-}]^2$ is not established.

Over a wide range of H^+ concentration, pH 6.0–8.5, and of total phosphate concentration, 3–80 mmoles per liter, and with the Ca^{2+} concentration kept constant, the minimum ion products at which calcification occurred in rachitic bone slices were determined.

These points were plotted against total phosphate concentrations and pH (Fig. 21). On the same plot were drawn curves representing $pK_{s.p.CaHPO_4} = 5.47$, and $pK_{s.p.Ca_3(PO_4)_2} = 23.1$, at varying concentrations of phosphate and varying pH. On the acid side of pH 7.3, the points at which calcification just occurred followed the curve for the ion product $[Ca^{2+}]^3 \times [PO_4^{3-}]^2$, while on the alkaline side, the points coincided closely with the curve for the ion product $[Ca^{2+}] \times [HPO_4^{2-}]$.

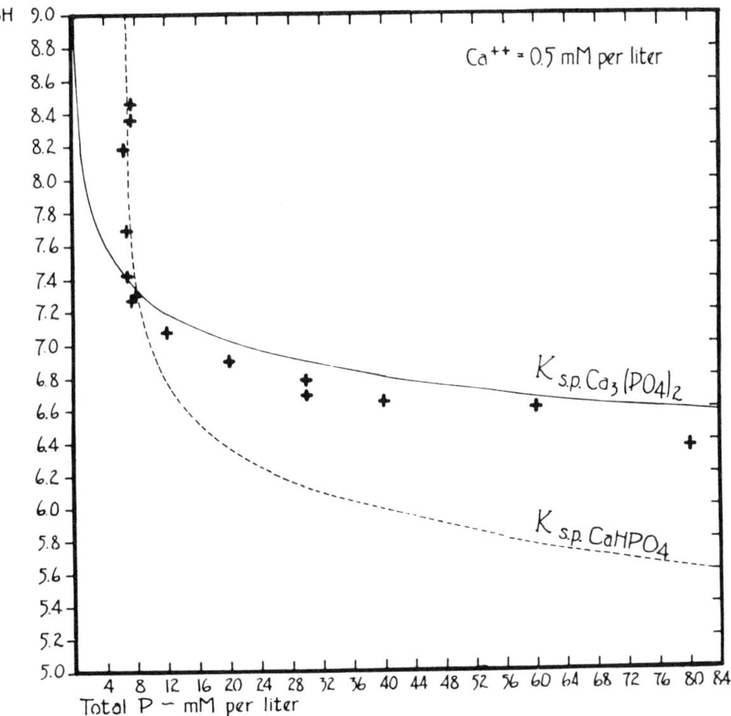

Fig. 21.—Relationship of calcium and phosphate concentrations and of ion products to calcification of rachitic cartilage *in vitro*. Total calcium (Ca^{2+}) 0.5 mmoles/l; pH and total phosphorus varied. Lines representing ion products drawn from $pK_{s.p.CaHPO_4} = 5.47$ (Shear and Kramer); $pK_{s.p.Ca_3(PO_4)_2} = 23.1$ (Logan and Taylor); + indicates minimum ion products at which calcification occurred. Note that calcification above 7.3 is correlated with solubility product constant for $CaHPO_4$; below pH 7.3 with solubility product constant for $Ca_3(PO_4)_2$. (From Fig. 3, McLean, Lipton, Bloom and Barron, Tr. Conf. Metab. Aspects Convalescence 14:33. Reproduced by courtesy of the publishers.)

The significance of the results on the acid side of pH 7.3 is not clear, partly because of the uncertainties concerning the ion product $[Ca^{2+}]^3 \times [PO_4^{3-}]^2$. In addition, the ionic strength of the solutions increases rapidly with increases in concentration of total phosphate. This has the effect of decreasing the activities of both Ca^{2+} and PO_4^{3-}; and if the proper corrections could be made, this might have the effect of bringing the experimentally determined points close to the curve representing $pK_{s.p.CaHPO_4}$. In spite of this uncertainty, the points are of interest because of their internal consistency.

On the alkaline side of pH 7.3 it appears that the ion product for $CaHPO_4$ is critical for calcification and that the end result is but little affected by an increase in alkalinity to pH 7.3 to 8.5. That increasing the alkalinity of the medium over this wide range does not increase its ability to calcify rachitic cartilage matrix is conclusive evidence that the ion product of $Ca_3(PO_4)_2$ does not play a decisive part in initiating and effecting calcification. Such a change in hydrogen ion concentration increases the PO_4^{3-} concentration by a factor of 10, but increases the HPO_4^{2-} concentration by a factor of only 1.1. At any point in this range of hydrogen ion concentration small amounts of added phosphate will lead to calcification, indicating that the pH itself is not critical. These observations are not compatible with the belief that the PO_4^{3-} concentration, or any ion product incorporating it, is critical for calcification. They are consistent with the view that the ion product $[Ca^{2+}] \times [HPO_4^{2-}]$ is a determining factor.

Neuman and Neuman (1958) have shown that the serum of normal adults, while supersaturated or metastable with respect to the mineral of bone, is undersaturated with respect to $CaHPO_4$. Their view is that the solubility product constant for this salt defines an upper solubility limit for calcium and phosphate ions in solution. Deposition of the bone mineral, by crystal growth, can and does occur at lower ion products; the *rate* of crystal growth depends upon collision frequency and is more rapid as the concentration of the ions increases. The ion product is important in defining the conditions under which calcification will occur; it also has a direct bearing on the dynamics of the process. Moreover, since the proportions of Ca^{2+} and of HPO_4^{2-} to the total Ca and total P are relatively constant, Howland and Kramer's empirical formulation (1921), Ca ×

P, is as reliable as is the ion product itself, or as the product of the activities of the ions.

The definition of an upper solubility limit for calcium and phosphate ions in the blood, without the need for this limit to be reached for deposition of the bone mineral to occur, may explain a finding that has puzzled investigators for some years. It is well known that the phosphate concentration in the serum of adult man is about half that of the infant; yet new bone formation occurs in both. The higher ion product in the infant makes for more rapid calcification; the lower ion product in the adult does not exclude calcification, albeit at a lower rate. There is still no explanation for the observation that, while in the rachitic infant the phosphate concentration in the serum is at the level normal for the adult, calcification ceases in the infant while it continues in the adult.

Calcifiable Matrix

Normally calcification occurs only in enamel, dentin, cementum, bone, and cartilage matrix where it comes in contact with hypertrophic cartilage cells. The matrix in which the mineral is deposited is elaborated by specialized cells, ameloblasts for enamel, odontoblasts for dentin, cementoblasts for cementum, and osteoblasts for bone. Under pathologic conditions, calcification may occur in tissues such as costal cartilage, tendon, muscle, stomach, lung, kidney, and skin, which do not contain cells specializing in matrix formation. When pathologic calcification is associated with bone disease and hypercalcemia, it is referred to as *metastatic;* when associated with degenerative changes in the tissue without hypercalcemia, it is termed *dystrophic.* In most instances, normal and pathologic, the calcium salt is an apatite mineral and the deposits always form inside the matrix to become an integral part of the fabric of the tissue. Thus, the meaning of the term matrix, as the intercellular substance of a tissue, is clearly applicable to the subject of calcification. How soft tissues can be devitalized, degraded, and transformed into calcifiable matrix is a question to be discussed further.

Calcification: Local Mechanism

A complex mechanism, including both enzymatic and nonenzymatic factors, brings about calcification, under favorable humoral conditions, by transforming ions in solution in the fluids of the body to the crystalline state in calcifiable tissues. What we call the local mechanism was first described by Robison (1930), in recognition of the inadequacy of his phosphatase hypothesis as set forth earlier (1923). He characterized it as favoring deposition of the bone mineral from supersaturated solutions. The mechanism was weakened, but not destroyed, by cyanide, by treatment of the hypertrophic cartilage with various solvents, or by desiccation. It was suggested that this mechanism is bound up with some labile structure of the tissue colloids, but that it does not depend for its functioning on the living cell. Robison left the nature of the mechanism in an unsatisfactory state but adhered to the view that it is enzymatic in character. This conclusion is strengthened by observation of the inhibitory effects of iodoacetate and sodium fluoride on calcification of cartilage matrix *in vitro.* Robison (1934) stated, however, that the conception of the local mechanism as an enzyme system did not preclude the possibility that factors of a different type, such as surface forces in the colloidal matrix, might also assist in the deposition of calcium salts.

At a later date it was shown by others that cartilage matrix may retain the property of calcifiability *in vitro* after all enzymes have been inactivated, although there are quantitative differences in the response to the conditions in the solutions in which they are placed. These differences may be due either to the absence of enzymes or to the effects of the methods used to destroy the enzymes upon the nonenzymatic components of the local mechanism. The local mechanism, or portions of it, sufficient to bring about characteristic calcification, will survive temperatures to 100° C, and will operate over a range in hydrogen ion concentration of at least pH 6.0–8.5, and is thus remarkably stable.

Further evidence of the stability of the local mechanism is derived from experiments in which calcification was produced *in vitro* and the cartilage slices were then decalcified in acetate buffer at pH 5.02–5.70. When they were again incubated in a calcifying solution, extensive calcification followed in every slice. Moreover, slices of cartilage aseptically removed and stored on moist gauze in a sterile Petri dish retained their ability to calcify for as long as ten days after removal from the animals.

In the present state of knowledge, the property of calcifiability cannot be attributed to any single factor. Instead, it is necessary to postulate a local mechanism, including both physical and chemical components, all of which act together in the living organism to bring about calcification; the property which we describe as calcifiability denotes that the tissue is prepared for nucleation or crystal seeding and has intermolecular spaces for crystal formation.

Nucleation

Calcification is crystal formation from nuclei arising inside the fabric of a tissue. The formation of nuclei is called *nucleation*. Nuclei are defined as the earliest conglomeration of calcium and phosphate ions in a geometric pattern to produce the crystal lattice of apatite. As with other chemical reactions, there is an energy barrier which must be overcome before crystallization is possible. The degree of supersaturation that must be attained before nucleation and crystal formation ensue is a reflection of the activation energy barrier. The critical cluster, the smallest possible crystallite, is the cluster of ions with maximum free energy. When the concentration of clusters, both ionic and molecular, becomes high enough, consolidation occurs. Nucleation is termed homogeneous when it occurs under ideal physicochemical conditions of purity of solutions. In biologic systems nucleation is by definition heterogeneous; that is, it occurs in the presence of impurities or catalysts, which lower the activation energy barrier. Catalyzing impurities are present in any and all solvents, reactants, or containers of a chemical reaction. In nucleation catalysis, therefore, the vital step takes place on the surface of substances and wherever there is reduction of the activation energy barrier.

While many different substances, such as extracted tendon, collagen, and rachitic cartilage, may lower the energy barrier and produce crystal formation of apatite from saturated solutions of calcium phosphate *in vitro*, the substance that performs this function in calcifying tissues in the living animal is unknown. There is now general agreement that the collagen fibers of tendon, bone, and cartilage play a dominant role in calcification. It is not fully known whether a change in the physicochemical composition and structure of collagen is responsible for localization of the deposits, and whether nucleation catalysis is the mechanism. Glimcher and associates (1957) maintain that phosphorylated collagen satisfies the requirements of a local mechanism for nucleation of apatite *in vitro*, but Taves (1966) argues that the hypothesis of nucleation catalysis involves a degree of simple diffusion that does not exist in living tissue and is insufficient to explain calcification. Sobel and his collaborators (1960) suggest that the complete system is more complex, and probably includes: (1) a specific form of acid-insoluble collagen; (2) a sulfated mucopolysaccharide or mucoprotein; (3) enzyme systems, such as adenosine triphosphate or uridine triphosphate; and (4) a system concentrating calcium and phosphate ions. They visualize the active nucleating center as a site or adjacent sites between the protofibrils of collagen, capturing a cluster of calcium and phosphate ions; the active center operates via a lock-and-key mechanism and is specific for conversion of the captured cluster of ions to a nucleus.

Still another approach to a possible inhibitor of nucleation is that of Neuman and his collaborators. Disturbed by the lack of a function to be provided by alkaline phosphatase, Neuman (1950) suggested some years ago that the enzyme might function, not to supply products, but rather to destroy a substance inhibitory to crystallization. Fleisch and Neuman (1961) have reported that ultrafiltrates from dog, beef, and human serum do, in fact, interfere with nucleation, and that incubation of dog serum with phosphatase removes this inhibitory action. These conclusions are based entirely on experimental evidence obtained from *in vitro* studies.

Calcification occurs *in vivo* in the presence or absence of alkaline phosphatase indiscriminately in collagenous and other fibrous proteins, such as elastin of arterial wall, proteins of the tubercle bacillus, uromucoid of kidney stones, bacterial mucoproteins, proteins of salivary calculi, and shell matrix proteins of a wide variety in lower animals. To investigate the manifold conditions responsible for calcification, it is necessary to consider pathologic processes in man, cartilage slices *in vitro*, rachitic tissues, vitamin intoxication or hyperparathyroidism, tendon in synthetic calcifying solutions *in vitro*, and transplants of various tissues in living animals.

The question underlying the occurrence of pathologic as well as normal calcification is whether there is a prenucleation phase change in the chemical composition of the tissue. Some investigators contend that calcium, and some contend that phosphorus, is the element that alters the structure of the protein that forms the nucleation site.

Enzymatic transfer of phosphate may provide such energy as may be necessary for initiation or seeding of calcification. Investigating the organic phosphorus compounds in collagen and enamel matrix proteins, Glimcher and associates hold that the presence of covalently bound phosphorus, including protein phosphokinases, would provide the bridge which links structural proteins to the inorganic crystals. Against the hypothesis that phosphorylation is the

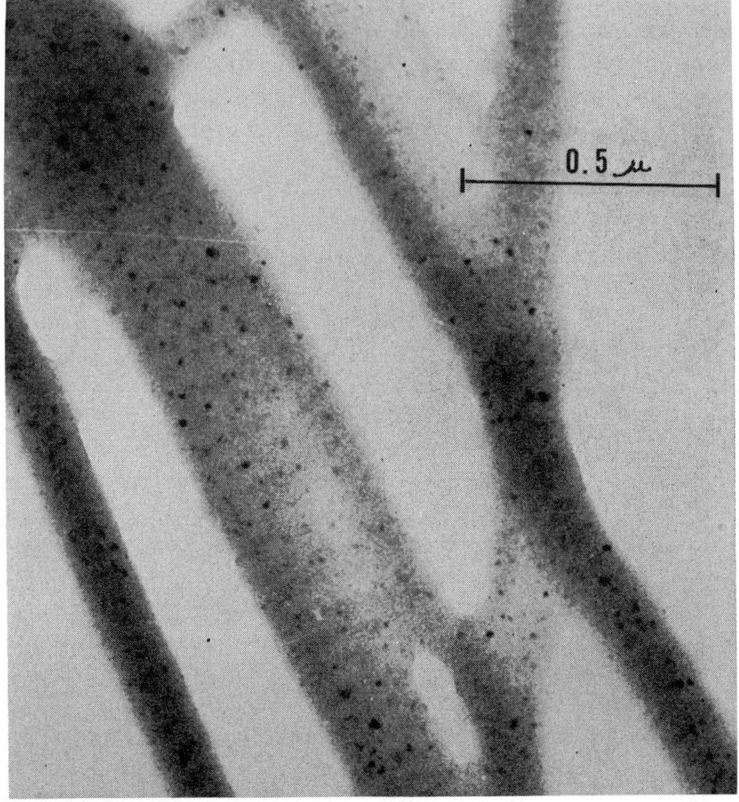

FIG. 22.—Unstained, unshadowed electron micrograph of an early stage of *in vitro* calcification of reconstituted collagen fibrils. Note periodic location of small, dense inorganic crystals, both longitudinally and laterally. ×66,600. (From original of Fig. 12, Glimcher, *in* Calcification in biological systems [Washington, D.C.: American Association for the Advancement of Science, 1960], p. 446. Reproduced by courtesy of the publishers.)

initial step in nucleation, Urist and associates (1964) state that tendon calcifies even after removal of 90 per cent of the organic phosphorus by ATPase, alkaline phosphatase, and acid phosphatase, and add the observation that phosphorylation of tendon with exogenous phosphate inhibits calcification.

A Triphasic Localization Mechanism

Urist and associates (1964), observing calcification in implants of tendon, decalcified bone, and other materials in the anterior chamber of the eye, and deposits of apatite in skin and muscle following injury, propose a theory of a triphasic localization mechanism in which the basic assumption is that the first ion to be bound is calcium. The idea began with Hofmeister in the nineteenth century and recently reappeared with support of strong, new experimental evidence. When uptake of calcium rises fourfold from 5 to 20 mmoles/kg in tendon, the fibrous protein diffracts X rays to produce a pattern more like elastin than collagen, and is termed *elastoid*. It is not elastin because it does not contain the characteristic large amount of the amino acid valine, but like calcium-saturated elastin it calcifies rapidly, even at the low Ca/P products of a normal adult animal. Hence it is proposed that calcium not only enters into the formation of the bone mineral, but is the activating principle in: (1) the formation of the calcifiable matrix; (2) the uptake of phosphate by ion association; (3) reduction of the activation energy barrier to nucleation; (4) efflux of protein and water to produce ultramicroscopic spaces in the tissue; (5) formation of a tripartite calcium-phosphate complex for the nucleation sites; (6) nucleation centers of apatite mineral by means of compartmentalized precipitation; and (7) crystal formation inside the fabric of the tissue. Because there is movement of some components out and others in, culminating in the formation of a crystalline solid phase in the interior of an organic matrix, the localization mechanism resembles *cire perdue*, a lost-wax process. *Cire perdue* is commonly employed in industry for casting metal objects too complex to be machined by power tools.

Quantitative chemical evidence to support the triphasic localization mechanism consists of a demonstration of the effects of a boost in the concentration of calcium ion locally by either endogenous or exogenous hypercalcemia and a simultaneous increase in the number of carboxylic and reactive groups in the tissue. Since calcification is both initiated and sustained under conditions of normal concentration of calcium ion in cartilage and bone, and in various dystrophic soft tissues, it is necessary to search for a fibrous protein polymer-depolymerase that is essential for matrix formation under physiologic conditions. It would act to produce a local increase in the number of reactive carboxylic acid groups for calcium binding. Under physiologic conditions *in vitro*, in the absence of exogenous enzymes, the uptake of calcium ions by tendon is associated with shrinkage, i.e., decrease in fiber length; imbibition or influx of water or swelling, i.e., increase in fiber width; efflux of proteinpolysaccharides and other neutral salt-soluble, nitrogenous substances; cleavage of collagen fibers to form fibrils and filaments, including tropocollagen in solution; ion disassociation and association; removal of hydrophobic groups; and rupture of interfibrillar cross linkages. Competitive reactions between organic or inorganic positively charged substances and carboxylic acid–reactive groups are involved and demonstrable with blocking reagents.

Crystal Growth

With the widespread acceptance of the principle of nucleation in the initial phase of the localization mechanism comes the obligation to deal with many details and ill-defined factors. We have considered what is known of nucleation, by which is meant formation of the initial fragments of the solid phase; following this, there is crystal growth until the crystals attain their full size.

A common misconception is the idea that the formulation for hydroxyapatite is the formula of a molecule; at the same time, it is frequently assumed that formation of the solid phase requires simultaneous collision of the eighteen ions in the diagrammatic representation of a unit cell. The formulation of hydroxyapatite, or of the related bone mineral, however, represents only the *ratios* of all of the constituent ions of the solid phase in terms of smallest whole numbers; the unit cell describes only the arrangement of these ions in space. In the actual crystal both the ions and the unit cells are repeated by the thousands or millions in the spatial configuration characteristic for the particular cells; to imply formation of a unit cell as a fully formed unit of structure is an error in interpretation of the terms used.

Another misconception, related to this, is identification of precipitation with crystal formation. Precipitation implies formation of a solid phase from a solution, generally in aggregates of molecules, but without the orderly array of ions associated with crystal structure. Crystal formation, on the other hand, emphasizes the internal structure of the crystal; attainment of this structure occurs by stepwise addition of ions to the nucleus being transformed into the final form and size of the crystal. Formation of mature bone mineral is properly to be regarded as crystal formation, in close relation to an organic matrix, rather than as simple precipitation within the matrix.

The internal structure of the crystals of bone mineral is determined by interionic forces, resulting in an array of ions characteristic for each particular mineral; it is not necessary to postulate a pattern or template which might pack each ion in its special location during the nucleation and subsequent growth of a crystal. *Orientation* of the crystals, with their long dimensions in the axis of the collagen fibers, with a co-oriented X-ray diffraction pattern of apatite and collagen, does, however, suggest a mechanism for the packing of the crystals. Such orientation is especially prominent in native bone but is not demonstrable when reconstituted collagen is calcified *in vitro*. Neuman and Neuman (1958) have suggested that the orientation of hydroxyapatite crystals can be influenced by epitaxy, defined as crystalline intergrowth or oriented overgrowth, and they state that the weight of evidence is that collagen, itself a crystalline substance, can produce such an epitactic growth and orientation of the crystals. Observers are agreed that in the remineralization of demineralized bone, the orientation of the crystals of mineral to collagen fibers resembles that in native bone.

Crystal Interior

The situation in the interior of the crystals of bone mineral is that the exact composition depends upon the conditions in the fluid from which they are derived, and that, once formed, substitutions and exchanges in the atomic structure are not readily brought about. Such substitutions and exchanges do occur, however, and there is continuous, although slow, movement of ions from the exchangeable to the nonexchangeable fractions of the mineral. It has been shown, for example, that following administration of ^{45}Ca

to rats, the greater part retained in the skeleton is transferred within a few weeks to the stable bone mineral. For the movement of ions to the interiors of crystals, three mechanisms have been proposed: (1) recrystallization, in the classic sense, requiring dissolution and re-formation of crystals, with incorporation of ions not previously within the crystal structure; (2) thermal diffusion or thermal vibration, analogous to the process by which movement occurs within the structure of other solids; and (3) intracrystalline exchange, comparable to the exchange of surface ions but occurring at a much slower rate. It is assumed that, for complete or partial solution of crystals to occur, mediation of a biologic nature, such as by the local effect of an osteoclast, may intervene. Simple solution of apatite crystals in the fluids of the body, except perhaps for very thin or partial crystals on the surface, should be the exception rather than the rule.

Surface Chemistry

The situation on the surfaces of the crystals is quite different from that in their interiors. Ca^{2+}, PO_4^{3-}, CO_3^{2-}, and OH^- ions are exposed to the hydration shell and to the surrounding body fluids; ion exchange takes place readily, especially in the more accessible and more reactive portions of the bone—that is, the metabolic bone in the new and partially mineralized osteons. Here the surfaces of the crystals are in contact with an aqueous medium in which they have a finite solubility. They are subject to constant ion exchange, as well as to other surface phenomena, and must be considered as a very dynamic system, with a labile structure. The surfaces are in equilibrium with their immediate environment; any attempt to describe them in static terms would lead to false impressions.

While this statement is generally acceptable with reference to the immediate environment of crystals—that is, the extracellular fluid in direct contact with their surfaces—there are recurring suggestions that the blood plasma and even the bulk of extravascular fluids are not representative of equilibrium with the crystals of bone mineral. Instead, there is postulated a gradient, or even a physical barrier, which maintains a differential between the pH at the surface of the crystal and that in the circulating fluids; the nature of such a hypothetical barrier or gradient has not been elucidated. MacGregor and Nordin (1960) postulate a hydrogen ion concentration corresponding to pH 6.8 at the surface of the crystals; Terepka *et al.* (1960) state that the pH in the immediate environment of the crystals must be lower than 6.8 and believe that the gradient between this and the hydrogen ion concentration in the circulating fluids in the body is maintained by the production of acid by the cells of bone. Borle *et al.* (1960) also support the concept that the concentrations of calcium and phosphate found in the extracellular fluid are the result of local pH changes at the bone mineral surface, determined by lactic acid formation.

The physiologic significance of such a pH gradient from the surface of the bone mineral to the blood would be that acid is essential for the solubilization of the mineral and for its movement from bone to blood. As will be seen later in connection with regulation of this transfer by the parathyroid hormone and vitamin D, it is further believed that this regulation is mediated by the control of production of acid in the glycolytic cycle. In support of this thesis, some observations purporting to show that the pH is low in areas of resorption of bone are quoted.

While we are prepared to accept the postulate that the *production* of acid in bone, and also the production of the citrate ion, play a part in the solubilization of the mineral, and hence its transfer from bone to blood, our view of the mechanism of this action is somewhat different from that of the authors just cited. We do not accept the idea that there is a pool of fluid, at pH 6.8 or below, surrounding the crystals in process of dissolution; in fact, we regard the concept of pH itself at the crystal surfaces as of doubtful validity. We are prepared to believe that hydrogen ions, liberated from the glycolytic cycle, may react with the crystal surfaces, as H^+ becomes available, in such a manner as to convert an insoluble salt of calcium and phosphate to soluble ions. Such a reaction, which we prefer to think of as occurring in a stepwise fashion, rather than in the presence of a pool of excess acid, might be represented as follows:

$$Ca_3(PO_4)_2 + 2H^+ \rightarrow 3Ca^{2+} + 2HPO_4^{2-} .$$

This question will be dealt with further under the topic of regulatory processes; here the attempt is to visualize the dynamics of reactions at the crystal surfaces.

It may be assumed that the conditions at the surfaces of the crystals in reactive or labile bone, such as that localized in the new and still incompletely mineralized osteons, are different from those in the more stable and completely mineralized bone of the older osteons and of lamellar bone. Our description of surface conditions applies primarily to reactive or metabolic bone; we assume that the surfaces of the crystals of stable bone mineral, while still capable of ion exchange, correspond to our description to a much lesser degree.

The special conditions at the surfaces of crystals include the effects of several forces, not mutually exclusive. The classic adsorption phenomena, in which the bonding is primarily the result of van der Waals forces and in which the adsorbed material may be present in multilayers, refer primarily to the adsorption of gases by solids; ions in solution are not known to undergo classic adsorption. Chemisorption refers to electrovalent or covalent bonding, in which the chemisorbed material is usually limited to a surface monolayer. Ions in solution are frequently chemisorbed. An excellent example is the adsorption of calcium and phosphate ions from serum shaken with lead phosphate; hydroxyapatite is also an effective chemisorber for these ions. Many attempts have been made to explain the uptake or exchange of ions by the bone mineral in contact with fluids of the body in terms of chemisorption. Currently, however, the emphasis is on exchange and transfer of ions between the body fluids and crystal surfaces. This concept has been subjected to careful quantitative studies, which have led to elucidation of stoichiometric relationships and to the conclusion that the dynamics of the behavior of ions at the crystal surfaces are best expressed in terms of ion exchange, without, however, eliminating the possibility of chemisorptive forces acting concurrently.

Ion Transfer and Ion Exchange

Strictly speaking, the term *ion exchange* implies a one-for-one exchange of ions between a solid and the fluid that bathes it. This exchange may be *isoionic,* the exchange of one ion for another of the same element, or *heteroionic,* exchange for a different ion. The rapid physiologic exchange between the bone mineral and the fluids of the body is almost entirely isoionic.

A more general term is *ion transfer,* which designates the movement of ions between bone and blood, without requiring an equal number in exchange. It is assumed that there is a pool of labile mineral in the reactive or exchangeable bone which can move rapidly into the circulating fluids when they are depleted; conversely, an excess of calcium in the blood is transferred rapidly to the labile pool.

This concept of labile calcium and of ion transfer that does not require any destruction of organic matrix bears a superficial resemblance to the older concept of *halisteresis*, which described a leaching of mineral out of bone, and may seem to contradict the assertion, now commonly made, that resorption of bone destroys mineral and matrix together. Halisteresis, however, was a term used to describe an older concept of rickets, which was that in the pathogenesis of rickets, mineral was dissolved from bone, leaving the organic matrix intact. This concept was disposed of by Pommer (1885), who first showed that in both rickets and osteomalacia there is a failure of organic matrix to calcify, resulting in the characteristic uncalcified osteoid tissue. The concept of labile calcium is simply that a portion of the calcium, variously designated as labile, exchangeable, metabolic, or reactive, is capable of moving in or out of bone, in response to a disequilibrium with the immediate environment, without any necessary disturbance of the organic matrix with which it may be associated. This, then, draws a sharp distinction between resorption and ion transfer; they occur in different places, under different conditions, and by different mechanisms.

For reactive bone, there is conceptually a choice of four positions in which a particular ion may be at any one time and still be in relation to hydroxyapatite. It may be in the interior of a crystal, and hence in a relatively stable position. Or it may be in a special relation in the surface, in one of three positions: (1) in the crystal surface; (2) adsorbed on the surface of the crystal, by chemisorptive forces; or (3) in solution in the hydration shell. Where the ions of hydroxyapatite or carbonate hydroxyapatite are concerned, Ca^{2+}, PO_4^{3-}, OH^-, and CO_3^{2-}, the distinctions at the surface are rather arbitrary. The system is in a dynamic state; the surface undergoes continual exchange; and its extension into the aqueous phase is blurred dimensionally and energetically. It is assumed that the degree to which this is true depends upon the maturity of the crystal and upon its environment; in no case, however, is it probable that mineral in bone exists in the state of stability of a dry crystal in contact with air.

Diffuse Activity and Long-Term Exchange

When ^{45}Ca or ^{226}Ra is taken up by bone, activity appears not only in exchangeable or reactive bone, undergoing appositional growth, but also in pre-existing bone, producing a *diffuse* and relatively uniform low level of darkening in an autoradiogram. This diffuse deposition, believed to represent a one-for-one exchange of ions, isoionic or heteroionic, with those present in compact bone, has been designated as *long-term exchange,* defined as an exchange process with time constants greater than a week. While a radioisotope taken up in this manner does not produce as striking a picture in autoradiograms as do radioelements taken up in newly forming bone, where strong images are produced, it is estimated that as much as 50 per cent of the total uptake of ^{45}Ca or ^{226}Ra may be in the form of the *diffuse component.*

The justification for referring to this phenomenon, regarded by some as an irreversible uptake, as long-term exchange is that observations of ^{45}Ca transfer indicate that a significant fraction of the total calcium turnover in the skeleton occurs as a result of such exchange, and that this may play an important part in the regulation of the serum calcium level. Evidence is accumulating that ^{226}Ra is removed slowly from the mineral, without the necessity of direct resorption, and apparently by the same exchange process that deposited it originally.

Localization of the diffuse component, in relation to the crystals of bone mineral, remains uncertain. It is assumed that the first deposition of the radioisotope is at the surfaces of crystals, in exchange for an equal number of Ca^{2+} ions. Beyond this, it is a reasonable assumption, in the present state of knowledge in solid-state physics, that any ions so deposited that are capable of substituting for Ca^{2+} in the crystal structure may, in time, find their way into the interior of the crystal. Whether this is the case for ^{226}Ra, which may be demonstrated in compact bone many years after the original uptake, has not been shown.

CHAPTER VII

Enzyme Systems and Metabolic Pathways in Bone and Cartilage

There is no doubt that enzyme systems participate in the phenomena characteristic of bone and cartilage, such as morphogenesis, intramembranous and endochondral bone formation and growth, calcification, and resorption. Exploration of the possible role of specific enzymes in the physiology of skeletal tissue, while yielding important information on the metabolic pathways of bone and cartilage, has failed to clarify many of the problems of this area of investigation. This is in part because many of the enzymes in bone and cartilage are common to the soft tissues as well, and because their primary functions are related to the metabolic activities of all cells. It seems desirable, therefore, to trace, insofar as is possible, the metabolic pathways of the hard tissues, and to attempt to define to what extent such pathways, with their associated enzyme systems, may participate in activity specific for these tissues.

Phosphorylative Glycogenolysis

The metabolic pathways that appear to be most closely related to the physiology of bone and cartilage are those of phosphorylative glycogenolysis. Except for the initiation of these sequences in the glycogen of hypertrophic cartilage cells, these pathways are identical with those of anaerobic glycolysis in muscle and other soft tissues. An abbreviated version of the major pathways of glycogenolysis and glycolysis is illustrated in Figure 23. Extended versions of these sequences are available in all textbooks of biochemistry and monographs on carbohydrate metabolism, and need not be reproduced here. It is sufficient to say that, in the replacement of cartilage by bone, phosphorylative glycolysis begins with the enzymatic phosphorylation of the glycogen of hypertrophic cartilage cells, with the formation of glucose-1-phosphate. Beyond this point the pathway joins the stream of utilization of glucose from the blood. Anaerobic glycolysis is characterized by a series of stepwise oxidations, with phosphorylated intermediates, all reactions being catalyzed enzymatically. The end products of glycolysis, as well as of glycogenolysis, are pyruvic acid and adenosine triphosphate (ATP); with their formation by pyruvic acid kinase the function of anaerobic glycolysis has been accomplished; no further ATP can be formed in this sequence. The part played by this system in the physiology of bone and cartilage may be examined

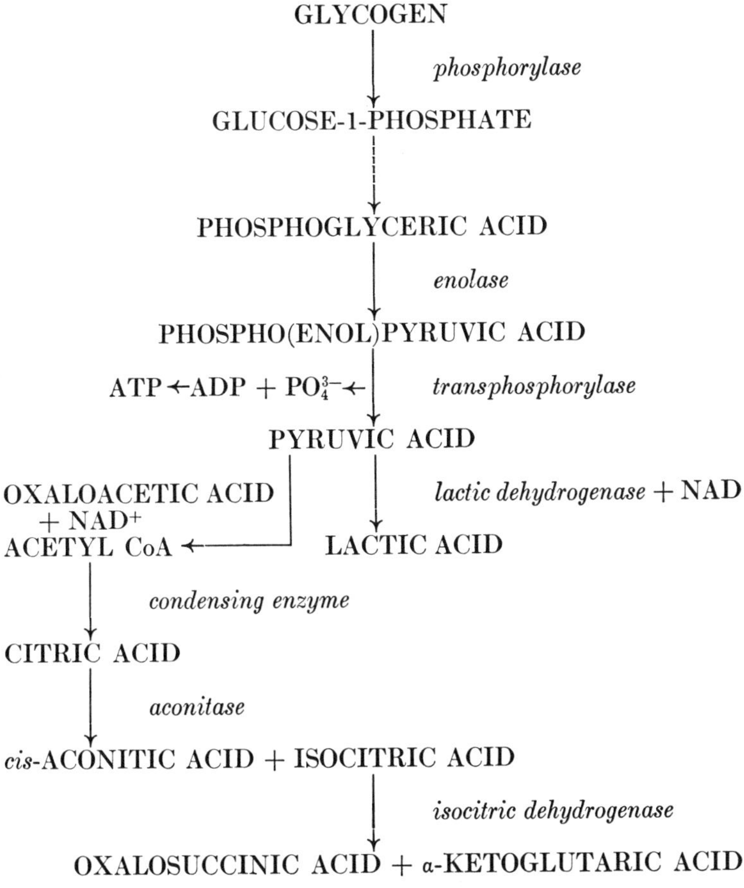

FIG. 23.—Abbreviated version of the glycolytic cycle in bone and cartilage (see pp. 92–97).

at this point, following which the aerobic fate of pyruvic acid, with its implications for the physiology of bone, may be considered.

Phosphorylase and Alkaline Phosphatase

Robison (1923) announced that he had found an enzyme in the ossifying cartilage of young rats and rabbits which rapidly hydrolyzes hexosemonophosphate esters of phosphoric acid. He suggested that this reaction, by adding to the local concentration of phosphate ions, might be a factor in bone formation. From this discovery it was an easy step to the assumption that the action of the enzyme is critical in calcification. To this was added the demonstration of glycogen in hypertrophic cartilage cells by Harris (1932), and of a phosphorylase in calcifying cartilage by Gutman and Gutman (1941). Following this there was an intensified effort to incorporate these observations into a unified system, with the major emphasis on the role of alkaline phosphatase in calcification of cartilage matrix and/or bone.

This effort has not proved successful, largely because no substrate has been found for the participation of alkaline phosphatase in adding to the concentration of inorganic phosphate (P_i) in the fluids of the body, and alkaline phosphatase, as such, does not appear in the glycolytic pathways. The history of this effort has been dealt with in detail in the second edition of this book (1961), and need not be repeated here.

Instead, attention is directed to the final step in anaerobic glycolysis, as shown in Figure 23, in which there is an enzymatic transfer of inorganic phosphate to adenosine diphosphate (ADP) to form ATP, and phospho(enol)pyruvic acid, by the loss of P_i, is transformed to pyruvic acid. Although there is some difference in designation of the enzyme systems active at this point, according to whether it is desired to emphasize transphosphorylation to form ATP from ADP or to an unidentified acceptor in the cartilage matrix, or to place the emphasis on the formation of pyruvic acid from phospho(enol)pyruvic acid, there is reason to believe that this is the critical point at which glycolysis may contribute to the calcification mechanism. Gutman attributed the transphosphorylation activity to alkaline phosphatase, and it has been suggested that the essential role of glycolysis, insofar as calcification is concerned, may be the generation of ATP, although there is a difference among the investigators in the field as to whether calcification may occur *in vitro* with ATP as the only source of phosphate. The generation of ATP continues in the stepwise oxidation of pyruvic acid, which is considered below.

Although Gutman and others have suggested the need for a source of energy in the calcification mechanism, it has not been demonstrated that this is a requirement for the deposition of bone mineral from solution. The possible role of glycolysis in calcification has been questioned, among others by us, on the ground that the P_i that enters the glycolytic cycle is not added to by the successive steps of glycolysis. It may be pointed out, however, that while P_i is incorporated into glucose-1-phosphate in the initial step of phosphorylative glycogenolysis, it is here held with a low-energy bond; it leaves the cycle to form ATP at various steps in glycolysis, with the high-energy bond characteristic of this compound. The free energy of hydrolysis $\Delta F°$ for phospho(enol)pyruvate (−11,000 cal. per mole at 25° C) is the greatest of all known naturally occurring high-energy phosphate compounds. The ATP yield from glycolysis amounts to a net of 14 moles per mole of glucose equivalent. Thus while glycolysis does not add to the P_i available for the formation of bone mineral, it does contribute significantly to the energy in the system for any purpose it may serve in calcification.

The Citric Acid Cycle

Pyruvic acid occupies a central position in metabolism, and occurs in several metabolic pathways, of which those of possible interest in the physiology of bone are illustrated in Figure 23. To pursue the role of ATP further, attention is directed to the citric acid cycle, and the contributions it may make to the physiology of bone.

The possible role of citric acid in the resorption of bone is considered below. Here we may note that the citric acid cycle in a respiring system adds 24 moles of ATP per glucose equivalent, making a total of 38 moles. Whether we are considering the local mechanism within the system which comprises hypertrophic cartilage cells in contact with calcifying matrix, or whether we look to the glucose of the intercellular fluid, which is an intermediate in the formation of glycogen and has a larger pool of carbohydrate and thus of potential energy, 38 moles of ATP per glucose equiva-

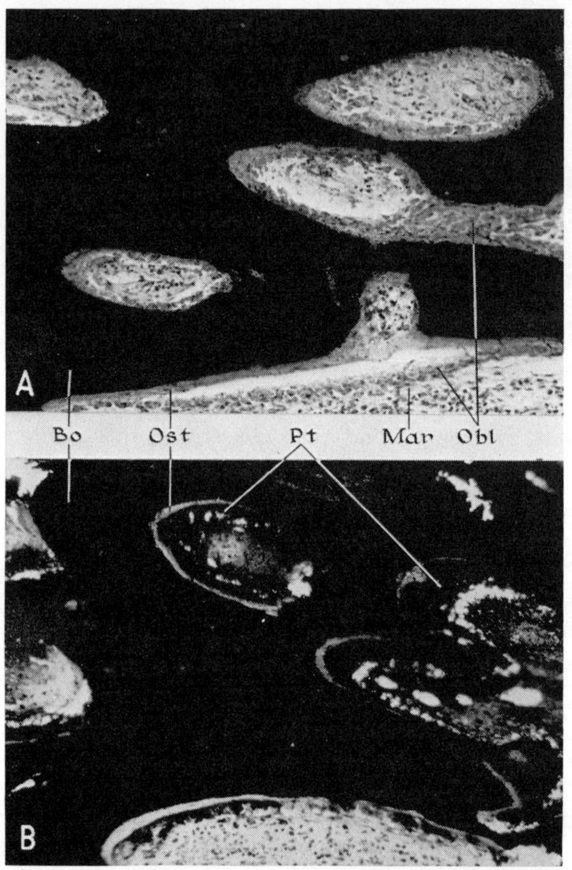

Fig. 24.—Sections illustrating distribution of alkaline phosphatase in bones of a puppy with minimal rickets. (*A*) Photomicrograph of an undecalcified longitudinal section through the shaft of a rib of a puppy fed control diet without vitamin D; *Bo*, indicates calcified bone; *ost*, borders of uncalcified osteoid tissue; *obl*, osteoblasts; *mar*, bone marrow. (*B*) Similar area of a section from the same block incubated with sodium glycerophosphate in presence of calcium before staining. *Pt* indicates heavy deposits in layers of osteoblasts, showing localization of phosphatase; other symbols as in *A*. Note borders of uncalcified osteoid tissue free from phosphatase. Alcohol fixation; silver nitrate–hematoxylin-eosin. ×100. (From original photomicrographs of Fig. 7, Freeman and McLean, Arch. Path. 32:401. Reproduced by courtesy of the publishers.)

lent afford a possibly critical factor in the calcification of cartilage matrix. It must be pointed out, however, that this line of reasoning does not lead to clarification of the mechanism of calcification of bone matrix, in which the stage of glycogen formation and storage is missing. It does, however, provide a source of ATP in the metabolic pathways of the cells of bone, more particularly of the osteoblasts.

The end product of anaerobic glycolysis, pyruvic acid, enters the organelles present in all respiring cells—that is, the mitochondria. Within these subcellular organelles is a highly ordered array of enzymes, which catalyze a series of transformations. The mitochondrion has been called the power plant of the cell, since, with its some 50 enzymes, it brings about the final degradation of the carbohydrate molecule, putting its energy to immediate use, or trapping it by synthesis of ATP.

ATP and Calcification

We have seen that the generation of ATP, with its entrapment of energy derived from the degradation of glucose, is an important product of both anaerobic glycolysis and of the sequences in the citrid acid cycle. It remains to be shown that ATP, which has been called *the unit of currency* in metabolic energy transformations, is in fact related to calcification.

Gutman and Yu (1950) reported that they were unable to induce calcification in rachitic cartilage *in vitro* when phosphate was supplied in the medium only in the form of ATP. They stated, however, that in view of certain technical difficulties, they were not in a position either to affirm or to deny that ATP played a significant role in endochondral calcification. Cartier and Picard (1955*a*) reported that, while inorganic phosphate or hexose phosphates led to very poor mineralization of embryonic cartilage *in vitro*, very heavy mineralization was induced if phosphate was supplied as ATP. This finding was confirmed by Perkins and Walker (1958) in the cartilage of rachitic rats. There are, however, some conflicting opinions concerning the role of ATP in calcification, particularly in the living animal.

ATP is subject to enzymatic breakdown at either of two places, yielding orthophosphate or pyrophosphate, respectively. Enzymes that catalyze transfer of phosphate from ATP to an acceptor are designated *kinases*, sometimes called *ATPase.* Since the formation of pyrophosphate by the activity of ATPase has been demonstrated in bone and cartilage, it is necessary to consider the transfer of orthophosphate and pyrophosphate separately. Krane and Glimcher (1962) demonstrated that the terminal phosphate of ATP may be bound to collagen in a manner similar to that demonstrated for inorganic pyrophosphate; their data suggested that the terminal phosphate was first split from the nucleotide and then bound to collagen partly in a covalent link. They also present evidence that the ATPase activity remained with collagen on purification, and appeared to be related to the structure activity of collagen itself.

Cartier (1952), on the other hand, demonstrated the presence of an enzyme in cartilage which he also calls ATPase, not necessarily identical with the ATPase of Krane and Glimcher. His view is that, under the influence of this enzyme, ATP transfers pyrophosphate to some component of the organic matrix, presumably by a reaction with the free amino groups of collagen, as follows:

$$\text{Collagen-NH}_2 + \text{ATP} \xrightarrow{\text{ATPase}} \text{Collagen-NH-P} \sim \text{P} + \text{AMP}.$$

This fixation of pyrophosphate, according to Cartier, leads to nucleation, followed by combination with calcium and formation of the bone mineral. Since the transfer of a pyrophosphate radical is not a frequent occurrence, Zambotti (1957) has suggested that this might be a reaction characteristic of preosseous tissue.

An opposing role for pyrophosphate, leading to *inhibition* of calcification of collagen, is strongly supported, particularly by Fleisch (1964). There are thus conflicting views as to the parts played by both ATP and by pyrophosphate in the calcification mechanism. This brings into question the inorganic *pyrophosphatase,* which is localized to the area of proliferating cartilage cells. Kuhlman (1965) postulates that during structural synthesis in the cyclic metabolic sequences that affect bone growth, metabolic fuel, such as glucose, is oxidized by epiphyseal cartilage cells to produce energy which is stored and transported in high-energy phosphate compounds such as ATP. At the same time these metabolic processes produce structural intermediates which, following activation by ATP, are synthesized into the structural elements of protein and into DNA. In these processes, pyrophosphate is elaborated, but the *pyrophosphatase* system restores the phosphate economy by making phosphate available for reutilization. In the primary spongiosa, however, where inorganic pyrophosphate is bound to the bone mineral, the binding of and destruction of ATP is prevented. Perhaps in some such manner the conflicting reports concerning the roles of ATP and of pyrophosphate, in nucleation and in inhibition of calcification, may be reconciled.

Citric and Lactic Acids and Resorption of Bone

Although the citric acid cycle is ordinarily described in terms of the final steps in the oxidation of glucose, we have above emphasized the importance of this sequence in the capture of energy as ATP. Here we are concerned with the organic compounds which appear as intermediates in the cycle, and with their possible significance in the resorption of bone.

Phosphorylative glycogenolysis, as above described, consists of a series of transformations by which each glucose molecule is oxidized into two molecules of pyruvic acid; these steps occur in the cytoplasm of cells. Pyruvic acid may then enter the mitochondria, where, by the cooperation of several enzymes and four cofactors present in a tightly knit complex, the sum of which constitutes *pyruvic acid dehydrogenase*, it is transformed into acetyl coenzyme A (acetyl CoA), with the formation of NADH (nicotinamide adenine dinucleotide, reduced form) by reduction of the oxidized form, NAD^+. By the activity of a *condensing enzyme*, acetyl CoA and oxaloacetic acid are combined to form citric acid, and a new cycle begins. Oxaloacetic acid, utilized in this initial condensation, is regenerated in the final stage of the cycle, permitting the process to operate in a continuous manner as long as pyruvic acid is supplied to the cycle as acetyl, and hydrogen atoms and CO_2 are removed.

Our concern with the citric acid cycle is with the citric acid, or citrate, formed by activity of the condensing enzyme and, converted by the activity of *aconitase*, to *cis*-aconitic acid and isocitric acid, which is then oxidized by *isocitric acid dehydrogenase* (ICD) to oxalosuccinic acid. At equilibrium the citric acid-*cis*-aconitic acid–isocitric acid system is represented by citric acid, forming 90 per cent of the total of the three products.

Citric acid is a powerful complexing agent for calcium, and this reaction, together with the liberation of H^+, has been believed to be responsible for solubilization of the bone mineral and for returning calcium to the bloodstream. Attention has been directed toward the effect of parathyroid hormone in increasing the local concentration of citrate in bone, either by increasing the rate of its synthesis or by promoting its accumulation, by blocking the activity of ICD. Not all of the evidence available favors this view, and this possible mechanism of the action of parathyroid hormone in favoring resorption of bone cannot be regarded as established.

Another important possibility of influencing resorption of bone, or more specifically of solubilization of the bone mineral, is by means of the production of lactic acid from pyruvic acid, under the influence of *lactic acid dehydrogenase*. Lactic acid does not complex calcium to any appreciable extent, but since, as an end product of glycolysis, it is formed much more abundantly in bone than is citric acid, the solubilizing effect of the H^+ formed is potentially much greater than that of the citric acid present.

There remains some doubt as to the validity of the concept that the H^+ liberated in bone in carbohydrate metabolism is an important factor in resorption of bone, but we shall return to the problem below in connection with other enzyme systems.

Lysosomes and Acid Hydrolases

De Duve (1963) described previously unrecognized subcellular particles obtained by subfractionation of the classic mitochondrial fraction into heavier and lighter components. It was shown that the lighter fraction lacked *cytochrome oxidase* but had a high concentration of *acid phosphatase*, and this fraction is now recognized as consisting of cell particles distinct from mitochondria. De Duve gave them the name *lysosomes*, because of their richness in *lytic enzymes*. Since all of these have maximum activity at acid pH, they have been grouped together as *acid hydrolases*. Those that have been demonstrated as associated with lysosomes in bone cells are: *acid β-glycerophosphatase*, *β-glucuronidase*, *β-N-acetylaminodeoxyglucosidase*, *acid ribonuclease*, *acid deoxyribonuclease*, and part of *acid phenylphosphatase*, with optimum activity around pH 5.0, together with *cathepsin*, *β-galactosidase*, and *hyaluronidase*, all with optimum activity around pH 3.6. The activity of all the lysosomal acid hydrolases shows structure-linked latency—that is, they are latent in fresh, untreated homogenates, and are released in closely parallel fashion in preparations subjected to graded activating treatments. In contrast with the lysosomal acid hydrolases, *cytochrome oxidase* and *alkaline phenylphosphatase* (in part) do not exhibit latency. The particulate fraction of *catalase*, which sediments together with the acid hydrolases during cell fractionation, occurs in partly latent form, requiring activation to exhibit full activity. The acid hydrolases play a decisive role in intracellular digestive processes and appear to be concerned also in the dissolution of extracellular material. Through their activity, engulfed necrotic materials are digested and perhaps reutilized.

It is usually stated that only two enzymes, isolated from bacteria, have been established as true *collagenases*. The products of digestion of collagen with these enzymes are peptides; free amino acids have not been produced. There is, however, recent evidence that the enzymatic degradation of bone collagen during active resorption produces peptides whose size and amino acid sequences are similar to those produced by bacterial collagenase. Such peptides may then be further degraded by other enzymes, so that the end product may be largely in the form of free amino acids. It has not been shown that this apparently specific collagenolytic activity originates from lysosomes.

The lysosomes, however, exhibit *protease* activity in the degradation of cartilage and bone; the relation of this to the collagenolytic activity just described is not clear. The lysosomes are also implicated in skeletal morphogenesis and in the resorption of bone. *In vitro* activation and/or release of the lysosomal enzymes has been demonstrated under the influence of parathyroid hormone and of vitamin D.

Lysosomes and Resorption of Bone

Current evidence indicates that there is a specific release of lysosomal acid hydrolases from osteoclasts under the influence of parathyroid hormone. It is postulated that this occurs by exocytosis—that is, by the extrusion of vacuoles containing lysosomes or their enzymes in concentrated form. The enzymes then exert a local eroding action on bone in the resorption lacunae, before slowly diffusing passively into the fluids of the body or, *in vitro*, into the surrounding medium. It is further assumed that organic acids, such as lactic and citric, are released in the same locations, and that they bring about a local pH shift toward the acid side, contributing to the solubilization of the bone mineral, and leaving the organic matrix uncovered and available to the digestive action of the hydrolases. Such a shift in pH would also create a suitable environment for the action of the acid hydrolases. This sequence of events, while still highly speculative, and which has been questioned earlier in this chapter, offers a reasonable explanation for integration of the effects of the glycolytic cycle, producing lactic acid; of the citric acid cycle, producing citric acid; of the lysosomal enzymes, effective at acid pH; and of the effects of the parathyroid hormone, which affords partial control of the resorptive mechanism.

Skeletal Morphogenesis

The lysosomes play an important part in morphogenesis by removing unwanted tissue, including the metaphyseal side of the epiphyseal plate during growth; formation of the primitive marrow cavity by cartilage excavation has also been attributed to cell death followed by removal, dependent upon the activity of acid hydrolases. The teratogenic effects of some agents—vitamin A, cortisone, and insulin, for example—are also believed to depend upon their actions on the lysosomes and their collection of hydrolytic enzymes.

Lysosomes and Calcification

While lysosomes have not been specifically implicated in the calcification mechanism, recent work on the degradation of the cartilage matrix suggests that preparation of the matrix for calcification may be brought about by the activity of lysosomal enzymes.

Robison (1930) postulated a "second mechanism" in the calcification of the matrix of hypertrophic cartilage. He assumed (1934) that this mechanism was enzymatic in nature, and his last words on the subject (1936) were that "the two mechanisms which have been empirically distinguished, namely phosphatase and the 'second mechanism,' which induces deposition from supersaturated inorganic solutions, may form one complex enzyme system by which phosphoric esters are synthesised from inorganic phosphate and subsequently hydrolysed for the precipitation of the bone salt." He identified alkaline phosphatase as an essential component of the enzyme complex, and concluded that the full calcifying mechanism is enzymatic in nature, but did not advance the subject beyond this point.

Dziewiatkowski (1966) has reported that an enzyme capable of degrading proteinpolysaccharides has been found in cartilage. This enzyme, at pH 4, behaves as a protease. From his work and that of others working in Honor B. Fell's laboratory, it seems probable that this enzyme is lysosomal in origin, and that its activity may be critical in preparing cartilage matrix for calcification. Present evidence indicates that the existence of Robison's second mechanism will be confirmed, although its nature will not be that postulated by him.

It is well known that initiation of calcification in cartilage matrix occurs only in a narrow zone in epiphyseal cartilage, referred to as the zone of provisional (or preparative) calcification, in contact with hypertrophic, degenerating cartilage cells about to be invaded by advancing osteogenic tissue. Robison's second mechanism was postulated only for this zone in cartilage, and never for bone. Moreover, embryonic chick cartilage, as well as other connective tissues in the embryo or in postfetal life, may be rich in lysosomal activity, but without exhibiting calcifiability.

We suggest that acid hydrolases, of lysosomal origin, are responsible for conferring calcifiability upon the matrix of hypertrophic epiphyseal cartilage; there remains the necessity of accounting for the limitation of this effect to a narrow zone of the cartilage matrix.

Alkaline Phosphatase and Calcifiability

Having indicated that acid hydrolases, of lysosomal origin, confer calcifiability on a narrow zone of the matrix of hypertrophic epiphyseal cartilage, we have stated that this mechanism does not appear to bring about calcifiable matrix in bone, which is calcifiable as it is formed. There are recurring suggestions in the literature that alkaline phosphatase, present in quantity in the osteoblasts, is responsible for the formation of a calcifiable matrix—the matrix of bone. There is abundant evidence that this enzyme takes part in the synthesis of mucoproteins and fibrous proteins in all connective tissues, calcifiable as well as noncalcifiable. Once a calcifiable matrix is formed, it remains calcifiable after all enzymes are inactivated; it is therefore not necessary to postulate that enzymes are directly involved in the calcification process itself.

CHAPTER VIII

Resorption of Bone

Resorption refers to the destruction or solution of the elements of bone. Our knowledge of the morphologic aspects of this process begins with a monograph by Kölliker (1873), one of the great early histologists, who wrote a clear description more than ninety years ago, still a classic in the subject. Kölliker not only described resorption, with its role in the growth and reconstruction of bone, but also described and named the osteoclast. He found that bone mineral and bone matrix are absorbed simultaneously, a fact repeatedly rediscovered in modern times, and he offered speculations concerning the mechanism of resorption to which relatively little has been added to this day. In many respects resorption is no more clearly understood now than it was when Kölliker left it.

Resorption is, in essence, the putting into solution of a complicated structure in such a fashion that it disappears, its end products entering the blood stream. Of the components of bone, a small fraction is already in fluid form, and hence easily disposed of; the remainder is in solid form, for the most part insoluble or soluble with great difficulty in the aqueous fluids that permeate it. For bone to be resorbed, it must be reduced to substances soluble in water, and these must then be transferred to the fluids of the body.

Components of Bone

Of the solid components of bone, three substances together make up the main bulk. These are: (1) the bone mineral; (2) a fibrillar protein, collagen; and (3) the ground substance, characterized by its content of one or more polysaccharides. The ground substance is closely related to the interstitial fluid, and its proteinpolysaccharides may be made soluble in water by a change in their state of polymerization. Since no enzyme specific for the depolymerization of chondroitin sulfate has been isolated, hyaluronidase is described as mediating this process.

Collagen may be rendered soluble rather readily. At the temperature and hydrogen ion concentration of the fluids of the body it can be dissolved by digesting or disintegrating its protein structure. This can be accomplished in the test tube by proteolytic enzymes, such as bacterial collagenase; collagenolytic activity, capable of degrading collagen to soluble peptide molecules, has been demonstrated in bone.

Kölliker (1873) concluded that the osteoclast erodes bone by chemical means, without further specifying the nature of the chemical action required. Later, others added the assumption that the action is a combination of that of an acid with that of a proteolytic ferment; the necessity for the presence of acid to account for the solution of bone mineral still dominates the literature on resorption. This situation has been changed, in theory at least, by the introduction of a group of compounds known as chelating agents, of which the prototype is ethylenediamine tetraacetic acid (EDTA).

Chelating Agents

Chelating agents are characterized by the formation of very poorly dissociated complexes with metallic ions. Together with this property, which involves the formation of ring structures with coordination linkages, chelate structures exhibit greatly increased stability and changes in the dielectric constant. These characteristics differentiate chelate structures from such complex ions as are formed by calcium with citrate; from the physiologic point of view the important difference is that the ability of a chelated complex to ionize in solutions is very much below that of calcium citrate.

It is now a common laboratory procedure to decalcify bones and teeth with chelating agents for histologic purposes; this is possible even in neutral or alkaline solutions. It may safely be assumed that the bone mineral may be dissolved whenever another substance with a stronger affinity for calcium in solution comes in contact with bone. This removes one of the obstacles to forming a hypothesis for the resorption of bone Such a hypothesis may now account for the solution of bone mineral, collagen, and ground substance, all at the hydrogen ion concentration of the body fluids.

Resorption of Bone

As noted above, it has been agreed for a long time that both the organic and the inorganic constituents of bone are resorbed together, leaving smooth surfaces at the loci of resorption. If it be assumed that there is continuously applied to the surface of bone a solution that will depolymerize mucopolysaccharides, digest collagen, and hold calcium in a firm and soluble combination, this constitutes the basis for a working hypothesis for the mechanism of the resorption of bone. Such a mechanism would require only certain enzyme systems and an organic substance to combine with calcium. This does not conflict with any known facts, but there is no positive evidence that it adequately describes the process. As suggested elsewhere in this volume (Chapter VII), if the acid hydrolases elaborated by the lysosomes of osteoclasts are responsible for the dissolution of the bone matrix, they would operate in a favorable environment, that is, at acid pH, which would also contribute to the solution of the bone mineral.

Role of the Osteoclast

It can no longer be doubted that osteoclasts play an active part in the resorption of bone. Whereas for many years the evidence to this effect was indirect, and dependent upon the study of fixed tissues, the studies of Gaillard (1961), of Goldhaber (1960), of Hancox and Boothroyd (1961), and others, all of whom have observed resorption of bone in tissue culture, making use of time-lapse motion pictures, have conclusively demonstrated the melting away of bone before advancing osteoclasts, which display very active ruffled borders and energetic *endocytosis*. The ruffled border as seen in tissue culture may correspond to a brush border or striated border between the osteoclast and the underlying surface of bone in fixed preparations.

The observations of living osteoclasts have also shed light upon the mechanism of osteoclastic resorption of bone. They leave little doubt that these cells have a secretory activity, and that this serves to fragment and loosen both the mineral and the organic matrix of bone. They do not, so far at least, give a final answer to the problem of the possible phagocytic activity of the osteoclasts. Their secretory activity results in the liberation of debris; some of this may be swept up by the undulating ruffled border and the amoeboid movements of the entire cells, accompanied by endocytosis. On the other hand, both *in vivo* and in tissue culture, there are large numbers of very active macrophages, seemingly adequate for phagocytosis of such debris as is present.

Phagocytosis

The above calls for a further review of the evidence for and against the concept of phagocytosis, by the osteoclasts themselves, as at least a part of the mechanism of osteoclastic resorption of bone. Such a suggestion has appeared in the older literature, reviewed by McLean and Bloom (1941). They studied the mobilization of bone mineral in a variety of animals under the influence of toxic doses of parathyroid extract, staining undecalcified sections of fixed bone tissue by the von Kóssa method, for visualization of the mobilized mineral. They found aggregations of mineral, particulate during the life of the animal, in the macrophages and megakaryocytes of the bone marrow, but found also that the osteoclasts were singularly free of these aggregates. They concluded that osteoclasts do not participate in the phagocytosis of the mineral liberated from resorbing bone (Fig. 25).

Subsequent observations, by the use of electron microscopy, require a reopening of this question. Rodlets of bone mineral lying within the osteoclasts of untreated animals have been found, and this has been interpreted as phagocytosis of the crystallites (Fig. 26). These observations have been repeated, but it has not been made clear that the crystallites are actually in the cytoplasm of the cells; they appear rather to be in the folds of the endoplasmic reticulum or in vacuoles, and they remain as discrete particles; they are not concentrated by the cells. Under these circumstances we prefer to use the term *pinocytosis*, or *endocytosis*, for a mechanism that can take up fragmented mineral, rather than to use the term *phagocytosis*, which implies active ingestion and concentration.

Osteolysis

Bélanger (1965) has studied a process somewhat similar to, but not necessarily identical with, osteoclastic resorption, which he has called *osteolysis*. He has defined this as an active physiologic phenomenon taking place within the intimacy of bone under the influence of the osteocytes, whereby bone matrix is modified and bone mineral is lost.

According to Bélanger, it is apparent that there is a normal mechanism of bone resorption occurring under the influence of mature osteocytes (osteolysis). The cells responsible for this produce alkaline phosphatase and protease; they are surrounded by matrix with a lower concentration of both mineral and organic matter con-

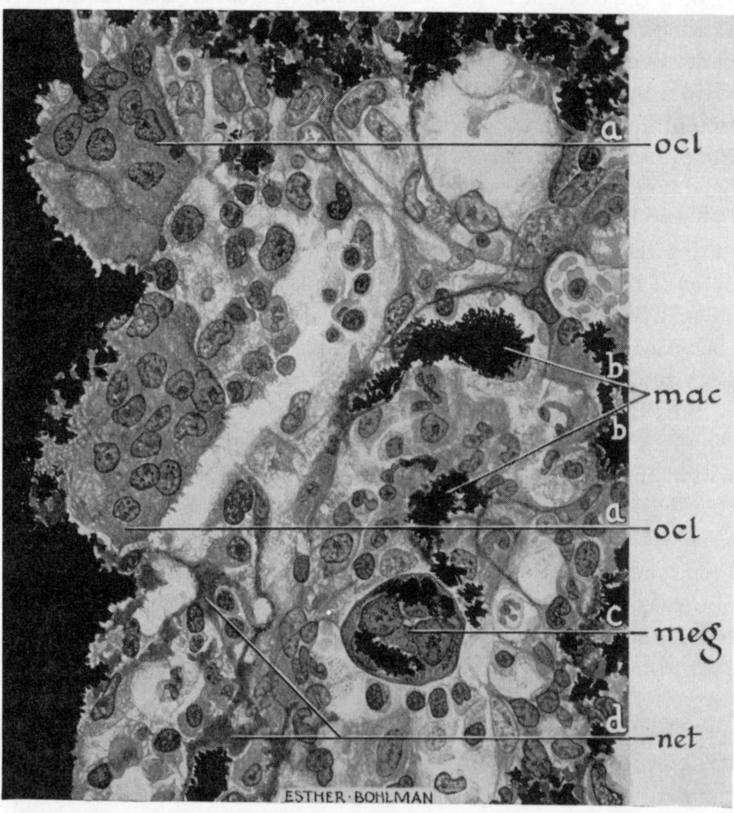

FIG. 25.—Mobilization of bone salt under the influence of toxic doses of parathyroid extract. High-power view from undecalcified section of a rib of a puppy 12 hours after injection of 200 U.S.P. units of parathyroid extract per kilogram of body weight. *a*, Osteoclasts, free from aggregated bone mineral; *b*, macrophages, packed with bone mineral; *c*, megakaryocyte, containing bone mineral; *d*, basophil network. Formaldehyde fixation; silver nitrate–hematoxylin-eosin; camera lucida. ×681. (From original drawing of Fig. 2*B*, McLean and Bloom, Arch. Path. 32:310. Reproduced by courtesy of the publishers.)

taining mucopolysaccharides stainable by the periodic acid-Schiff reagent, and which induces toluidine-blue metachromasia. The rapid maturation of the small osteocytes, accompanied by production of protease, and the presence of adjacent low-density bone, not in the vicinity of osteoclasts, lead to the conclusion that there is a relation between osteocytic activity and the rapid passage of calcium into the blood, as well as between this activity and the release of collagen breakdown products. Osteolysis, while occurring in the bones of normal, untreated animals, is enhanced by a variety of stimuli, notably those associated with hyperparathyroidism; it appears to contribute to the regulation of the serum calcium con-

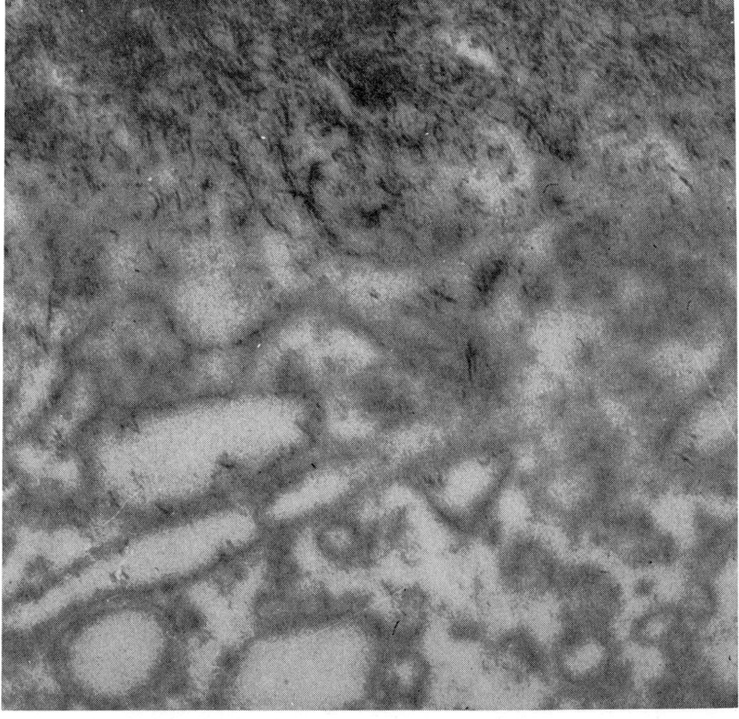

FIG. 26.—High-resolution electron micrograph showing mineral crystals from resorbing bone within the cytoplasmic vacuoles of an osteoclast. ×66,600. (From original of Fig. 18, Scott and Pease, Anat. Rec. 126:495. Reproduced by courtesy of the publishers.)

centration. There is now wide acceptance of the view that the osteocytes play a more active part in the metabolic activity of bone than had formerly been believed.

Control of the Resorption of Bone

Assuming that the osteoclasts resorb bone, and that the osteocytes perform a similar function, there remains the very important subject of the control of these activities, which certainly do not occur spontaneously or at random. Resorption of bone, accompanied by the presence of osteoclasts, begins with the very earliest stages of ossification in the embryo and continues throughout life, although there are marked differences in the location and rapidity of resorption, according to the physiologic and structural needs of the moment. The influences that evoke and control osteoclastic and osteocytic activity must be looked for, and these may be found either generally, throughout the organism, or locally, in circumscribed areas.

Even under humoral control there are differences in the responsiveness of particular bones or particular locations in bones to the stimulus carried in the blood. Of the humoral mechanisms for control, that studied most intensively is the action of the parathyroid hormone. In both clinical and experimental hyperparathyroidism the appearance of osteoclasts is a prominent feature of the histologic picture. Cell transformations have been frequently observed and have added strength to the belief that osteoclasts may arise from other cells characteristic of bone and may return to their former states or be transformed to reticular cells in the bone marrow.

Later in this volume the evidence for parathyroid control of resorption of bone, as a part of the homeostatic regulation of the plasma calcium level, will be reviewed. It may here be stated, however, that recent evidence indicates that the resorption incident to the growth and remodeling of bone is only partially under the control of the parathyroid hormone. Jowsey *et al.* (1958) have shown that the internal remodeling of compact bone, essential for the maintenance of the organism's complement of reactive bone, continues after parathyroidectomy in puppies, although perhaps at a reduced rate. Moreover, young animals subjected to parathyroidectomy continue to grow, and the resorption incident to growth in the length of the long bones is accompanied by osteoclastic activity.

Similarly, Lindquist *et al.* (1960) have found that while resorption of the trabeculae of the spongiosa in the long bones of young rats is inhibited by administration of estrogen, as had previously been shown, the resorption incident to the growth and remodeling of the bone is not significantly interfered with by administration of this hormone; this suggests that resorption, in this instance, is under the control of more than one regulatory mechanism.

Another situation in which widespread osteoclastic resorption occurs without parathyroid control is exhibited during the egg-laying cycle of birds. In the pigeon, in which the separate phases of the cycle are clearly marked, resorption of intramedullary bone, formed during the preovulatory period, is initiated when the first egg enters the oviduct and begins to undergo calcification of the shell. Nothing is known of the mechanism that brings about the rapid reversal from osteoblastic formation of bone to osteoclastic resorption. The complex series of events occurring during the egg-laying cycle is given detailed consideration in a later chapter, in connection with the influence of estrogens on bone.

The observations on control of osteoclastic resorption of bone are in keeping with the currently accepted view that hormones in general do not initiate metabolic processes, but rather exert their influence by regulating the rates of specific reactions. Moreover, it is clear that osteoclastic resorption of bone is not under the exclusive control of any one hormonal activity. Resorption serves structural as well as metabolic and homeostatic needs, and osteocytic osteolysis is concerned predominantly with local events, and with the transfer of fluid and dissolved substances between bone and blood. It seems likely that resorption and osteolysis are controlled in different ways.

Local Factors in Resorption

The influences of local factors in the resorption of bone are most easily seen during its growth, when the metaphyses of the long bones are singled out for reconstruction. Such reconstruction invariably includes a considerable amount of osteoclastic resorption, followed by appositional bone formation, with the result that the size and shape of the bones progress toward the adult state. Organization and regulation of these phenomena, affecting most of the bones of the body simultaneously, is a part of the overall growth, and must be under genetic control. Some of the factors, at least, are local, especially those related to the strains and stresses to which a particular bone is exposed. It has been suggested that osteocytes act as strain gauges or mechanoreceptors, leading to formation or resorption of bone tissue, and that they play a large part in mediating the effects of the local and mechanical factors contributing to the reaction of individual bones to environmental factors.

CHAPTER IX

Regulatory Processes and Bone

A. Bone Matrix

Consideration of the regulatory processes affecting bone, or in which bone plays an important part, requires attention to the interplay of the physiologic factors in the growth, mineralization, turnover, and maintenance of the integrity of skeletal tissues. And since bone is so closely linked with the homeostatic control of the composition of the internal environment, especially of its content of calcium and phosphate but including sodium and magnesium as well, it is not possible to consider the factors influencing the mineral of bone without attention to the bone-blood relationships; these are influenced by both vitamins and hormones.

Growth Hormone

Of the hormones known to influence growth, including androgens, estrogens, adrenocortical hormones, thyroid, and insulin, only the growth hormone of the anterior lobe of the pituitary gland exhibits a specific effect upon the growth apparatus by means of which growth in length of the long bones continues up to closure of the epiphyses.

The anterior lobe of the pituitary gland secretes, among other hormones, a growth or somatotropic hormone that exerts an influence on skeletal growth. Until recently, the hormone has been prepared mainly from bovine sources, and the test object has usually been the rat—intact or hypophysectomized.

In the long bones, prior to closure of the epiphyses, growth in length occurs by a continuous invasion of the proliferating cartilage by capillaries and osteogenic cells and its replacement by diaphyseal bone. The net result is that the cartilage disk remains at approximately constant thickness, while the diaphysis increases in length. The growth of the bone is dependent upon proliferation of the cartilage; but unless the mechanism that we have referred to as the *growth apparatus* functions as a whole, physiologic growth cannot occur.

Hypophysectomy of the immature rat leads to prompt cessation of growth, both in weight and in length. The epiphyseal disks of the long bones soon show evidence of inactivity. Within two weeks the thickness of the cartilage disk is far below the normal for the age of the animal; the cartilage cells of the disk decrease in size; the osteoblasts become spindle-shaped; and the primary spongiosa disappears. Eventually the epiphyseal cartilage disk becomes sealed from the marrow by a lamina of bone. As a result of the premature arrest of growth, the disk resembles that of the adult rat.

If the growth hormone is administered to such an animal while the growth apparatus is quiescent, increase in weight and in skeletal size occurs promptly. Growth in the epiphyseal cartilage and in the adjacent spongiosa is resumed, and there is removal of the sealing lamina of bone, with reestablishment of invasion of the cartilage. The histologic appearance of the entire growth mechanism is again that of the growing animal. Similarly, if growth hormone is administered to a rat at the age of approximately five months, at a time when the growth curve has reached a plateau, reactivation of the growth apparatus is demonstrable. There is a large volume of literature upon the effects of growth hormone on metabolic activity, both in man and in other animals. Most of this is of uncertain applicability to the subject of the growth in length of the long bones, to which our attention is restricted. For our present purposes, we are concerned with the growth apparatus as a primary target for the action of the hormone.

The results of the administration to man of growth hormone derived from bovine or porcine sources have been disappointing; large doses administered to patients with panpituitary dwarfism have had little effect. More recently, preparations of the hormone from primate sources, including human pituitary glands, have demonstrated the importance of species specificity. Purified human growth hormone (HGH), administered to children with anterior hypopituitarism or with possible isolated growth-hormone deficiency, given as replacement therapy in weekly dosages of 2.5 to

5 mg, has proved effective in achieving normal or accelerated growth velocity for the maturational age.

It was reported by Rosenbloom (1966) that the growth-promoting effects of human pituitary growth hormone have been described in more than fifty short-statured patients probably deficient in growth hormone. The usual replacement doses of HGH have not promoted growth in conditions in which growth failure was not associated with HGH deficiency; for this reason, and in view of the extreme scarcity of the hormone from human sources, the use of HGH in children without such deficiency is not regarded as justifiable. In 1964, the National Institutes of Health, through the National Pituitary Agency, in Baltimore, Maryland, organized the collecting of human pituitary glands and the distribution of HGH to investigators.

Thyroid Hormone

Cretinism, a form of dwarfism and mental deficiency resulting from thyroid insufficiency, has been observed for centuries. It did not become a well-established entity, apart from other forms of dwarfism, until the function of the thyroid gland was discovered; it then became known that lack of the internal secretion of this gland causes a general retardation of skeletal development and growth.

Removal of the thyroid gland in young rats leads to a marked slowing of growth. The skeleton resembles those of hypophysectomized rats in its small size, but there are important differences. The epiphyseal cartilages are not sealed by bony plates; some erosion continues; and the primary spongiosa retains its characteristic appearance. Normal growth is resumed when thyroid hormone is administered. Growth in thyroidectomized rats can also be elicited by injection of growth hormone, although they are relatively insensitive to this treatment. Thyroxin injected into normal rats causes no increase in body length, but it has a synergistic effect when administered together with growth hormone. All these observations point to a nonspecific effect upon the growth of bone; they may be interpreted as reflecting indirect effects of the action of the thyroid secretion on metabolism in general.

Overdoses of thyroxin in experimental animals may lead to premature closure of the epiphyses and consequent cessation of growth. The same effects may follow administration of thyroid to children in an effort to promote growth. A temporary increase in the rate of growth may occur, but the final result may be undesirable. Retardation of growth of the long bones has also been reported in clinical hyperthyroidism.

The thyroid hormone with the highest biologic activity, amounting to from five to ten times that of thyroxin, is 3,5,3′-triiodothyronine; it represents 5–7 per cent of the total iodine in the gland. The mixture of four iodothyronines, of which thyroxin is the most abundant, may be considered as the physiologic hormone, since all are present and each has biologic activity.

Insulin and Glucagon

There is interest in the role of *insulin* in promoting growth, and an insulin-like action of growth hormone has also been described. By using a slow-acting insulin in gradually increasing doses, an average increase in weight of 36 g in 15 days has been attained in completely hypophysectomized rats. Control rats ate less of the same diet and did not grow. These findings are interpreted as demonstrating that insulin may stimulate growth, and they strengthen the possibility that decreased liberation of insulin may be one of the factors limiting growth in hypophysectomized animals.

On the other hand, an effect on glucose uptake of the diaphragm from a normal rat, similar to that observed with insulin, has been demonstrated under the influence of growth hormone. The effect is absent when the rat is made diabetic, but it returns when diabetic rats are treated with insulin. It has been proposed that the anabolic effect of *human growth hormone* is made effective by the presence of insulin, while the diabetogenic effect of the hormone is dominant in the absence of insulin.

Intravenously administered *glucagon* causes an increase in the blood levels of insulin and glucose. The results demonstrate a direct effect of glucagon on insulin secretion. The suggestion has been made that the insulinogenic effect of glucagon is physiologically important and is due to accelerated β-cell glycogenolysis. It is further suggested that glucagon secretion, in α-cells adjacent to β-cells, may, in conjunction with changes in glucose levels, determine insulin secretion. The observations of the interrelationships between insulin, glucagon, growth hormone, and glucose are interpreted to afford evidence that insulin secretion under the influence of glucagon may influence growth, including that of the skeleton, by enhancing the effectiveness of growth hormone.

Androgens and Gonadotropins

The chief source of gonad-stimulating hormones is from the placenta; these hormones appear in large amounts in the urine during pregnancy. Because of their origin, they are called *chorionic gonadotropins*. Their effects are similar to, but not identical with, those of hormones elaborated by the anterior lobe of the pituitary gland. When they are administered to male animals, including man, they have certain effects upon the growth of bone resembling those of the male hormones or androgens. Since the effects of the gonadotropins are the result of increased production of androgens, the two groups of substances will be considered together.

The long bones of rats castrated at the age of twenty-one days and killed when one year of age are significantly shorter than those of control rats. Large doses of androgens depress growth or have no effect. In the human male the influence of the gonadotropic hormones of pituitary origin is correlated with the growth that occurs normally at the age of puberty. In the female, gonadotropin is not often used to induce growth; testosterone may be used instead.

The chorionic gonadotropins are considered by some to be the most reliable growth-promoting substances available. They have an accelerating effect upon growth during childhood, as well as at puberty, but give rise to premature development of secondary sex characteristics. Induction of sexual maturity with chorionic gonadotropins may be useful in preparation for the administration of growth hormone. Reports that they lead to early closure of the epiphyses are now discounted.

Dwarfism

There are probably few cases of dwarfism, apart from cretinism, in which the retardation or cessation of growth is attributable to the absence of any one hormone. Interest has been centered largely on dwarfism ascribed to insufficiency of the anterior lobe of the pituitary gland. The syndrome of hypopituitary dwarfism, however, frequently includes genital retardation or infantilism and may include cryptorchidism; this syndrome is known as *panpituitary dwarfism.*

Stunting of growth resulting from hypothyroidism is easily recognized, and the treatment is specific. The differentiation between hypopituitary dwarfism, *primordial dwarfism,* and constitutional delay of growth and development is difficult in childhood; the diagnosis is often established only toward the end of the period in which growth is possible. The hypopituitary dwarf has marked delay in epiphyseal ossification and fusion, but differs from the hypothyroid dwarf in that the skeletal proportions assume the mature type and that epiphyseal dysgenesis does not occur. The primordial or *genetic dwarf,* represented by the pygmy, has relatively normal epiphyseal development and exhibits no gonadotropic or other hormonal deficiency. The dwarfism that occurs as the result of *ovarian agenesis* resembles the primordial type.

As indicated above, growth hormone from human pituitary glands has produced linear growth and retention of nitrogen, calcium, sodium, and potassium in human subjects. Species specificity has been demonstrated, and the efficacy of the hormone from primate sources no longer remains in doubt. Further progress in this respect will depend upon developing adequate sources of material that can be used in patients with pituitary dwarfism.

Chorionic gonadotropin and preparations of gonadotropin from pituitary sources are in use for treatment of sexually immature dwarfs; thyroxin and androgens are also of practical value. Gonadotropins, when applicable, are preferable to sex hormones for young patients because they stimulate rather than depress gonadal function; as a rule, testosterone is preferred in females. Synthetic hormones, such as diethylstilbestrol, are as effective as natural female sex hormones; when administered in cycles they are helpful in dwarfism associated with ovarian agenesis.

Because of the undesirability of inducing secondary sex characteristics prematurely, gonad-stimulating therapy should not begin until the patient is about fourteen years of age. The consensus now is that premature epiphyseal closure following administration of gonadotropins need not be feared; contrary results are reported after testosterone.

Hormonal Regulation of Integrity of Organic Matrix of Bone

Since physiologic turnover affects both the mineral and organic constituents of bone, it follows that there must be continuous destruction and rebuilding of the organic matrix. It appears that collagen itself is only slightly, if at all, subject to metabolic turnover; it requires replacement only when destroyed by resorption. Once resorption has occurred, rebuilding follows; this is best seen in the haversian remodeling of compact bone. There is a belief that this rebuilding is under hormonal control and, indeed, that there exists an antianabolic as well as an anabolic factor. A current view is that the sex hormones—androgens and estrogens—provide the anabolic factors, and that the adrenocortical hormones—cortisone and hydrocortisone—are antianabolic in their effects. According to this view, there is a balance between the production of the sex hormones and the adrenocortical hormones, which under normal circumstances results in a balance between matrix destruction and matrix rebuilding.

The integrity of the organic matrix, as well as its normal growth and development, depends also upon an adequate intake of vitamins A and C. For this reason the influences exerted by these vitamins upon bone are considered together with those of the hormones.

Estrogens and Bone

Steroid hormones, both natural and synthetic, which are capable of producing estrus, also lead in certain experimental animals to specific effects upon bone. Many compounds with estrogenic activities are known, of which estradiol and estrone have been isolated from the ovaries and are the prototypes for the group.

Present knowledge concerning the relationship of estrogens to postfetal osteogenesis is obscure in all animals except birds. Kyes and Potter (1934) observed that female pigeons, during the preovulatory phase of the egg-laying cycle, produce a secondary system of spongy bone arising from the endosteum and growing into the marrow cavity. These intramedullary deposits of new bone, a secondary sex characteristic, develop under the influence of estrogens, and serve the purpose of storing calcium to be used later for calcification of the eggshell. Intramedullary bone develops naturally in the females of all avian species studied; it may also be produced in either males or females by administration of estrogens. In mice a similar reaction can be produced by estrogen injections, but it does not occur naturally during reproduction. Still another reaction to estrogen, that of inhibition of resorption of the spongy bone of the metaphysis, can be seen in the growing rat.

The role of estrogen in the regulation of calcium and bone metabolism is more highly developed and easier to study in the domestic chicken than in any other animal. In the laying hen estrogen controls, simultaneously, the formation of phosphoprotein and its transport together with calcium for the developing egg yolk, as well as the formation and calcification of intramedullary bone for later use in the calcification of the eggshell. During the initial fourteen-hour phase of the egg-laying cycle, the plasma calcium may rise to three times the normal level. The calcium added to the serum is bound to a phosphoprotein (X_1) as a nonionized, nonultrafilterable complex. This is produced by the liver, in association with a lipoglycophospholipid lipoprotein (X_2). The two proteins are very large molecules in transport in the plasma and serve as precursors to the granules of the egg yolk. These proteins do not exist in the plasma without a large complement of calcium, and they are dependent upon calcium for transportation from the liver to the yolk sac in the form of osmotically inactive units. The hypercalcemia of X_1-X_2 proteins is also found during egg production or following estrogen treatment in the plasma of fish, frogs, turtles, and viviparous snakes (Fig. 27).

It is the diffusible and not the protein-bound fraction of the plasma calcium that is concerned with calcification of the eggshell. During the final ten hours of the egg-laying cycle, especially at night when the bird is not feeding, the egg rests in the uterus for deposition of the calcified eggshell. During this time, by some stimulus that is not known, but not by action of the parathyroid hormone, the calcium is mobilized from the intramedullary bone, which undergoes extensive resorption. The calcium is transferred from the skeleton to the eggshell and is redeposited as calcium carbonate; the phosphate is excreted in the urine.

It is easy to follow the transformations of the cells in pigeons during the rapid and extensive changes in the bone marrow under the influence of estrogen. During the preovulatory bone-forming period, reticular cells become osteoblasts and then, in turn, osteocytes. In the bone-destroying phase after ovulation of the first egg, osteoblasts and liberated osteocytes become osteoclasts; the osteoclasts may turn into osteoblasts during the second period of bone formation. In the postovulation period, osteoblasts and osteoclasts again become reticular cells.

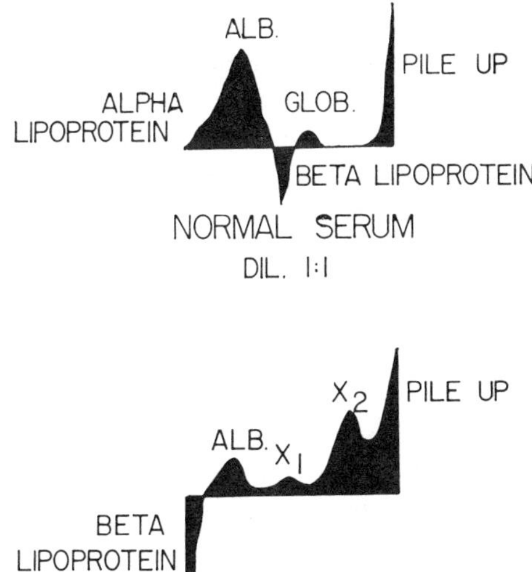

FIG. 27.—Composite schlieren patterns of the serum (*above*) of a normal rooster, and (*below*) of a heavily estrogenized rooster. X_1 and X_2 are new components secreted by the liver into the plasma in the form of complexes with calcium. (From original of Fig. 1, Urist, Schjeide, and McLean, Endocrinology 63:573. Reproduced by courtesy of the publisher.)

When estrogens are administered to mice, a similar, although not identical, reaction begins in the spongy bone of the metaphysis and grows into the marrow cavity by direct extension. Newborn mice do not respond, but after ten days of growth and until senility the skeleton is always capable of producing large amounts of endosteal bone. Within the limits of tolerance of the animal to the hormone, the yield of new bone is proportional to the dose and the period of administration; it may eventually fill the entire marrow cavity (Fig. 28). There is no inhibitory or synergistic action by progesterone, deoxycorticosterone, or testosterone, or by anterior pituitary growth hormone, gonadotropic hormone, or adrenocorticotropic hormone. Experiments with ^{14}C-labeled estrone indicate that there is a selective deposition of the hormone in the endosteum; its further fate is not known.

The formation of endosteal bone in the mouse under the influence of estrogen has not been shown to reflect any physiologic function. Bone formation is not followed by rapid resorption, as it is in the bird; when administration of the hormone is discontinued, there is gradual removal of the excess bone. During pregnancy, when large amounts of estrogens are being excreted in the urine, neither the fetal nor the maternal skeleton exhibits medullary bone formation. Nor has it been possible to induce new-bone formation in either mature or immature mice by stimulating the animal's own ovaries by large doses of gonadotropic hormones. Moreover, estrogens implanted in the bones, in the form of pellets, produce only the usual systemic effects, with no special local reaction. During the period of new-bone formation the serum calcium, inorganic phosphate, and alkaline phosphatase levels remain within normal limits.

Administration of estrogens to young, growing rats leads to superficially similar, but essentially different, effects from those seen in birds and in mice. No formation of new bone is observed, but the resorption of metaphyseal bone is inhibited, with the result that for a distance of several millimeters in the marrow cavity there is an elongated core of unresorbed spongy bone (Fig. 29). The effects of estrogens on the bones of the rat are limited to this specific action upon one part of the growth apparatus, concerned only with endochondral growth. Consequently, as is to be expected, no demonstrable effects are found in adult rats, and intramembranous ossification is not affected at any time.

Lindquist *et al.* (1960) have shown, by a combination of autoradiography and the *kinetic analysis* of Bauer, Carlsson, and Lindquist (1955), that the inhibition of resorption by estrogen in the young rat affects only the cores of secondary spongiosa, as observed in the long bones; the resorption incident to growth in length and the accompanying remodeling is not influenced by the hormone (Fig. 30).

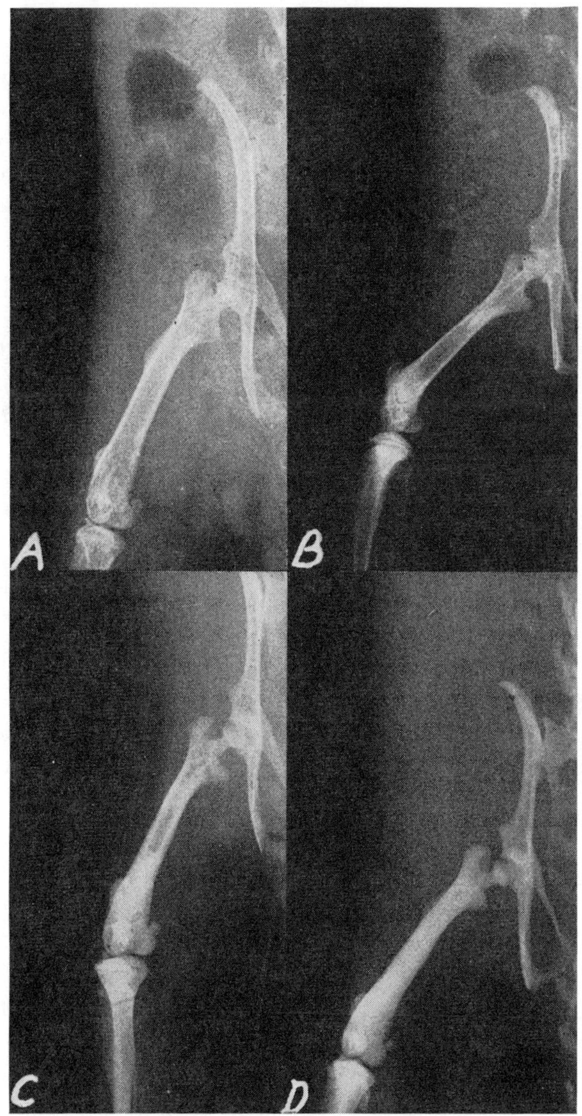

Fig. 28.—Roentgenograms of femurs of mice to illustrate formation of new bone within marrow cavity under influence of substances with estrogenic activity. Littermate CF_1 mice treated with large doses of diethylstilbestrol in corn oil. (*A*) Control, injected with 0.4 ml corn oil. (*B*) 6.0 mg in 5 weeks. (*C*) 14.0 mg in 15 weeks. (*D*) 16.0 mg in 17 weeks. The volume and distribution of the new bone can be determined as accurately by roentgenograms as by histologic sections. (From originals of Fig. 3, Urist, Budy, and McLean, J. Bone Jt. Surg. 32A: 146. Reproduced by courtesy of the publishers.)

Guinea pigs, hamsters, rabbits, kittens, and puppies have failed to show any specific skeletal response to administration of estrogens. Administration of these hormones to man, particularly in the presence of *osteoporosis*, has led to equivocal results; there seems to be no basis for extrapolating the effects on birds, mice, and rats to man or to any species other than those named.

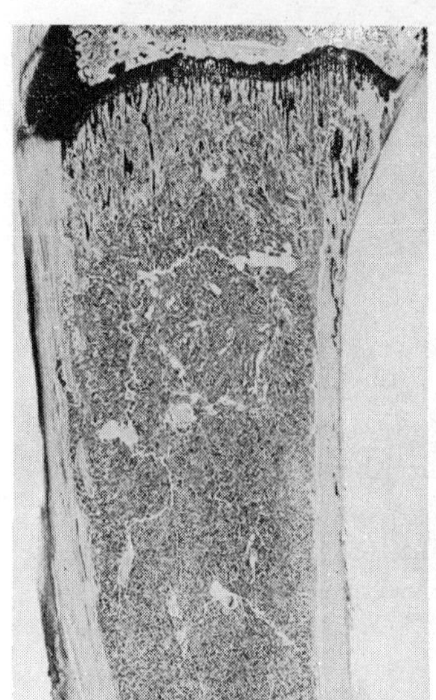

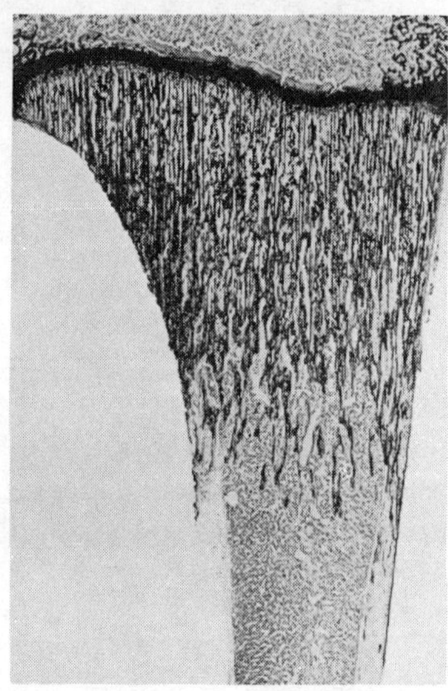

Fig. 29.—Sections to illustrate inhibition of resorption of spongiosa, with consequent increase in length, following administration of estrogens to immature rats. Photomicrographs of the proximal ends of tibias. *Left*, control; *right*, increase in the length of the spongiosa up to 6–8 mm resulting from administration of 8.0 mg of 17-β estradiol benzoate over a period of 5 weeks. Hematoxylin-eosin-azure II. ×9.6. (From original of Fig. 2, Urist, Budy, and McLean, Proc. Soc. Exp. Biol. N.Y. 68:325; and Figs. 1 and 4, Budy, Urist, and McLean, Amer. J. Path. 28:1157 and 1163. Reproduced by courtesy of the publishers.)

Corticotropin (ACTH) and Adrenal Cortical Steroids

Many steroids, some with biologic activity, have been isolated from the adrenal cortex; others, with similar activities, have been synthesized and are widely used in medicine. Those concerned in gluconeogenesis are classified as glucocorticoids; they have systemic regulatory physiologic effects. The naturally occurring glucocorticoid with the most important action on the skeleton in man is *hydrocortisone* (17-hydroxycorticosterone). Elaboration of this substance by the adrenal cortex, as well as of *cortisone* (11-dehydro-17-hydroxycorticosterone), is under the control of the anterior lobe of the pituitary gland, mediated by secretion of the *adrenocorticotropic hormone* (corticotropin; ACTH). Production of glucocorticoid hormones by the adrenal cortex continues after hypophysectomy, but at a reduced rate.

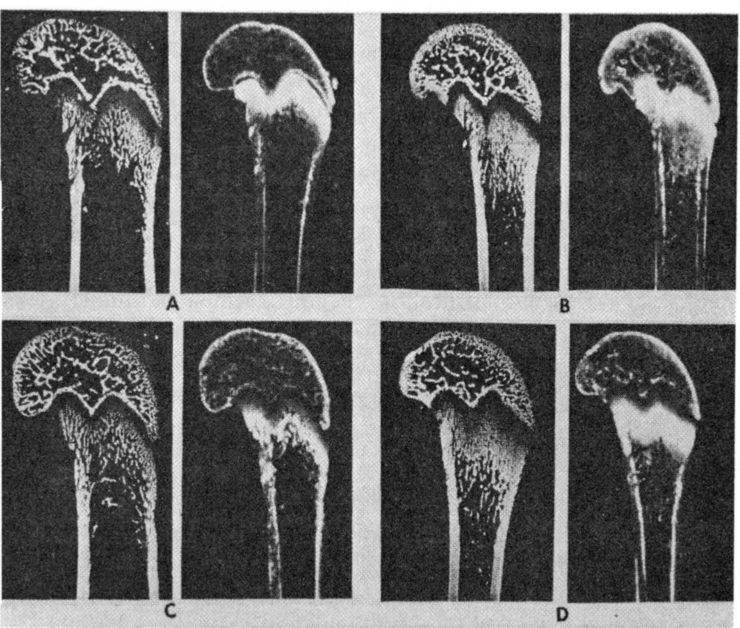

Fig. 30.—Microradiographs (*left*) of sections and their autoradiographs (*right*) of control and estrogen-treated rats after administration of ^{45}Ca. The sections were made from the distal ends of left femurs. Note the unresorbed spongiosa in the estrogen-treated rats. The uptake of ^{45}Ca at 1 hour is identical in control and estrogen-treated rats. At 8 days there is retention of radioactivity in the estrogen-treated rat despite new endochondral growth below the cartilage plate, whereas in the control rat the corresponding activity has been removed by resorption of the spongiosa. *One hour post-injection:* (*A*) Control and (*B*) estrogen-treated. *Eight days post-injection:* (*C*) Control and (*D*) estrogen-treated. (From Fig. 5, Lindquist, Budy, McLean, and Howard, Endocrinology 66:110. Reproduced by courtesy of the publishers.)

Insofar as the adrenal corticosteroids affect the growth of bone, the effects apppear to be nonspecific and secondary to the systemic regulatory functions of the hormones. Overdosage, either of ACTH or of the glucocorticoids, leads to loss of nitrogen in the urine and feces, attributed to an interference with the metabolism of proteins. In young growing animals there is also an adverse effect upon the growth apparatus, resulting in a slowing of growth. Similarly, retardation of healing of experimental fractures in animals as a result of administration of glucocorticoids is attributed to depression of osteoblastic activity.

The adrenal glucocorticoids assume major importance in relation to the skeleton in *Cushing's syndrome* (*hypercortisonism*), in which there is hypersecretion of the corticosteroids. This was originally attributed to a basophil adenoma of the pituitary gland, but overactivity of the adrenal cortex may result from other causes or may be associated with a primary hyperplasia or tumor of the cortex itself. The condition has a characteristic constellation of symptoms; the effect upon the skeleton is a marked loss in the mass of bone (*osteoporosis*, *osteopenia*), often accompanied by fractures. Similar effects are reported following long continued administration of exogenous corticosteroids, either natural or synthetic, although there is not a one-to-one correlation between dosage and skeletal effects. There are continuing efforts to modify the steroid molecule in such a way as to enhance the desirable physiologic or therapeutic effects, while reducing the undesirable side effects, such as osteoporosis; in no instance has it been demonstrated that the risk of osteoporosis can be lessened by use of newer compounds. The relationship of the corticosteroids to osteoporosis is treated at length in a subsequent chapter.

The adrenal cortex also secretes substances with mineralocorticoid activity, of which the most important is *aldosterone;* its role in mineral metabolism is considered in connection with homeostasis and control of the electrolyte pattern of the internal environment.

Vitamin A

Vitamin A is a product solely of animal metabolism from precursors that are metabolic products only of plants. These precursors are carotenoid pigments, yellow and red, widely distributed in the plant world, over the range from bacteria and diatoms to garden fruits and vegetables. Of such pigments, at least twelve, called provitamin A carotenoids, can form vitamin A in the animal organism. They are also known as carotenes, and the most widely distributed member of this group is β-carotene; one international unit (IU) of vitamin A is equivalent to 0.6 μg of crystalline β-carotene, itself a precursor of a colorless material with vitamin A activity.

Vitamin A is a lipid-soluble alcohol and forms esters with fatty acids; most of the vitamin A in the livers of both mammals and fish is present in esterified form. Vitamin A alcohol is subject to oxidation to the aldehyde and the acid forms. The acid replaces vitamin A for all functions other than vision and maintenance of reproduction; it cannot be reduced to the aldehyde or alcohol; it can neither be stored nor excreted. The ultimate metabolic fate of the vitamin is not known. Vitamin A acid has been found to be at least as potent in its effects on embryonic chick cartilage models as is vitamin A alcohol, and it is also active in preventing vitamin A deficiency in animals.

Utilization of vitamin A involves cellular metabolism, particularly in epithelial cells; its formation from precursors; absorption, mobilization, and transport; and its specific function in vision. It is essential for the activities of epiphyseal cartilage cells, for without it they cannot carry out the sequence of growth, maturation, and degeneration of the growth apparatus; this failure results in suppression of endochondral growth of bone. Remodeling sequences also cease to operate; appositional growth of bone of periosteal origin continues. These effects lead to abnormalities in the shapes of the bones; the failure of certain bony foramina to enlarge brings about pressure on various nerves.

Excessive amounts of vitamin A lead to fragility and subsequent fractures of the long bones. The mechanisms of these changes have been studied in detail *in vitro* by Fell (1964), using organ cultures of limb rudiments from chick embryos (see chapter VII). Under the influence of an excess of vitamin A, acid hydrolases are released from lysosomes, and their proteolytic activity results in the breakdown of the protein component of the proteinpolysaccharide of the matrix; these effects are inhibited when hydrocortisone is added to the medium. Vitamin A thus increases the fragility of the lysosomal particles, while hydrocortisone enhances the stability of the lysosomes, with consequent reduction in hydrolytic activity.

Fragments of crystalline vitamin A acetate have been attached to small pieces of parietal bone and implanted into the cerebral hemispheres of litter-mate rats. Resorption of the grafts, accompanied by numerous osteoclasts and often leading to perforation of the bone, was apparent within fourteen days. This is interpreted to indicate that vitamin A, like parathyroid hormone, has a local action on the osteoclastic resorption of bone; this is not accompanied by any effect on the serum calcium level.

Information about tissue changes resulting from vitamin A deficiency is based on observations on infants and young children, where previous storage of the vitamin is limited; it is not usually a simple deficiency state. Avitaminosis A rarely occurs in adults, and then only in association with a prolonged intake of inadequate and unbalanced diets deficient in many dietary essentials. Since the effects of vitamin A deficiency may be prevented by very small amounts of the vitamin in the diet, avitaminosis A is not a frequent occurrence. On the other hand, it has been emphasized that the hazards of vitamin A poisoning from the routine prophylactic feeding of vitamin concentrates to healthy infants and children are considerably greater than the hazards of vitamin A deficiency when vitamin concentrates are not given. There are reports of acute poisoning in adults, attributed to the eating of the liver of the polar bear, which contains exceptionally large amounts of vitamin A.

Vitamin C

Vitamin C, or *ascorbic acid,* is widely distributed in the plant and animal kingdom; it is present in abundance in many fresh vegetables and fruits but is entirely lacking in the common cereals and grains. All pure vitamin C used in pharmaceutical products is prepared synthetically. It is a dietary essential for man, other primates, and the guinea pig, but can be synthesized by other species. In animal tissue the highest concentration of the vitamin is found in the adrenal cortex, eye lens, and liver tissues.

The metabolic consequences of experimental vitamin C deficiency in susceptible animals are restricted to tissues of mesenchymal origin and are characterized by failure of formation and maintenance of intercellular materials. All intercellular substances of the supporting tissues—bone, cartilage, fibrous connective tissue, and dentin—have in common a matrix largely made up of collagen, and it is this material that in *scurvy* either is not produced or is produced in defective form. As to bone, deposition of the matrix ceases and osteoblasts assume the form of reticular cells. The mechanism of calcification itself is not affected, but abnormal connective tissue formed in bone during vitamin C deficiency is not calcifiable. The effects of the deficiency are reversible and are rapidly corrected when ascorbic acid is supplied. There is no evidence that the vitamin has any deleterious effects when supplied in excess, and there is no rationale for its use in any condition other than its deficiency.

CHAPTER X

Regulatory Processes and Bone
B. Vitamin D–Parathyroid Complex

Higher organisms are possessed of systems which comprise mineralization and resorption of bone in addition to exchange of the ions of the bone mineral with the fluids of the body. Closely allied with these physiologic activities is the homeostatic control of the calcium ion concentration in the blood plasma and in the other extracellular fluids. In the functioning of these systems, the organism controls absorption of calcium and phosphate and their excretion, making use of the gastrointestinal system and the kidneys, both for conservation of needed elements and for elimination of any excess. Operation of such complex and interrelated functions requires integration of regulatory mechanisms, under central and humoral control. Of the controls, the most important, insofar as the metabolism of calcium and phosphate is concerned, are vitamin D, both endogenous and exogenous, and the parathyroid hormone. So closely interrelated are the functional activities of the parathyroid hormone and of vitamin D that it will serve our purposes to regard them both as component parts of an integrated system, which exercises control over the mechanisms required for proper functioning of the organism as a whole.

It was suggested very early that the vitamin and hormone might act by influencing each other; this, however, has never been demonstrated, and it is now assumed that each makes its own contributions to the regulatory processes. To state these briefly, the parathyroid glands monitor the calcium ion concentration in the plasma and apply the necessary corrections, mainly by influencing the mobilization of calcium from the skeleton; the parathyroid hormone also exercises control over the excretion of phosphate by the kidneys and aids in influencing the absorption of calcium in the gastrointestinal tract. Vitamin D, on the other hand, is the major influence upon the absorption of calcium; by this means it controls the mineralization of bone by assuring an adequate supply of the necessary materials. Vitamin D also exerts an effect upon mobilization of mineral from bone, complementing the action of the parathyroid hormone in this respect. An oversimplified version of current views would be to say that vitamin D influences mobilization in proportion to its formation and intake, and that the parathyroid glands are called upon to balance the interplay between dietary intake, absorption, urinary and fecal excretion of calcium, and the regulatory effect of vitamin D. In support of the view of a synergistic action of vitamin D and the parathyroid hormone it may be mentioned that both promote the formation of citrate in bone, and that both thus contribute to whatever effect bone citrate may have upon the transfer of calcium from bone to blood.

The enlargement of the parathyroid glands observed in rats on diets deficient in both calcium and vitamin D, and believed to result from the deficiency in calcium, has been attributed by others to the deficiency in vitamin D, since hypertrophy of the parathyroids does not occur when rats are fed diets very low in calcium but with an adequate supplement of vitamin D. Bloom *et al.* (1960), however, have reported that hypertrophy of the parathyroid glands occurred when laying hens were placed on a diet low in calcium but adequate in all other components, including vitamin D. While the state of the parathyroids in the two species cannot be correlated with the vitamin D intake, there is good correlation between the plasma calcium levels and the size of the parathyroids. In the rats the serum calcium was maintained at near normal levels by the action of vitamin D, at the expense of the skeleton; in the hens, however, the serum calcium was markedly depressed, in the presence as well as in the absence of vitamin D. The conclusion seems warranted that hypertrophy of the parathyroids was the result of a low plasma calcium level, rather than a direct result of a deficiency in vitamin D.

Vitamin D

Numerous contributions on the role of vitamin D in calcium metabolism, and on the mode of its action, are now appearing, including studies at the cellular level. Vitamin D, whether endogenous or exogenous, may be regarded as essential to the total system that includes calcium metabolism and mineralization of bone; its effects are made manifest in a variety of ways.

The term vitamin D was originally applied to the factor in cod-liver oil responsible for its antirachitic potency. It is now used to refer to two or more lipid-soluble sterols with antirachitic activity and also the ability to elevate the serum calcium level, by influencing the mobilization of mineral from bone. Two forms of vitamin D are well characterized chemically. Vitamin D_2, or calciferol (ergocalciferol), is obtained as one of the products of activation of ergosterol. Vitamin D_3 (cholecalciferol) is the naturally occurring antirachitic factor in cod-liver oil; it can also be prepared by activation of 7-dehydrocholesterol. These two forms of vitamin D possess equal antirachitic potency in man. Dihydrotachysterol is closely related to calciferol; it has negligible antirachitic potency but has calcemic activity. The current trend is to regard it as a form of vitamin D. Since there are now several sterols possessing antirachitic and calcemic properties in varying proportions, chemical identification and characterization should be the basis for nomenclature.

The antirachitic activity of vitamin D, in prophylactic doses, is effected mainly by its influence upon intestinal absorption of calcium. In very large doses, 50,000 IU or more daily, vitamin D exhibits a marked calcemic effect, resulting in an increased concentration of calcium in the blood plasma—an effect similar to that produced by parathyroid extract. This subtoxic action of the vitamin and of other chemically related sterols is made use of to raise the level of serum calcium in hypoparathyroidism. In even larger doses the effects are manifestly toxic and result in *hypervitaminosis D.* This is associated with resorption of bone, comparable to that induced by large doses of parathyroid extract. In the young rat there follows a marked increase in the trabeculae of the spongy bone of the metaphysis. This new bone is calcified poorly or not at all, in spite of hypercalcemia and a consequent elevation of the Ca × P product; this is the result of production of an uncalcifiable matrix and has been designated as *hypervitaminosis D rickets.*

Parathyroid Hormone

The parathyroid glands supply an internal secretion, the parathyroid hormone, intimately concerned with the regulation of the calcium ion concentration in the blood. The primary target of the hormone, in this respect, is the skeleton; regulation of the plasma calcium level is also indirectly aided by an effect upon tubular reabsorption of phosphate by the kidneys. Enhancement of active transfer of calcium across the gut wall by parathyroid hormone has been demonstrated *in vitro;* there is also an influence of the hormone upon the secretion of calcium by the lactating mammary glands of rats. A further extension of parathyroid activity to connective tissue in general throughout the organism, with its chief effect upon the mucopolysaccharides of the ground substance, has been postulated; this effect, if it exists, is poorly understood. While a primary effect of the hormone is upon mobilization of calcium from the bone mineral, there is no evidence that it influences deposition of the mineral.

Ablation of the parathyroid glands leads to hypoparathyroidism, with a lowering of the calcium ion concentration in the blood, frequently accompanied by tetany. An excess of parathyroid hormone, either endogenous or exogenous, leads to an increase in the calcium ion concentration in the blood and may produce profound changes in the skeleton.

The parathyroid hormone acts rapidly and has a short half-life. Melick *et al.* (1965), using the hormone labeled with ^{131}I, have found a half-life of 22.3 minutes in normal rats, 24.3 minutes in parathyroidectomized rats, and 27.6 minutes in parathyroidectomized rats given excess carrier hormone. These data support the conclusion that circulating parathyroid hormone is rapidly destroyed.

Nature of Parathyroid Hormone

The chemical properties and structural requirements for biologic and immunologic activity of the parathyroid hormone have been treated exhaustively by Potts and his co-workers (1965). They have isolated bovine PTH in pure form, free from detectable nonhormonal constituents. The material obtained after carboxymethyl cellulose chromatography was resolved into a major (90 per cent) and a minor (10 per cent) component, both biologically active, immunologically similar, and differing only slightly in covalent structure. It is suggested that each component represents a genetically determined molecular variant of the hormone; the two forms were derived from parathyroid glands from many animals, pooled before the hormone was extracted.

The pure hormone is a single-chain polypeptide, with a molecular weight of 8,500, yielding 84 amino acid residues on hydrolysis, and containing no cysteine, but with 2 methionine, 1 tyrosine, and 1 tryptophan residue, and a single end-terminal amino acid, alanine. A short region of the polypeptide near the COOH- terminus is concerned with both biologic and immunologic activity; this region includes a sequence of 19 amino acids, or slightly less than one-fourth of the molecule. The pure preparation has both calcium-mobilizing and phosphaturic activities; there is now no support for the view that the parathyroid glands elaborate separate hormones for their two principal activities.

Evocation of Secretion of Parathyroid Hormone

The homeostasis of calcium constitutes a special case among the cations of the blood plasma. Homeostatic control of the concentrations of other cations of the fluids in the body, and of their retention or excretion by the kidneys, is exerted by integration of neural and hormonal factors. The parathyroid glands, so far as is known, act as the receivers of information concerning the calcium ion concentration in the plasma, and make any necessary correction by an increase or decrease of secretion of the parathyroid hormone. Their function is thus accomplished without participation of the central nervous system, the adenohypophysis, or the adrenal cortex; the existence of a parathyrotropic hormone, elaborated by the anterior lobe of the pituitary gland, is not supported by any evidence, and the idea of such a link between the pituitary and the parathyroids has disappeared from modern endocrinology. Patt and Luckhardt (1942) were able to demonstrate, by perfusion of the parathyroid glands with serum depleted of calcium, that these glands respond directly to a lowered concentration of calcium in the plasma by increased activity. All current evidence supports this observation.

Some have believed that the concentration of inorganic phosphate in the plasma also exerts an influence upon the secretory activity of the parathyroid glands; current evidence does not support this view, and now that it has been demonstrated that the parathyroids secrete one hormone with both calcemic and phosphaturic activities, the case for a second stimulus, originating from the phosphate in the plasma, is still further weakened.

Mode of Action of the Parathyroid Hormone on Bone

Almost from the discovery of the active principle of the parathyroid glands and of the influence of hyperparathyroidism on the skeletal system there was a considerable difference of opinion concerning the mode of action of this hormone on bone. One view was that the effect on bone is secondary to an increased excretion of phosphate in the urine; the other was that the hormone acts specifically on bone, leading to resorption with solution of the bone mineral.

These differences may now be regarded as resolved. The parathyroid hormone acts directly *both* on bone and on the kidneys. Current effort is directed toward elucidating the effects of the hormone on cells and on metabolic pathways, and toward integration of the major effects into a single system responsible for the primary function of the parathyroids—that is, homeostatic control of the blood calcium level. In view of the intimate association between the physiologic activities and functions of vitamin D and the parathyroid hormone, such an integrated system must incorporate both the vitamin and the hormone.

The conclusion that there is a direct action of the hormone on bone rests on: (1) histologic examination of the bones of animals treated with parathyroid extract; the changes in the bones, described as characteristic of the toxic action of the hormone, are observed even when the kidneys of the animals have been previously removed; (2) observation that in dogs treated with parathyroid extract the serum calcium continues to rise after a Ca $\times$ P product in the plasma is attained sufficient to induce calcification in rachitic cartilage *in vitro* (Fig. 31); (3) demonstration of a direct effect of parathyroid transplants on bone in contact with them; and (4) demonstration of a direct effect of parathyroid hormone on surviving bone in tissue culture.

Evidence for an action of the parathyroid hormone on the renal tubules is equally convincing; the net result is an increase in the excretion of phosphate in the urine. The possibility that this is the result of a hemodynamic effect on glomerular filtration has been excluded by observations with the pure hormone; the purified hormone has been shown to be devoid of the hemodynamic effects often observed following administration of crude parathyroid extract. The effect on excretion of phosphate has been attributed to decreased tubular reabsorption; an effect on tubular secretion has not been excluded.

Cellular and Subcellular Action of Parathyroid Hormone on Bone

There is agreement that the influence of the parathyroid hormone on bone, as well as its effects on such other tissues as kidney tubules, intestinal epithelium, and the mammary glands, depends on an action upon cellular constituents; there is now no suggestion that the hormone *directly* influences the solubility of the bone mineral in the fluids of the body. In bone, an action could be upon any one or more of the cells of bone—mesenchymal cells, osteoblasts, osteocytes, or osteoclasts. Moreover, there is an increasing

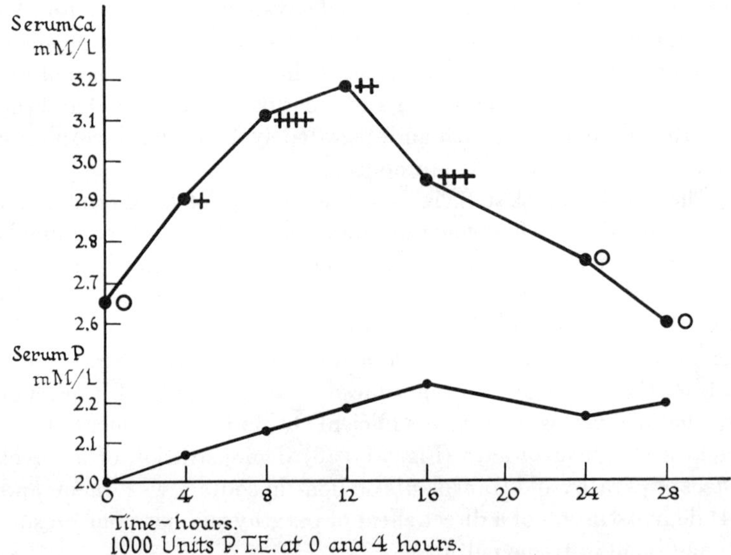

Fig. 31.—Influence of concentrations of serum calcium and serum phosphate of a dog treated with parathyroid extract upon calcification of cartilage of a rachitic rat when incubated with serum. The dog was given 1,000 U.S.P. units of parathyroid extract at 0 hour and again at 4 hours. Serum of blood withdrawn at 0, 24, and 28 hours produced no calcification of rachitic cartilage *in vitro;* serum of blood withdrawn at 4, 8, 12, and 16 hours produced +, ++++, ++, and +++ calcification, respectively. (From Fig. 4, McLean, Lipton, Bloom, and Barron, Tr. Conf. Metab. Aspects Convalescence 14:34. Reproduced by courtesy of the publishers.)

body of evidence concerning the nature and mechanism of actions of the parathyroid hormone at the subcellular level, affecting perhaps every cell in the body.

At a symposium on the parathyroids held in Holland in 1964, increasing attention was given to the metabolic pathways of biologic oxidation as observed in skeletal tissue, and in the possible role of the parathyroids in the resorption of bone. The emphasis was on the pathways that include citric, lactic, succinic, and carbonic acids; many believe that these acids may be important in solubilization of the bone mineral, and hence in the resorptive process. This topic is given further consideration elsewhere in this volume.

At the same symposium Neuman (1965) who with Terepka and Dowse (1960) had previously introduced a unifying concept of parathyroid hormone action, concluding that all aspects of the action of the hormone could be explained in terms of its ability to enhance the transport of P_i into cells, with an associated increase in acid production by glycolysis in bone, reported further on their studies. Neuman summarized the status of the problem as follows: (1) parathyroid hormone increases the entry of ^{32}P into various tissue cells; in bone *in vivo*, and in kidney and intestine both *in vivo* and *in vitro;* (2) high concentrations of P_i in the *in vitro* medium mask or mimic the parathyroid effect.

At this point the reports on the mode of action of the parathyroid hormone were carried to a subcellular level, referring back to reports of hormone-stimulated formation of calcium phosphate deposits in isolated mitochondria. It was reported by DeLuca and Sallis (1965) that: (1) calcium is taken up by mitochondria mainly as a phosphate salt; (2) it is deposited as an amorphous precipitate (not hydroxyapatite) in granules in the mitochondria; (3) this translocation is powered by the energy of oxidative phosphorylation. The physiologic significance of these observations remains in doubt. Osteoclasts do, in fact, accumulate the amorphous combination of Ca and P_i, but that this is not specific for osteoclasts is shown by electron micrographs of rat-liver mitochondria, loaded with Ca and P_i. It was further shown that vitamin D plays a basic role in the transport of Ca and P_i across cellular and subcellular membranes; and the mitochondrial membrane was treated as a model for a study of Ca and P_i transport as influenced both by vitamin D and PTH. There was also extended discussion on the control of energy utilization in mitochondria by parathyroid hormone. While the discussion did not clarify the systemic effects of the hormone at the subcellular level, it is of great interest that the parathyroids have a marked influence on cellular, subcellular, and membrane events.

Homeostatic Regulation of Calcium Ion Concentration in Blood

The parathyroid glands play a decisive part in the homeostatic regulation of the calcium ion concentration in the blood plasma. There is a direct correlation between the calcium levels in the body fluids and the state of activity of the parathyroid glands. At all levels, however, a rapid exchange of calcium and phosphate occurs between the blood and bone; in young animals this may amount, for calcium, to 100 per cent of the blood calcium per minute; in adult man about one calcium ion out of every four has been said to leave the blood every minute. In spite of this rapid turnover, the plasma calcium is maintained at a remarkably constant level; even in the absence of the parathyroid glands a relatively constant, although low, concentration of calcium ions is maintained in the blood. Thus while the parathyroid glands are responsible for monitoring the calcium ion concentration, and for correcting deviations from the normal, other factors enter into the regulatory mechanism and must be taken into account.

Cybernetic Aspects of Homeostasis of Calcium Ions

The Ca^{2+} concentration in the blood is itself the stimulus to which the parathyroid glands respond; the condition being regulated activates the regulatory mechanism, feeding back information about the output to an earlier stage so as to influence its action and thereby control the output. This is a clear-cut example of *negative feedback*, in terms of *cybernetic* or *control-system theory*, and will be treated as such.

The term *cybernetics*, as now used, includes the whole field of *control and information theory*, both in the machine and in biologic systems. The word itself is derived from a Greek word meaning "steersman." *Information theory*, in the biologic sense, refers to the type of information that is transmitted by nervous or humoral pathways and is capable of eliciting a physiologic response. In such a system, the deviation from the normal is called the *error.* The term *negative feedback* refers to reduction of the error and may operate, in the case of Ca^{2+}, to correct a concentration that is either too high or too low. A *closed-cycle system,* such as that under consideration, is also called a *servo system.* There are many servo systems in living organisms.

A servo system characteristically includes three parts: (1) an *error-sensing device;* (2) a *feedback transducer,* which translates the *error signal* from one form to another, such as, a chemical signal to a change in the rate of output of an internal secretion; and (3) a *control-signal transducer,* which brings about a further change in the nature of the signal in such a fashion as to affect the *output.* In biologic systems, two of these functions may be included within a single physiologic unit.

In many explanations of homeostatic control in biologic systems, the common thermostatic control of temperature has been cited as an analogy. In such a system there are only two possible settings for corrective action—on and off. This is called *directed correction.* It is unlikely that such a crude type of control ever exists in a biologic system. A second type of control is called *proportional control;* the action of the control mechanism is proportional to the deviation from the norm, i.e., proportional to the error. This is the simplest type of control commonly found in biologic systems.

A third type of control makes use of proportional control, but adds *derivative control,* in which the action is proportional to the rate of change of the error and is useful in preventing overshoot. This is used in gunfire control to anticipate the location of the target on the basis of its present velocity. Derivative control is postulated for biologic systems in which overshoot, possibly leading to oscillation, would be an unfavorable consequence of regulatory action.

A fourth type of control includes proportional and derivative control and adds *integral control,* sensitive to the accumulation of error with time. Some degree of integral control is doubtless present in most of the biologic systems required for physiologic regulation.

Aubert and Bronner (1965) have developed a symbolic model as an attempt at a unifying expression for the regulation of the blood calcium level by bone metabolism in normal and thyroparathyroidectomized rats. They state that in thyroparathyroidectomized rats the control is of the proportional type, whereas in normal animals an integral control resulting from the physiologic action of the parathyroid hormone is added to the proportional control. They do not take into account the possibility of a second hormone; the addition of a second hormone to the system will be considered below.

Figure 32 is a diagram, in terms of control theory, of the control mechanism responding to a deviation in the Ca^{2+} concentration in the blood as mediated through the parathyroid glands. The parathyroid glands act first as error-sensing devices, and then as feedback transducers by translating the stimulus received from the Ca^{2+} concentration into variations in output of the parathyroid hormone. The hormone is then carried in the blood to the bones, where it influences the mobilization of Ca^{2+} by cellular action. The cells participating in this action should be regarded as control-signal transducers, since they respond to control by hormones. Such a response to parathyroid hormone occurs from both osteoclasts and osteocytes. *In vitro* studies with ^{14}C-glycine yield some evidence of participation by the osteoblasts; collagen synthesis is impaired in cultures of bone in the presence of parathyroid hormone. It is postulated that calcitonin takes part in the homeostasis of the Ca^{2+} concentration in the blood plasma, but the degree to which it does so, the pathways by which information is carried, and the target cells acting as control-signal transducers still remain uncertain; for these reasons no attempt is made here to delineate the cybernetic aspects of the physiologic action of calcitonin, which is reviewed elsewhere in this chapter.

Role of Parathyroid Glands in Homeostasis

Once it was established, only a generation or so ago, that the parathyroid glands regulate the release of calcium from the bones into the blood, it was commonly believed that this relatively slow-acting mechanism was adequate to maintain a physiologic level of calcium ions in the plasma. Introduction of tracer methods, however, and increasing understanding of the fine structure of bone have made it clear that the parathyroid mechanism, while responsible for hour-to-hour or day-to-day adjustments, is not alone adequate for the minute-to-minute interplay between blood, interstitial fluid, and bone. Especially revealing in this respect is the demonstration that in young animals the equivalent of the total amount of calcium in the blood may be replaced every minute.

As pointed out by Rasmussen (1961) any integrated concept of the role of the parathyroid glands in homeostatic control of the calcium ion concentration must take into account not only the direct effect of the parathyroid hormone on osteoclastic resorption

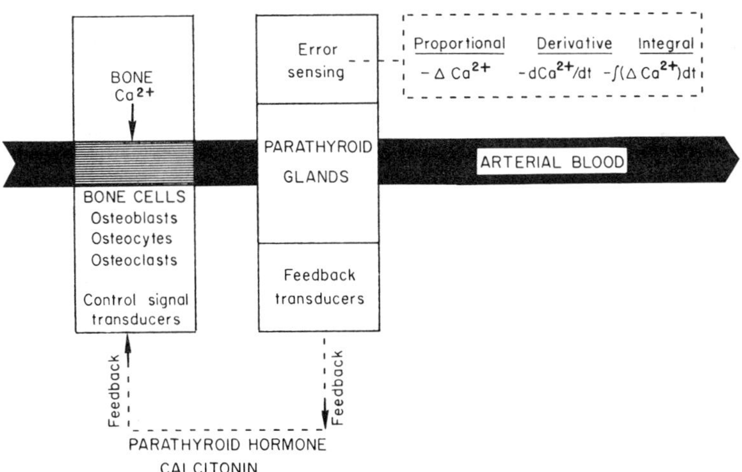

FIG. 32.—Diagram of control system that regulates calcium ion concentration in the blood. (From Fig. 1, McLean, J. Bone Jt. Surg. 45-A:1314. Reproduced by courtesy of the publishers.)

of bone, but also the other mechanisms and controls used by the organism to effect the fine adjustment required. Of the mechanisms under parathyroid control, Rasmussen has redirected attention to the kidneys, and to the effect upon calcium ion activity in the plasma of the changes in ion activity brought about by renal excretion of phosphate; he believes that the rapid action on the kidneys has a buffering effect upon fluctuations that would be corrected more slowly by the direct effect upon bone. The effect of the hormone on absorption of calcium by the gastrointestinal tract undoubtedly aids homeostasis. It is important also to emphasize the buffering effect of the extracellular fluids; calcium from this source is the first to reach the blood plasma in the event of depletion; this operates also in the opposite direction, and any excess of calcium in the plasma is rapidly transferred first to the extravascular fluid.

Dual Mechanism

Except for the action of the hormone on bone, liberating calcium into the blood by control of osteoclastic resorption, the most important factor in maintaining the stability of the calcium ion concentration in the plasma is the pool of exchangeable calcium of the bone. Transfers between the blood and bone, buffered by the extravascular fluids, are effected rapidly in both directions.

To account for the rapid turnover of calcium between blood and bone, in both directions, and for the ability of the organism to maintain constant calcium ion concentrations in the blood plasma, we have introduced the concept of a *dual mechanism.* The slow-acting part of this mechanism—that mediated by the parathyroid glands by control of osteoclastic resorption—is a clear example of a self-regulating process. The parathyroid glands are sensitive to the concentration of calcium ions in the blood; a deficiency in calcium ions leads to an increased activity of the glands, while an excess leads to decreased activity (Fig. 33). The control normally maintains the plasma calcium level at approximately 10 mg per 100 ml. When the parathyroids have been removed, the mechanism for release of calcium into the blood is absent. When there is a hyperfunctioning adenoma, there is no evidence that it responds to the increased calcium ion concentration in the plasma; it appears rather that the regulatory system goes out of control.

The rapidly acting part of the dual mechanism requires ion transfer between blood and bone and is able in the absence of the parathyroid glands to maintain the plasma level of calcium at approximately 7 mg per 100 ml. One view is that the bone acts as an ion exchange column, taking up calcium ions from the blood and returning others by passive physicochemical mechanisms. According to this, the labile or reactive bone mineral is in equilibrium with the ions in the fluid in contact with them. If the equilibrium is disturbed by removal of calcium ions from the blood, additional ions are transferred from the labile stores until the physiologic level has again been reached; if calcium is added to the blood, the excess is promptly transferred to the labile stores. This is, of course, subject to the conditions that the first line of defense, in either direction, is the extravascular fluid, and that diffusion through this fluid must occur before the pool of labile calcium in the bones is reached.

If we regard the parathyroid hormone as regulating osteoclastic

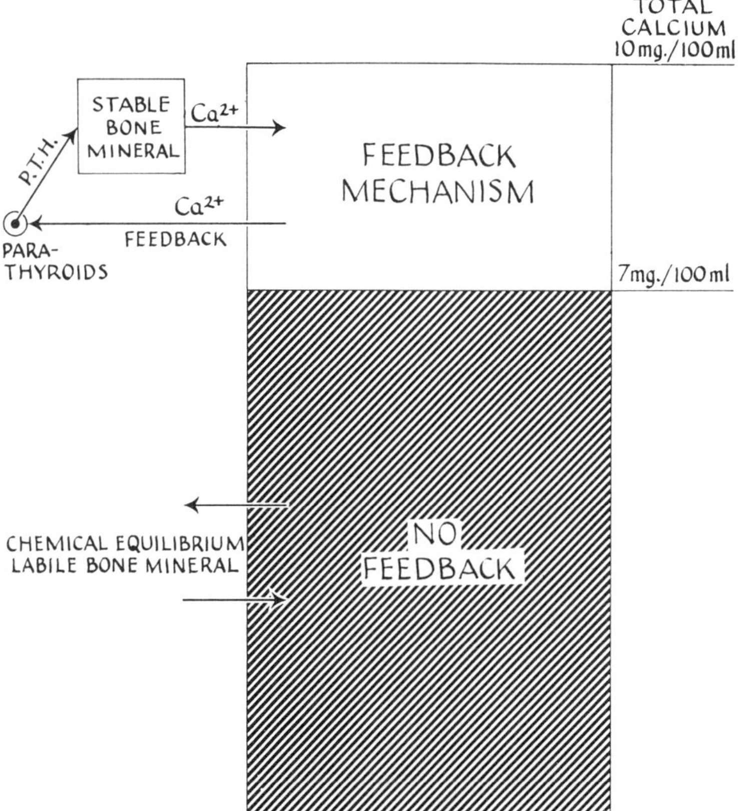

FIG. 33.—Diagram to illustrate mechanism of exchange of calcium between blood plasma and bones. Chemical equilibrium with labile fraction of bone mineral is independent of parathyroid glands and is adequate to maintain plasma calcium level at 7 mg per 100 ml. Parathyroid activity is under control of feedback from Ca^{2+} concentration in plasma and regulates release of calcium from stable hydroxyapatite crystals of bone mineral. This results in maintenance of plasma calcium at normal level of 10 mg per 100 ml. (Redrawn from original Fig. 14, McLean and Urist, Bone: an introduction to the physiology of skeletal tissue [Chicago: University of Chicago Press, 1955], p. 77.)

resorption of bone by a direct action upon the osteoclasts or their precursor cells, it becomes clear that this part of the dual mechanism has access to a portion of the bone not accessible to passive ion transfer; Woods and Armstrong (1956) have provided direct evidence to support this statement. Osteoclasts are found only on the surfaces of bone and exert their effects upon resorption accordingly. The dual mechanism, then, affects the mobilization of calcium both from the labile fraction of bone, by ion exchange or transfer, and from the stable bone mineral, by resorption.

Calcitonin

Copp and his collaborators (1962) have demonstrated that a hypocalcemic factor is released by high calcium perfusion of the thyroid and parathyroid glands of the dog. They attributed this factor to the parathyroids and called it *calcitonin.* It soon became evident that the factor was released from mammalian thyroid glands. Hirsch *et al.* (1963) reported the extraction of a potent hypocalcemic material from the rat thyroid and named it *thyrocalcitonin* to indicate the source of the material and its possible relationship to calcitonin.

Calcitonin activity has been demonstrated in thyroid tissue from all mammals studied. Potts *et al.* (1967) have reported isolation of a highly purified, potent, and homogeneous peptide, which approaches the composition of a pure hormone. It is a straight chain peptide with 43 amino acid residues and a molecular weight of 4,500. Its activity has been found to be 200 Medical Research Council (MRC) units per milligram.

Copp *et al.* (1967) have presented evidence for the ultimobranchial origin of calcitonin. The ultimobranchial bodies are paired follicular glands which arise from the ventral floor of the sixth pharyngeal pouch in a relation similar to the origin of the parathyroids from the floor of the third and fourth pharyngeal pouches. In fish, amphibia, reptiles, and birds they exist as distinct glands, but in mammals the ultimobranchial tissue becomes intimately associated with the thyroid gland. Copp and his associates (1967) have found the ultimobranchial glands of the chicken to yield calcitonin activity 100 times greater than that from whole hog thyroid, while only a trace of the activity is found in the chicken thyroids. It thus seems clear that in all species calcitonin activity is produced by cells of ultimobranchial origin and that the association with thyroid tissue in mammals is an accident in embryonic development. Calcitonin and thyrocalcitonin are identical, and there is no reason to perpetuate the accidental association with the thyroid gland in mammals in the name of the hormone.

Although calcitonin is characterized by its hypocalcemic activity, and it is tempting, and indeed logical, to assume that precise calcium homeostasis depends upon the opposing actions of two hormones, there is no direct evidence in support of this view. The situation is analogous to that of homeostasis of the blood glucose concentration. Two hormones, insulin and glucagon, are produced by the islands of Langerhans in the pancreas; the physiologic significance of glucagon is still in doubt.

It has been stated by Rasmussen (1961) that a simple feedback mechanism, involving the parathyroid hormone alone, would tend to oscillate. All regulatory mechanisms which depend upon negative feedback require oscillation to be effective. Such oscillation around the norm is damped by proportional, derivative, and integral controls, and it is not safe to assume that calcitonin is required for regulation of the calcium level in the blood plasma. Further investigation will doubtless clarify the relation of calcitonin to hormonal regulation of calcium metabolism.

Vitamin D and Calcium Homeostasis

It has been indicated above that vitamin D plays a part in the homeostatic control of the calcium ion concentration in the blood; the mechanism of this action has not been fully clarified.

Vitamin D exerts an influence on the citrate content of bone; this effect has been attributed to a more rapid conversion of pyruvate to citrate in the tricarboxylic acid cycle. Vitamin D elevates the citrate content; vitamin D deficiency reduces it. Until recently, it was postulated that production of citrate was an important factor in the transfer of calcium from bone to blood, and that parathyroid hormone and vitamin D, although acting at different points in the glycolytic cycle, were synergistic in this respect. Now that the emphasis has been shifted to acid production in bone, and especially to lactic and pyruvic acids, and since acid production occurs before vitamin D is believed to exert its influence on glycolysis and on citrate production, the possible role of vitamin D is less clear.

This does not deny an effect of vitamin D on mobilization of bone mineral, even though it does not provide a mechanism for such action. It has been suggested that this action of vitamin D is essential to calcium homeostasis, and that the maintenance of blood levels of serum calcium as high as 7 mg per 100 ml in the absence of the parathyroid glands depends upon this action. It was demonstrated as early as 1930, however, that both dogs and rats can survive in the absence of both vitamin D and the parathyroid glands. There is no evidence that vitamin D liberates H^+ in glycolysis. For the present, although we accept the evidence for mobilization of calcium under the influence of vitamin D, the details of such an action remain obscure.

It has been noted above that vitamin D plays a basic role in the transport of Ca and P_i across cellular and subcellular membranes; the mitochondrial membrane has been treated as a model for a study of Ca and P_i transport as influenced by both vitamin D and PTH.

At the subcellular level, vitamin D, whether given *in vivo* or added *in vitro*, greatly stimulates the release of calcium phosphate from mitochondria. Parathyroid hormone added *in vitro* acts synergistically with vitamin D. The hormone also stimulates the release of calcium, but only in mitochondria isolated from rats receiving vitamin D. In the absence of vitamin D, the hormone has no effect whatsoever, even at the highest concentrations tested. This adds weight to the statement at the beginning of this chapter that the parathyroid hormone and vitamin D may be regarded as component parts of an integrated system that exercises control over the mechanisms required for proper functioning of the organism as a whole.

CHAPTER XI

Mineral Metabolism

Internal Environment of Bone

Bone tissue shares the internal environment with the other tissues of the body. This includes the circulating blood plasma and the intercellular fluid—a total of approximately 20 per cent of the weight of the body. An even larger amount of fluid, 50 per cent of the body weight, is intracellular; a small proportion of this is in the cellular elements of bone.

There is an extremely rapid exchange of water and dissolved substances between the various compartments of the body; this serves not only to bring oxygen to and take carbon dioxide away from the cells, but also to transfer and exchange fluids and electrolytes. It is by the movement of water and dissolved substances that the minerals essential to the bones are brought to the locations at which they are to be deposited and are released when needed to maintain the physiologic constancy of the composition of the body fluids.

The important cation of the internal environment, from the standpoint of bone, is calcium. Of this element, a man weighing 70 kg has approximately 280 mg in the circulating plasma, of which half, or 140 mg, is in the form of calcium ions. This does not exchange, to any considerable degree, with the contents of cells, but it does exchange freely and rapidly with the 10 liters of intercellular fluid, which contains about 500 mg of calcium, nearly all in the ionized form. The plasma plus the intercellular fluid forms the *calcium compartment*, amounting to 15–20 per cent of the weight of the body and containing, in a 70-kg man, 525–700 mg of calcium ions.

This amount of calcium, in the ionized form, is seemingly insignificant when compared with 1,200 g of calcium in the skeleton. Moreover, in view of the very rapid exchange of calcium between the calcium compartment and the bones, it is remarkable that the organism is able, by means of homeostatic mechanisms, to maintain a constant level of calcium ions in the body fluids, especially when an individual ion may stay in the plasma for only a matter of minutes.

Of the anions in the fluids of the body, the most important for the maintenance of osmotic pressure are Cl^- and HCO_3^-. From the standpoint of the mineral constituents of bone, the most important is inorganic phosphate, mainly as the ions HPO_4^{2-} and $H_2PO_4^-$. Since these ions exchange to some degree with the contents of cells, the space available to phosphate in the body is larger than the calcium space, but the phosphate ions exchange as rapidly as the calcium ions.

The term *internal environment* was adopted by Claude Bernard (1878) to indicate that, as organisms become mobile and independent, they carry with them the constant and closely regulated environment necessary for the survival of their cells. As minute sea organisms move through the water, they modify the composition of the sea by an exchange of elements; but whereas the composition of the sea changes relatively slowly, owing to the enormous volume of water, the internal environment is under the constant influence of rapid exchange with the cells. The net effect of such exchange is that the conditions of life for the cells are kept constant.

Homeostasis in Mineral Metabolism

Until recent years it was customary to regard the kidneys as functioning in an automatic fashion, with built-in mechanisms responding to alterations in the composition of the blood plasma to conserve elements in short supply and to eliminate those in excess. But recently it has become apparent that the ability of the kidneys to act automatically is limited, and that increasing importance must be ascribed to central and hormonal control. We have advanced the hypothesis that the major cations of the blood plasma—Na^+, K^+, Ca^{2+}, Mg^{2+}, and H^+—are subject to such extrarenal control. In some cases the evidence is clear; in others it is only suggestive. On the whole the generalization seems permissible, at least as a working hypothesis, that the concentrations of all of these cations in the blood are centrally or hormonally controlled.

It is further proposed that for regulation of the cations of the blood plasma, the organism is supplied with a number of *information centers*, of which the respiratory center is one; each of these responds to information as to a particular state of affairs. The centers then relay this information, through a *chain of command*, to the organs whose function it is to apply the necessary corrections.

For the major anions of the blood plasma—Cl^-, HCO_3^-, $H_2PO_4^-$/HPO_4^{2-}, and SO_4^{2-}—the situation is quite different. As against the generalization that the cations of the blood are subject to central or hormonal regulation, the contrary statement may be made for the anions—that the control of none has been shown to depend upon information transmitted from a higher center, and that the existence of a feedback mechanism has been found for none.

With respect to homeostatic regulation of the cations of the blood, a major advance in recent years has been the discovery and partial elucidation of the control system that regulates the concentration of sodium in the body fluids. The system includes an extrahypophyseal diencephalic regulatory center, located in the hypothalamus, or perhaps in the region of the pineal body; this responds primarily to the level of serum electrolytes, either directly or by way of chemoreceptors. Neurosecretory cells of the regulatory center produce a tropic substance, called *aldosteronotropin* or *glomerulotropin*, which finds its way to the adrenal cortex, either directly by a humoral pathway or indirectly through the pituitary stalk and the adenohypophysis. This tropic substance in turn controls the output of *aldosterone*, which then influences the reabsorption of sodium by the renal tubules. This complex mechanism fulfils all of the criteria for an information center, coupled with a chain of command that eventually leads to the corrections that must be made by the kidney. The kidney, while actually performing the functions that result in homeostasis, is far from doing so automatically, insofar as sodium is concerned.

Aldosterone, the sodium-retaining hormone elaborated by the adrenal cortex, is a *mineralocorticoid*. Its properties are also exhibited by other adrenocorticoids, but aldosterone is many times more effective than any other known natural steroid. The existence of a supraoptic information center that controls the output of aldosterone is well established, but many details of the control system remain in doubt.

We have shown above that while calcium homeostasis is subject to hormonal control, it constitutes a special case, in that the parathyroid glands serve both as information centers and as the source of the hormone that controls the release of calcium from the bones to the blood. Homeostatic control of the calcium ion concentration in the plasma, mediated by the parathyroid glands, is also influenced by vitamin D.

Calcium of Fluids of the Body

All or nearly all of the calcium in the blood is in solution in the plasma; the amount in the red blood cells is negligible. In normal man the concentration of calcium in the plasma is usually between 9 and 11 mg per 100 ml, with 10 mg per 100 ml (2.5 mmoles per liter) a representative figure. This is in constant exchange with the calcium of the extracellular fluid and of the bones; the homeostatic mechanism that maintains the constancy of the concentration in the plasma is the function of the parathyroid glands. In the absence of the parathyroid glands, the plasma calcium may fall to 7 mg per 100 ml or even lower. In clinical or artificially induced hyperparathyroidism the figure may reach a level of 15 mg per 100 ml or higher.

It has been known since early in the present century that the calcium in the plasma is separable into two major and roughly equal fractions—diffusible and nondiffusible. It has also been known that the nondiffusible fraction is associated with the plasma protein. For some years, however, there was a difference of opinion concerning the diffusible fraction. It was held by many that a major portion of this fraction is in the form of a complex with the citrate ion or with some other comparable substance. These uncertainties have been resolved, and the relationship of calcium to the plasma protein has been incorporated in a formulation that describes the plasma as a solution of a weak electrolyte, calcium proteinate, the ionization of which may be represented by the equation:

$$\mathrm{CaProt} \rightleftharpoons \mathrm{Ca^{2+}} + \mathrm{Prot^{2-}} \tag{11.1}$$

and by the mass-law equation:

$$\frac{[\mathrm{Ca^{2+}}] \times [\mathrm{Prot^{2-}}]}{[\mathrm{CaProt}]} = K_{\mathrm{CaProt}} = 10^{-2.22}. \tag{11.2}$$

From these two equations and from the expressions [Total Ca] = [CaProt] + [Ca^{2+}], and [Total Prot] = [$CaProt^{2-}$], there may be derived a general equation from which the calcium ion concentration of the plasma or serum may be calculated from analyses for total calcium and total protein—quantities easily determined in the laboratory:

$$[\text{Total Ca}] = \frac{[Ca^{2+}] \times [\text{Total Prot}]}{[Ca^{2+}] + K} + [Ca^{2+}] . \quad (11.3)$$

The calculation is facilitated by the use of a nomogram, constructed from equation 11.3, shown in Figure 34, which illustrates the

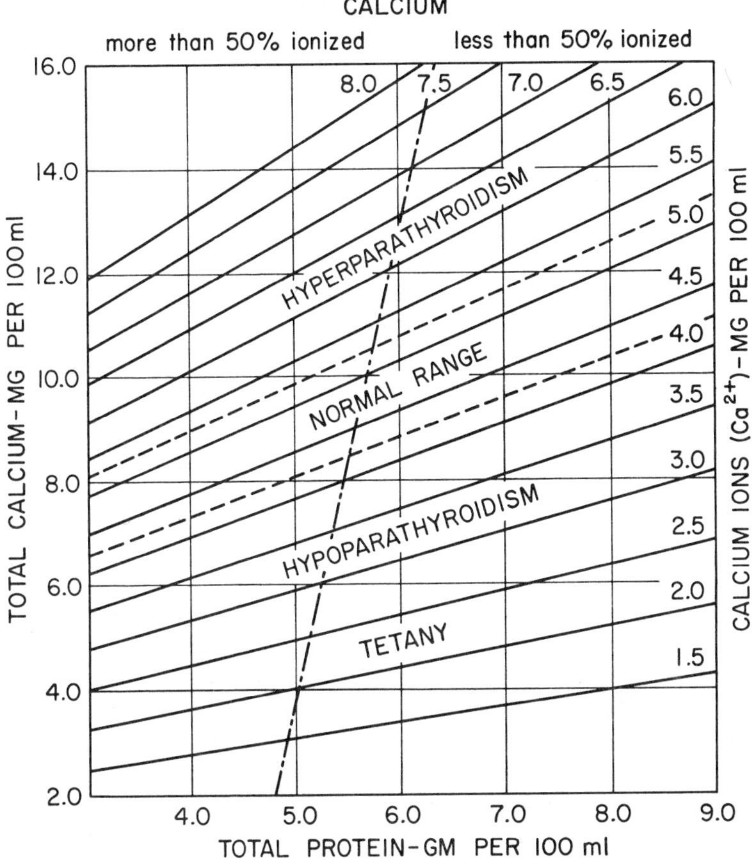

FIG. 34.—Nomogram for calculation of Ca^{2+} concentration from total protein and total calcium of serum or plasma. Constructed from mass-law equation $[Ca^{2+}] \times [Prot^{2-}]/[CaProt] = K$. (From Fig. 2, McLean and Hastings, Amer. J. Med. Sci. 189:606. Reproduced by courtesy of the publishers.)

relationships of the ionized and un-ionized fractions of calcium at varying protein and calcium levels.

At normal protein levels, about half the plasma calcium is in the ionized form, the other half being mainly in an undissociated complex with protein. Since this is an ionization phenomenon, shifts from the ionized to the un-ionized form occur instantaneously; the un-ionized calcium is not in firm combination with protein. Moreover, the formulation does not describe a static system; it does describe a system in dynamic equilibrium.

According to the mass-law equation 11.2, the ratio $Ca^{2+}/CaProt$ is determined by the concentration of protein. When the total calcium falls, as in hypoparathyroidism, or when it rises, as in hyperparathyroidism, the ratio of ionized to un-ionized calcium should remain approximately constant, with only a small correction for a shift in the $CaProt/Prot^{2-}$ ratio, unless the concentration of protein changes or there is some qualitative change in the ability of the protein to complex calcium. That the relationship predicted by the mass-law equation is approximated over the entire range in serum calcium levels from hypoparathyroidism to hyperparathyroidism was reported by McLean, Barnes, and Hastings (1935), their calculations being based on direct observation of Ca^{2+} concentrations by the frog-heart method.

Freeman and Breen (1960, see chapter X), using the ultracentrifuge to separate protein-bound and free fractions of plasma calcium, and Lloyd and Rose (1958), using ultrafiltration for the same purpose, have found that while the amount of calcium complexed by protein is correlated with changes in the total calcium concentration, the quantitative results have not conformed to the simple mass-law equation 11.2; the discrepancies are attributed by Lloyd and Rose (1958) to an influence of the parathyroid hormone on the affinity of the serum proteins for calcium, while Freeman and Breen (1960) believe that they are correlated with the serum calcium concentration, and only indirectly with parathyroid activity.

Others have reported further discordant and still unexplained results. In our opinion the more recent findings, with different methods, do not invalidate the concept of calcium proteinate as a weak electrolyte, dissociating in accordance with a mass-law relationship; further refinement of methods, and further attention to variables other than total calcium, total protein, and calcium ions, seem to be required for resolution of the differences in observations and interpretations.

Differences in the affinity of serum albumin and serum globulin for calcium have also been reported, although current literature supports the view that these proteins, in the serum of normal individuals, have approximately the same calcium-binding capacity. This statement does not hold true for certain forms of hyperglobulinemia. That serum albumin combines in normal blood with more calcium than does serum globulin depends upon the higher concentration of albumin in the plasma.

This description, which takes into account only calcium ions and the un-ionized calcium proteinate fraction, ignores a small amount of calcium in other combinations. Calcium forms un-ionized fractions with the ions of phosphate, bicarbonate, and citrate, but the aggregate of all un-ionized complexes in the blood, with the exception of proteinate, can hardly account for more than 5–10 per cent of the total calcium. When serum is subjected to diffusion or to ultrafiltration, these fractions appear in the diffusible portions. For this reason the total diffusible calcium is slightly higher than the calcium ion concentration. Since the concentration of citrate in the blood is correlated with parathyroid activity, the calcium-citrate complex may account for a part of the discrepancies observed in the calcium-protein relationship.

In the protein-poor fluids of the body, such as the cerebrospinal and the intercellular fluids, the state of calcium approximates that in an ultrafiltrate of plasma. In such fluids the concentration of calcium is generally about 5 mg per 100 ml (1.25 mmoles per liter), virtually all in the diffusible form. Again, a fraction of this may be in the form of un-ionized, diffusible complexes; these have little or no physiologic significance. The distribution of the total calcium in the plasma is illustrated in Figure 35.

When calcium is to be deposited in the bones, it moves first from the plasma to the intercellular fluid and then is deposited in locations prepared for calcification. Under such circumstances the plasma requires replenishment to maintain calcium ion concentrations at physiologic levels; such replenishment ordinarily comes from the diet, but the skeleton itself is the principal depot for the storage of reserve supplies in the organism. Thus it frequently comes about that as calcium is being deposited in one or more places in the skeleton, it is being withdrawn from other places; the entire system *plasma–intercellular fluid–bone* remains in a state of dynamic equilibrium.

Physiology of Calcium Metabolism

REQUIREMENTS

The requirements of calcium under varying conditions have been the subject of much study. The recommended dietary allowances, as revised by the Food and Nutrition Board, National Academy of Sciences–National Research Council (1964), are given in Table 5.

All these recommended allowances are well above minimum maintenance levels and provide for a liberal margin of safety. Except for the special conditions of pregnancy and lactation, when calcium should be added to the diet, the requirements are met or exceeded by the drinking of one quart of milk daily, if the diet is

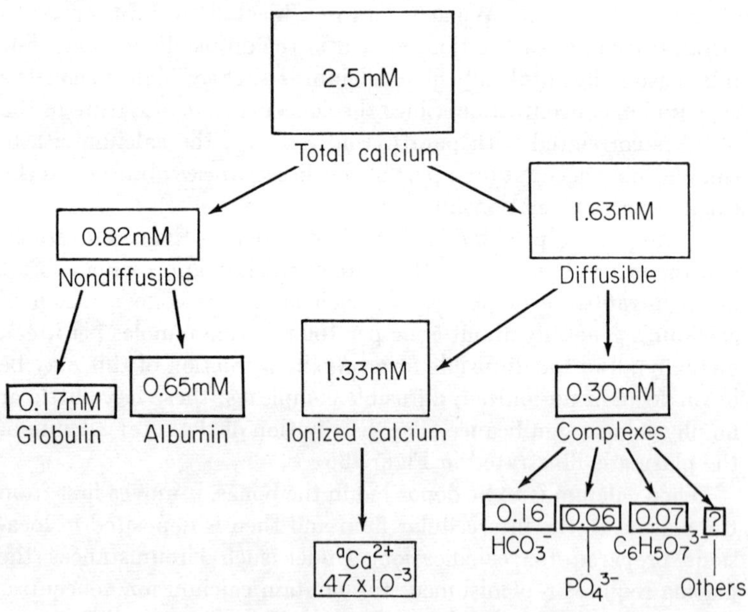

FIG. 35.—The state of calcium in normal serum as calculated from ultrafiltration data and formation constants; mM designates mmoles/liter. (Redrawn from Fig. 1.5, Neuman and Neuman, The chemical dynamics of bone mineral [Chicago: University of Chicago Press, 1958], p. 18. Reproduced by courtesy of the publishers.)

otherwise adequate. Many adults who do not drink milk are able to maintain themselves in calcium balance with intakes of calcium at 10 mg per kg per day, or 0.5–0.8 g daily.

ABSORPTION AND EXCRETION

The absorption of calcium takes place chiefly in the upper part of the small intestine, in both the duodenum and the jejunum. A large and variable part of the ingested calcium passes through the alimentary tract unabsorbed. Moreover, a considerable quantity of calcium, having been absorbed, is secreted with the digestive juices; the greater part of this is reabsorbed; a smaller portion appears in

TABLE 5

RECOMMENDED DAILY DIETARY ALLOWANCES (CALCIUM)

	Grams
Adults (men and women)	0.8
Pregnancy (2d and 3d trimester)	1.3
Lactation	1.3
Infants—to 1 year	0.7
Children—1 to 9 years	0.8
Boys	
9 to 12 years	1.1
12 to 18 years	1.4
Girls	
9 to 12 years	1.1
12 to 18 years	1.3

the feces. From the standpoint of *net absorption,* normal adults may utilize as little as 20 per cent of the calcium ingested. In rickets the net absorption is greatly reduced and may even fall to negative values, indicating a loss rather than a gain.

The most important single factor in the absorption of calcium is vitamin D. Absorption of calcium is unfavorably influenced by *oxalate* and *phytate* ions, and by failure of absorption of fatty acids from the intestinal contents, in the condition known as *steatorrhea;* in each case calcium passes through to the feces in an insoluble, nonabsorbable form. There is a widespread belief that acids and acidifying substances influence the absorption of calcium favorably and alkaline substances unfavorably. Experimental evidence indicates that such influences are too small to be of physiologic significance. The calcium intake markedly influences the net absorption of phosphate from the alimentary tract; the corresponding influence of phosphate upon the net absorption of calcium is negligible.

Loss of calcium from the body takes place through two channels, the alimentary canal and the urinary tract. Under ordinary conditions there is more calcium in the feces than in the urine, and under conditions of low intake it may exceed that in the food. It is no longer believed that there is any regulated excretion of calcium into the intestinal contents. The effect of increased ingestion of calcium upon net absorption is variable. Most healthy adults are able to adapt to low intakes of calcium, provided that there is no deficiency of vitamin D. Moreover, while extremely low intake of calcium (less than 200 mg daily) may be presumed to lead to continuous negative balances, there is no agreement as to when this results in an unphysiologic condition, so long as the plasma calcium is maintained within normal limits. In infants the absorption and utilization of added calcium is, within wide limits, proportional to the intake. Calcium administered parenterally or mobilized from the skeleton by parathyroid extract appears in the urine to the extent of approximately 80 per cent of that excreted; the remaining 20 per cent appears in the feces.

In adults the utilization of calcium is judged by the difference between ingested and fecal calcium. In infants and growing children the term is used in the sense of retention in the organism to meet the needs of growth, particularly of the skeletal system.

There is no food or drug that yields calcium as freely as milk. Calcium is in milk in what may be called a physiologic solution, together with phosphorus and with the protein to be utilized for the building of bone tissue. For these reasons milk is generally more effective than calcium phosphate or lactate or than any other single substance in providing for the needs of growth or repair of bone—even more effective than bone meal itself. The calcium of breast milk is no better utilized than that of cow's milk. Evaporated or dried milk is a satisfactory substitute for whole milk in promoting retention of calcium and the formation of bones in children. The utilization of dietary calcium varies inversely with the adequacy of the body's stores.

BALANCE

The calcium balance represents the net excess or deficit of retention of the element, as compared with the intake. The normal condition for a growing child is a substantial positive calcium balance, representing the retention necessary for skeletal growth. A daily storage of 10 mg per kg of body weight in children from 3 to 13 years of age is a desirable condition. For the adult the normal condition is calcium balance; a large proportion of the adult population is usually in negative balance, owing to insufficient intake. Negative calcium balances may be observed in women during early lactation, in spite of large intakes.

Calcium-balance studies have been useful in the clinic. They have revealed a negative balance in patients with hyperparathyroidism at stages and in forms of the disease in which there were no bone changes demonstrable by X ray; they are informative in clinical investigations in which it is necessary to determine whether therapy is effective without having to wait for gross and unequivocal evidence of improvement. An outstanding example is the discovery that a mixture of citric acid and sodium citrate will spare serious loss of calcium in patients with certain types of acidosis

KINETICS OF CALCIUM METABOLISM

Chiewitz and Hevesy (1935) first showed that there is a rapid interchange of phosphate between bone and blood. As radioisotopes became more readily available, they came into use for study of their disappearance from the blood and their appearance in the skeleton. Norris and Kisieleski (1948) demonstrated a rapid fall in the specific activity of the blood following intravenous injection of ^{45}Ca in mature rats, with a rapid rise in that of the bones. Armstrong and his collaborators (1952) published blood-disappearance curves for ^{45}Ca in dogs, and found that the curves could be expressed as a series of four exponentials. Thomas and his co-workers (1952) published similar data obtained from rabbits. Hansard, Comar, and Davis (1954) studied the effects of age upon the physiologic behavior of ^{45}Ca as a tracer isotope, and Bronner with his co-workers (1956) studied the disappearance of ^{45}Ca in nine boys and one young adult, again describing the curves by a series of four exponentials. By 1956 the disappearance of ^{45}Ca from blood following a single intravenous injection had been well described for dogs, rabbits, cattle, and man.

Bauer, Carlsson, and Lindquist (1955) related the disappearance of ^{45}Ca from the blood to its uptake by bone by a series of equations that made it possible to calculate the rates of accretion, resorption, and exchange reactions in the skeleton—parameters previously inaccessible to analysis. The methods for studying the kinetics of calcium metabolism and of the bone mineral have since been extended and refined, in large part by the original authors, but also by contributions from others.

The original method, as published by Bauer, Carlsson, and Lindquist (1955), depended upon (1) determination of the ^{45}Ca content of samples of bone and of the specific activity of the serum (plasma) calcium in rats at intervals following injection of a single dose of ^{45}Ca, and (2) upon the following basic equations:

$$^{45}Ca_{Obs} = {}^{45}Ca_E + {}^{45}Ca_A - {}^{45}Ca_R \qquad (11.4)$$

where

$^{45}Ca_{Obs}$ = total amount of ^{54}Ca present in a calcified tissue
$^{45}Ca_E$ = amount of ^{45}Ca present in the exchangeable fraction of the bone mineral
$^{45}Ca_A$ = amount of ^{45}Ca incorporated into the nonexchangeable fraction of the bone mineral through accretion
$^{45}Ca_R$ = amount of ^{45}Ca removed through resorption.

In more recent publications, while adhering to the same principles, Bauer and his co-workers (1961) have made changes in the symbols and in the methods of calculation to conform with common usage; the treatment here will follow that presently used by these authors.

Their general scheme for the kinetics of skeletal calcium, as indicated by tracer studies in animals, is as follows:

If the period of observation is shorter than the life span of the tissue examined, two types of movement appear to be detectable: (1) a rapid *exchange* between the plasma calcium and a fraction of the bone calcium, and (2) a one-way movement of calcium from plasma to bone (*accretion*). When the period of observation is longer than the life span of the tissues examined, a third process enters the picture: loss of calcium from the tissue, caused by *resorption* (bones) or *attrition* (incisors of rodents). This summary is derived from studies on the skeletons of animals, chiefly rats, but the same principles are applicable to study of the entire body, including that of man.

Curves derived from experimental observations may be expressed as follows:

$$*B_t = k_1 {*S_t} + k_2 \int_0^t *S(t)\,dt \qquad (11.5)$$

where

$*B_t$ = the amount of radioisotope in tissue B (bone) at time t

$*S_t$ = the specific activity of the element (i.e., activity per unit weight of the element) in serum at time t

$\int_0^t S(t)dt$ = the integrated serum activity; i.e., the area under the specific activity curve of the element in serum between $t = 0$ and time $= t$, and k_1 and k_2 are constants.

The authors arrive at the conclusion that, within acceptable limits, k_1 may be taken as equal to the amount of exchangeable bone calcium in the sample with the symbol E. Similarly, k_2 is taken as equal to A, or the rate of accretion. With these stipulations, equation 11.5 may be written as follows:

$$*B_t = E{*S_t} + \int_0^t *S(t)dt\,. \qquad (11.6)$$

This equation now contains two constants, E and A, and two variables, $*B_t$ and $*S_t$. These two variables can be determined experimentally, and the two constants can then be computed by using the data observed at two time intervals.

When longer time intervals are chosen, k_1 and k_2 are found to be time dependent, and a correction is introduced for the resorption of bone containing ^{45}Ca. The curve for the apparent loss by resorption is represented by the equation:

$$*R_t = *E_t + *A_t - *B_t \qquad (11.7)$$

in which $*R_t$ represents the amount of ^{45}Ca removed by resorption.

The above equations were originally derived from experiments on animals and required the analysis of samples of blood and bone. For extension to the study of whole man, serial blood samples have been analyzed and $*B_t$ in equation 11.7 is taken to represent the amount of isotope retained in the entire skeleton (i.e., dose administered minus excretion) at time t. The value of E then includes both extraskeletal and intraskeletal exchangeable calcium, and corresponds to the miscible calcium pool referred to below. Bauer *et al.* (1961), from their own data and those of others, calculated the accretion rate (A) of calcium in adult man as approximately 0.5 g per day and the total exchangeable calcium at about 5 g.

Alternative methods are described for calculation of values for A and E (equation 11.6), and each gives a somewhat different result. A simplified method, applicable under certain circumstances and with appropriate reservations, is by extrapolation of one of the exponentials characterizing the blood-disappearance curve to $t = 0$. The use made of this method by other authors is described below.

Bauer and Ray (1958) studied the kinetics of ^{85}Sr metabolism in man. The use of strontium in tracer amounts gives data on the metabolism of bone comparable to those obtained by the use of isotopes of calcium. Bauer and Ray used an electronic analog computer to simulate the plasma and excretory activity curves observed during 120 hours following injection of ^{85}Sr in five adult men. Bauer and his collaborators also pioneered in the utilization of a gamma-emitting isotope of calcium, ^{47}Ca, in the study of the kinetics of calcium metabolism in man by employing external scanning of the skeleton with collimated scintillation counters.

Heaney and Whedon (1958) have made similar studies on man, with similar results. In studying adult human subjects, they made the simplifying assumption that the miscible calcium pool, despite its theoretical complexity, behaves as a single compartment. They made use of extrapolation of one of the exponentials, as referred to above, but bypassed a possible source of error by extrapolating only from the portion of the curve representing the postequilibration-activity data. They expressed their results in terms of bone-formation rate (BFR), corresponding to the accretion rate (A), and as the miscible calcium pool (E) of Bauer, Carlsson, and Lindquist. They also introduced the term θ, defined as the time required for recycling of the isotope through the shortest lived species of bone, as determined by an abrupt change in the slope of the isotope-disappearance curve.

An innovation has been the use of stable isotopes of calcium, ^{46}Ca and ^{48}Ca, for the study of calcium metabolism. The method uses activation analysis, by neutron bombardment, followed by measurement of the induced radioisotopes, ^{47}Ca and ^{49}Ca, by gamma spectrometry. This gives results comparable to those obtained by the use of radioisotopes, but avoids exposing the subject or patient to radioactivity; this is particularly desirable in children.

Heaney (1963) has published a critical review on the evaluation and interpretation of calcium kinetic data in man, with special attention to the limitations and pitfalls inherent in the methods in use. He concludes that, except for external counting methods, the extreme simplification necessary for diagnostic purposes all but

TABLE 6

CALCIUM ACCRETION IN BONE DISEASE

HIGH
- Paget's disease
- Fracture
- Tumor
- Hyperparathyroidism
- Hyperthyroidism
- Vitamin D–resistant rickets treated with massive doses of vitamin D

NORMAL
- Osteopenia (osteoporosis) of unknown origin
- Vitamin D–resistant rickets
- Vitamin D–deficient rickets after treatment with vitamin D

LOW
- Osteopenia of unknown origin
- Hypoparathyroidism
- Hypothyroidism
- Vitamin D–deficient rickets

renders kinetic techniques valueless. On the other hand, for investigative purposes there is no substitute for kinetic analysis. The reading of his review is essential for anyone wishing to embark on the use of the principles and practice of the kinetics of calcium metabolism. In spite of these reservations, Table 6 is presented as an indication of what is to be expected in various skeletal disorders, in terms of the A values of Bauer, Carlsson, and Lindquist or the BFR of Heaney and Whedon.

THE POWER FUNCTION

As noted above, the kinetics of the bone mineral has generally been studied by the use of exponential functions in which time t appears in the exponential. An exponential function is also used to illustrate the kinetics of the decay of radioactive elements. The exponential function was characterized by Lord Kelvin as the law of compound interest, by means of which interest is compounded continuously instead of at arbitrary intervals. An exponential function appears as a straight line when plotted on semilog graph paper.

A second method used in the study of the alkaline earth radioisotopes is the *power function.* This is an expression in which the independent variable is raised to a constant power. For present purposes, this has the form t^{-b}, where t is the time and b is a positive fraction between zero and one. When such an expression is plotted versus time on log-log graph paper, the result is a straight line.

Norris *et al.* (1958) applied the power function to the retention of radioactive bone seekers and found that it provides a satisfactory empirical description of the retention of several radioisotopes preferentially deposited in skeletal tissue. Marshall (1964) has extended the usefulness of the power function by showing its general applicability to the study of the metabolism of the bone-seeking alkaline-earth radioisotopes with the use of only three adjustable parameters —accretion rate, excretion rate, and a very small constant added to t to prevent the failure of the power function at very short times after administration of the isotope, when it increases without limit as t approaches zero. Figure 36 illustrates a log-log graph of the specific activities of the whole body and of the serum in the dog for a period of three years following a single injection of ^{226}Ra.

Heaney (1963) has pointed out the applicability of the power function in certain special cases, in particular for the expression of long-term–retention data involving major fractions of an organism's life span, and thus contending with aging. It will be noted, for example, that the curves in Figure 36 represent data extending over a period of three years, and that many exponentials would be required to describe them.

Phosphorus

Inorganic phosphate is present in the fluids of the body in the form of the ions of orthophosphoric acid, H_3PO_4, chiefly as HPO_4^{2-}. The plasma of the infant, under conditions of active deposition of bone mineral, contains approximately 6 mg per 100 ml of total phosphorus as inorganic phosphate (2 mmoles per liter). In the plasma of the adult the inorganic phosphate level is reduced to approximately half that of the infant. It is characteristic of the rachitic infant that the concentration of inorganic phosphate in the plasma is at a level normal for the adult. The excretion of phosphate through the kidneys varies within wide limits, according to the intake; this has the effect of maintaining the blood phosphate at a relatively constant level; the part played by the parathyroid hormone in homeostatic regulation of the blood level of phosphate is imperfectly understood.

The transport of phosphate within the animal organism is a function of the circulating blood and of the intercellular fluid. Since

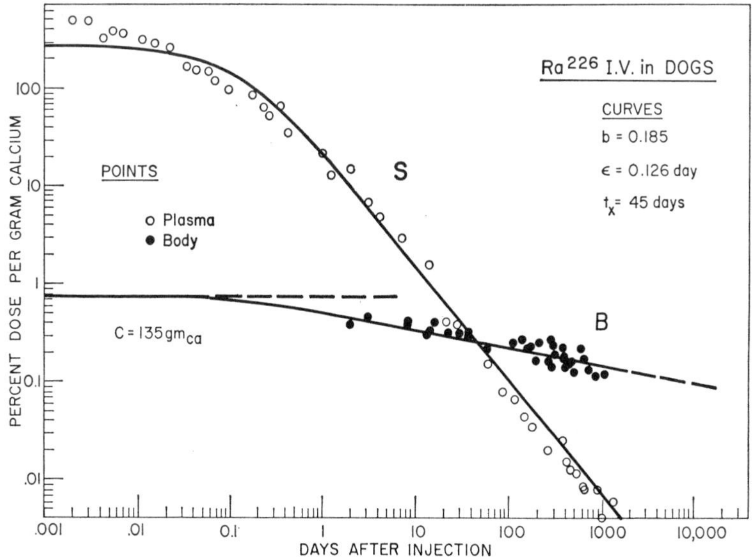

FIG. 36.—Log-log graph of specific activities of whole body and of serum of dogs, for 3 years after a single injection of ^{226}Ra. Data from several groups of beagles about 1.3 years of age at the time of the intravenous injection. (From J. H. Marshall, J. Theoret. Biol. 6:386–412, 1964. Recalculated from Van Dilla *et al.*, Radiat. Res. 8:417. Reproduced by courtesy of the publishers.)

phosphates have a manifold role in the organism and are closely related to many metabolic functions, as well as to calcification, they are found in many forms and in many locations. In the blood, in addition to the inorganic phosphate of the plasma, a variety of organic, acid-soluble compounds of phosphorus is present, mainly in the red blood cells; only about 0.5 mg per 100 ml of phosphorus is carried in the plasma as phosphoric esters. The movement of phosphate within and between the fluid compartments of the body and between fluid and bone occurs constantly and as rapidly as that of calcium.

So far as is known, the inorganic phosphate of the fluids of the body of higher vertebrates is virtually all in the form of free ions. Various attempts have been made to establish the presence of phosphate in a bound form, analogous to the un-ionized fraction of calcium. At present there seems to be no reason to accept a working hypothesis that accounts for any physiologically significant fraction of the inorganic phosphate of the blood as being present in an un-ionized complex.

METABOLISM OF PHOSPHORUS

An examination of the multiple role of phosphorus in the animal organism is beyond the scope of this volume. Except for a brief recapitulation of the types of phosphorus compounds found in the organism, this section will be concerned with the relationship of the metabolism of phosphorus to the skeleton.

TABLE 7

DISSOCIATION OF H_3PO_4

$H_3PO_4 \rightleftharpoons H^+ + H_2PO_4^-$,	$K_1' = 1.22 \times 10^{-2}$,	$pK_1' = 1.915$,
$H_2PO_4^- \rightleftharpoons H^+ + HPO_4^{2-}$,	$K_2' = 2.19 \times 10^{-7}$,	$pK_2' = 6.66$,
$HPO_4^= \rightleftharpoons H^+ + PO_4^{3-}$,	$K_3' = 1.66 \times 10^{-12}$,	$pK_3' = 11.78$.

All or almost all of the compounds of phosphorus, inorganic or organic, found in the body are derivatives of orthophosphoric acid, H_3PO_4, or of pyrophosphoric acid, $H_4P_2O_7$, itself a condensation of two molecules of orthophosphoric acid.

Of approximately 700 g of phosphorus in the adult human body, about 600 g are in the skeleton; the presence of this large amount of phosphorus in the bones depends upon the ability of orthophosphoric acid to form difficultly soluble compounds with calcium.

Orthophosphoric acid is a weak tribasic acid. Its dissociation constants, corrected for the ionic strength of serum, are given in Table 7. From these constants it may be calculated that, at pH 7.4, approximately 85 per cent of the total inorganic phosphate of the plasma is in the form of the divalent ion HPO_4^{2-}, while 15 per cent is monovalent $H_2PO_4^-$, and only 0.0035 per cent is trivalent PO_4^{3-}.

A major factor in the metabolism of phosphorus is the ability of the organism to synthesize all the organic compounds of phosphorus from inorganic phosphate. This is not to say that it can synthesize all the organic substances with which phosphate is united. But given thiamine, the organism can transform it into the active form thiamine pyrophosphate. Moreover, phosphate ingested in organic combination is for the most part split off and absorbed in the same manner as if it were ingested as inorganic phosphate. The biosynthesis of the large number of phosphorus-containing catalysts and intermediates requires additional enzyme systems, many of which themselves contain phosphorus. Phosphorus provides the linkage between the nucleotides that compose ribose and deoxyribose nucleic acids, and thus contributes to the structure of chromosomes and the processes of growth and heredity. It participates in the formation of numerous intermediate compounds and coenzymes essential to the metabolism of carbohydrates, as well as to many oxidation-reduction reactions and other intracellular processes.

Until recently *pyrophosphate* had been found in mammalian tissues in only very small amounts, in such organic compounds as thiamine pyrophosphate. Cartier and Picard (1955*b*), however, found that when phosphate was supplied to embryonic sheep cartilage in the form of ATP, approximately 80 per cent of the phosphate deposited in the cartilage was pyrophosphate. The corresponding figure for rachitic rat cartilage was found by Perkins and Walker (1958) to be only about 5 per cent; they attributed the discrepancy to a difference in the inorganic pyrophosphatase activity of the two tissues. Perkins and Walker also reported, for the first time, the finding of pyrophosphate in normal bone, and they found that the deposit formed *in vitro* on incubation of rachitic cartilage with a calcifying medium does not contain pyrophosphate unless ATP is added to the substrate; then the proportion of pyrophosphate attains the same order as that in normal bone. These findings seem to relate ATP, which has been called the *unit of currency* in metabolic energy transformations, and pyrophosphate to the calcification process, although the nature of this relationship is by no means clear. No one has as yet shown that energy, supplied locally, is essential to the deposition of bone mineral, although the possibility is receiving increased attention. If this could be demonstrated, the presence of ATP in calcifying systems would assume new significance.

SOURCE, REQUIREMENTS, AND ABSORPTION

As phosphorus is present nearly everywhere in the animal organism, so is it present nearly everywhere in nature. Ultimately, the source of the phosphorus in the animal is the sea or the soil. For marine plants and animals, phosphorus is always in short supply, 40 μg per liter of sea water; this small concentration must be turned over very rapidly to support life. Indeed, the population of living organisms in aquatic habitats appears to be limited as much by the supply of phosphorus as by any other single element of nutrition. For man the flow is first to the plant foods, then either direct to the human organism or indirectly by way of the animal tissues consumed by man. Fertilization of the soil consists in supplying it with phosphorus, as well as with nitrogen—two elements without which most plants cannot grow. A deficiency of phosphorus in the soil may limit both plant and animal life.

The daily requirement for phosphorus in the adult human organism is in the neighborhood of one gram; it is even higher in the growing child. In American diets phosphorus is so universal that a deficiency in the intake of this element scarcely constitutes a problem in nutrition. If the dietary requirement for calcium is met from milk, the phosphorus intake will be adequate, as it will be from other protein-rich foods. Certain borderline diets are deficient in phosphorus, but the importance of this is overshadowed by other concomitant deficiencies. The phosphorus content of mother's milk is much lower than that of cow's milk; this may be the limiting factor in the rapidity of mineralization of the skeleton in breast-fed infants. This cannot be regarded as a true deficiency. A deficient absorption or utilization of phosphate, in the presence of an adequate intake, is commonly associated with the low retention of calcium in rickets. The total effect is as though there were an actual deficiency of both calcium and phosphorus in the diet.

In view of the competing demands for phosphorus to serve its manifold functions in the organism, it is important to note that the first effect of a deficient assimilation of phosphorus is a failure of calcification of the bones, and that this failure, by removing the largest requirement for the element, usually leaves an amount adequate for all other purposes, except under the most extreme conditions.

COLLOIDAL CALCIUM PHOSPHATE

Increase in the product Ca $\times$ P to a point beyond the solubility product constant of $CaHPO_4$ not only is critical for deposition of the bone mineral, but also determines the formation of a colloidal calcium phosphate in the plasma. This substance, although in particulate form, is not precipitated from the blood, owing to the protective action of the plasma proteins. It is quickly removed from the blood by the histiocytes of the liver and spleen and is returned to the circulation in solution. It has not been shown that the formation and disposal of this substance are of physiologic importance or that it plays any part in the formation of the bone mineral.

Bone as a Reservoir of Minerals

The bones serve as a reservoir of calcium and phosphate, holding them available for the other needs of the body as well as for deposition in other parts of the skeleton when they are needed. Moreover, other mineral elements may be deposited in bone and may remain there throughout the life of the organism. As a rule they serve no known physiologic function, although sodium and magnesium may be mobilized when needed by the soft tissues. In growing animals when the bones respond to changes in intake of calcium and phosphorus or of vitamin D, profound changes in the state of mineralization of the bones may occur.

EFFECTS OF INTAKE OF CALCIUM AND PHOSPHORUS UPON BONE

Sherman (1947) investigated the calcium requirements of the laboratory rat and introduced the concepts of *adequate* and *optimum* diets. An adequate diet is one that will support normal growth, health, reproduction, and lactation, generation after generation; an optimum diet will produce increased growth, earlier maturity, higher adult vitality as indicated by superior breeding records, a longer period between the attainment of maturity and the onset of senility, and an increase in the average length of adult life. These concepts have been useful in guiding experimental work and in interpreting the conflicting results in the literature concerning the calcium requirements of man.

The bones of rats on diets classified as adequate in calcium intake may be seen to have: (1) a relatively short metaphysis and therefore a relatively short supply of stored calcium; (2) great osteoblastic and osteoclastic activity, reflecting the need for maximum turnover and utilization of the dietary calcium; (3) osteoid borders on the trabeculae, indicating that calcium is not being stored to the maximum capacity of the bone structure; and (4) a porous shaft, similar to that of very young animals.

The bones of rats on diets classified as optimum, on the other hand, have: (1) a relatively long and dense metaphysis, providing for the maximum storage of calcium; (2) diminished osteoblastic and osteoclastic activity, indicating minimum turnover and maximum conservation of bone mineral; (3) bone trabeculae calcified to the maximum density with no osteoid borders, evidence of an abundant and continuous supply of calcium and phosphorus in the diet and body fluids; and (4) a very dense shaft, similar to that of adult animals.

CITRATE

It has been known, since the report of Dickens (1941), that 90 per cent or more of the citric acid of the body is in the skeleton and that as much as 1 per cent of the fresh weight of bone may be accounted for as citrate.

The occurrence of citrate in the mineral portion of the skeleton forms one of the strongest arguments for the belief that such substances are held on the surfaces of apatite crystals, since the size of the citrate molecule clearly excludes it from the apatite structure itself. Whether citrate is present in bone as the citrate ion or whether it is combined in a complex form with calcium is still not clear. That portions of citrate may be dissolved from powdered bone only with difficulty, while other portions are readily soluble, suggests either that more than one form of citrate exists in bone or that portions of the citrate are held on entrapped surfaces.

Present interest in citrate centers upon its functional significance in bone. It is probable that at least part of the citrate in the circulating blood originates in the skeleton and is metabolized by the kidney. Moreover, the increase in the citrate in bone and in the blood, as induced by either the parathyroid hormone or vitamin D, or by both acting together, offers presumptive evidence that citrate plays an important role in the solubilization of the bone mineral and the transfer of calcium from bone to blood. It is not yet clear, however, how citrate is related to calcium metabolism; Terepka *et al.* (1960) now put more emphasis on the production of acid in the glycolytic cycle, with a consequent increase in the local concentration of hydrogen ions, than on the complexing of calcium by the citrate ion. Consideration has been given to these problems in an earlier chapter.

STORAGE OF CALCIUM AND PHOSPHATE

Except for the secondary system of medullary bone formed in birds during the egg-laying cycle, such storage of calcium and phosphate as occurs in the skeletal system is limited to the bones that also have a supporting function. Mammals have no special storage mechanism to meet the needs of pregnancy and lactation; skeletal calcium and phosphorus are, however, readily given up to meet the needs of the soft tissues. This enables homeostatic regulation of a normal calcium level in the plasma to be maintained over long periods of time, at the expense of a negative calcium balance; it also gives the manifold requirements of phosphate in the soft tissues a priority for the assimilation of the phosphate in the diet. Except under extreme conditions, such as in the Middle European countries in World War I and in underdeveloped countries, where the drain of pregnancy on the skeleton, coupled with a deficient intake of calcium and of vitamin D, may lead to severe osteomalacia, the organism is able to adapt to a low intake of calcium without demonstrable pathologic changes. The possible relation of calcium deficiency to osteoporosis is discussed in a later chapter.

STORAGE OF OTHER ELEMENTS

In addition to calcium, the skeleton contains other cations, some of which are foreign to the needs of the organism and have been ingested fortuitously. Of the additional cations found in the bone mineral, two are of physiologic importance: sodium and magnesium. For these the skeleton may be regarded as a storage reservoir, aiding in the maintenance of physiologic levels of these elements in the blood. Potassium has no special affinity for bone.

A number of foreign cations are found as contaminants of the bone mineral, having been deposited after reaching the bloodstream. Of these the most important are radium, strontium, and lead, any of which may substitute for calcium in the crystal structure of hydroxyapatite. Much recent attention has been directed to the harmful effects of radioactive elements when incorporated within bone; this is given consideration in the following chapter.

SODIUM

Some 46 per cent of the total body sodium is present in the mineral substance of bone, at a concentration approximating 400 mEq/kg of bone mineral. The effective concentration of sodium at the crystal surface is probably higher. Some 40–45 per cent of the total sodium of the skeleton is rapidly exchangeable and available to the fluids of the body; an additional 6–13 per cent can be mobilized in the adult, in response to various stimuli. In acute sodium depletion, the ability of bone to release sodium ions to protect the hydrogen ion concentration of the extracellular fluids appears to be dependent upon parathyroid secretion. The portion of the bone sodium not accessible to the body fluids is associated with the stable fraction of the bone mineral. Bone can also serve as an acceptor of Na^+, up to 8 per cent of the normal crystal content.

Vincent has studied sodium metabolism in the skeleton at the histologic level, employing two isotopic methods (1959; 1960). He has induced radioactivity in ground sections of bone by exposing them to a neutron flux, which activates ^{23}Na to form the radioisotope ^{24}Na, with a half-life of 15.06 hours; he has also administered ^{22}Na, with a half-life of 2.6 years; in both instances sections of bone were studied autoradiographically and by means of microradiograms.

Bauer (1954) gave ^{22}Na to growing rats, and killed them from one to twenty-five days later. By means of autoradiograms he showed that during growth sodium is incorporated in the nonexchangeable fraction of the bone sodium, from which it is not removed until the bone structure is reached by resorption. In another series of experiments with ^{22}Na, assuming that the sodium of the extracellular water of bone is freely exchangeable with the serum sodium, he concluded that 30–40 per cent of the excess sodium of bone is exchangeable with the extracellular water sodium. In short-term experiments in which the dynamics of sodium deposition in bone was studied after administration of ^{22}Na, Vincent (1960) found that rapid-exchange mechanisms predominate; no accumulation of sodium was observed either in the sites of osteogenesis or in the less calcified osteons. Radioactivity disappeared on decalcification but was retained in ethylenediamine-treated sections; the sodium was linked to the mineral of bone. In longer experiments, four to six weeks following injection of ^{22}Na there was concentration of the radioisotope in osteons in which bone mineral was being deposited at the time of injections; this is evidence for accretion of new sodium during initial mineralization. After immersion in a solution of $^{22}NaCl$, compact bone is uniformly labeled.

MAGNESIUM

Magnesium is believed to be chemisorbed on the surface of the crystals of bone mineral and is readily available to the fluids of the body, at least in large part; the complex $MgOH^+$ has also been proposed as a surface ion. No homeostatic mechanism for regulation of the exchange of magnesium between blood and bone is known. About a third of the skeletal magnesium can be mobilized in severe magnesium deficiency; this is accomplished by ion transfer from the labile stores in the skeleton to the circulating fluids.

FLUORIDE

One of the most avid of all bone-seeking substances is the fluoride ion. Approximately half of a dose of F^-, administered orally as NaF to an animal not previously treated, will be deposited in the skeleton. F^- is simultaneously eliminated in the urine and deposited in the skeleton. Young animals deposit and retain greater proportions of daily F^- than do adults. The mechanism works three ways: (1) by exchange of F^- for OH^- in the surface layers of the existing crystals of mineral of bones, teeth, and enamel; (2) by incorporation of F^- in the lattice of new crystals in place of OH^-; and (3) by incorporation of F^- in both surface and lattice structure of new crystals deposited in new bone mineral in parts of the skeleton undergoing haversian remodeling. When the F^- intake is low and the skeletal load is small, the bone mineral converts apatite to fluorhydroxyapatite (also called fluorapatite), and protects the body fluids and cells against the toxic effects of high concentration. The concentration of OH^- in blood is normally so low that it is readily exchanged for F^- and deposited in bone by isomorphic substitution. F^- and OH^- are almost exactly the same size and have the same charge. In chronic fluoride intoxication, the concentration of F^- in the serum is high, and phosphate is liberated from the mineral. Crystals of calcium fluoride can form on the surface of the particles of francolite, but this is rapidly replaced with more stable fluorapatite; no calcium fluoride crystals form in bone.

Roholm (1937) described fluorosis in industrial workers in plants processing cryolite (Na_6AlF_3). Years after their employment there was ended, the urinary fluoride was high, owing to slow resorption of fluorapatite and turnover of diseased bone. Laying hens and other animals that turn over large amounts of bone at a rapid rate and are able to shunt large amounts of F^- into the mineral phase seem to be able to elude the toxic effects of fluoride ion on the bone cells. The capacity of apatite for incorporating F^- is so large that if a man were to consume one milligram a day for a lifetime, not all of the mineral would be converted.

The disease known as *crippling fluorosis* in cattle and man is characterized by hyperostosis, an increase in mass and thereby also radiodensity of the bone. It begins in the spinal column and extends into the long bones. Exostoses form at the attachments of broad ligaments near joints, and subperiosteal bone spurs grow inside the origins and insertion of muscles. Johnson (1964) noted that the dense bone of victims of fluorosis is due to an abnormal pattern of bone matrix and a disarray of bone cells.

Fluoride is of great interest because NaF is present naturally in the water consumed by over three million people, and is added to drinking water in many urban areas of the United States, in amounts as small as one part per million, to reduce the incidence of dental caries. Four kinds of evidence for the effect of fluoride on dental caries are: (1) more perfect teeth in form and structure; (2) more resistant crystal structure; (3) lower solubility of mineral; and (4) reduced production of bacterial acid. In large amounts, 20–60 mg per day, NaF is given to patients with osteoporosis and Paget's disease, but the efficacy of such treatment is not established. In very large amounts, 100 mg per day, fluoride can produce gross increase in radiodensity within a year in the vertebral bodies of some victims of multiple myeloma. Factors related to species characteristics, age of the individual, and dosage of F^- influence the development of bone fluorosis.

CHAPTER XII

Radiation, Isotopes, and Bone

Neither radiation itself nor the metabolism of radioactive isotopes has any place in the normal physiology of bone. Within the last half century, however, and more especially in the last three decades, these subjects have assumed increasing importance, with the skeleton playing a major role. Excessive doses of X ray to the bones may be harmful, particularly during growth, and these effects have been studied experimentally. Early studies of the effects of internal radiation of the bones were confined to the damage caused by radium. Accidental poisoning by radium, usually from exposure some years ago, especially in radium-dial workers and in patients given radium therapeutically, continues to receive attention. The occurrence of osteogenic sarcoma was attributed to radium as early as 1929.

The introduction of the *cyclotron*, the subsequent development of *nuclear reactors*, and the exploitation of these and other instruments for the production of radioactive isotopes and even of new elements have increased both the hazards of radiation and the opportunities for the study of its effects. Concurrently, analysis of physiologic mechanisms by use of tracer quantities of radioactive material has been made possible and has come into extensive use. Metabolic studies of the rare elements, as well as of calcium and phosphorus, have been facilitated, and information not otherwise obtainable has appeared in the literature. Understanding of the biologic applications of radioactivity depends upon the advances made in nuclear physics.

Atomic Nucleus

NUCLEAR STRUCTURE

The nucleus of the atom represents all of the properties that distinguish the individual atom and by far the greater part of its mass. Around it revolve electrons, common to all atoms, each carrying the negative electronic charge *e*. It is not within the scope of this volume to enter into the details of nuclear structure, but certain features are essential to orientation in the subject matter of this chapter.

The nucleus contains two kinds of elementary particles, *protons* and *neutrons;* either serves as the unit of mass; to each is assigned mass number 1. The important difference between them is that each proton carries a positive charge, equal in magnitude to the negative electronic charge *e*, while the neutron carries no charge. Each element in the periodic table has a different number of *protons* in its nucleus; this is its Z or *atomic number*, which characterizes the element.

The *neutron*, also a constituent particle of the nucleus, adds to mass in proportion to the number present and thus contributes to the nuclear mass, but not to its charge. The sum of the number of protons in a nucleus plus the number of neutrons is the A or *mass number;* this together with the atomic number or nuclear charge characterizes the *nuclear species*.

An *isotope*, or *nuclide*, is a single nuclear species of a particular element. A given element may have as few as three or as many as fifteen or more isotopes; all have the same atomic number, contributed to by the protons constant for each element, but different mass numbers, determined by the sum of protons and neutrons. An isotope, or nuclide, may be *stable* or *radioactive*.

RADIOACTIVITY

Radioactivity depends upon the emission of energy in the form of *radiation;* this results from a condition of instability in the nucleus, which seeks a level of stability. Emission of energy from a given nucleus is in one or more of three forms: (1) *alpha particles;* (2) *beta particles*, or electrons, either negatively or positively charged; and (3) *gamma rays*, or electromagnetic radiation. Alpha or beta radiation is associated with *decay* of the element, resulting in spontaneous *transmutation* to another element. The *physical half-life* of a radioelement is the time in which the amount of a radioisotope is reduced by decay to half its initial value. Gamma radiation, while originating from isotopes undergoing alpha or beta decay, is not itself a part of decay or transmutation, since it represents neither loss of mass nor loss of charge.

Alpha particles carry two positive charges and are composed of two protons and two neutrons; they are identical with the nucleus of a helium atom. Their emission represents *alpha decay*, which occurs predominantly in elements with atomic numbers greater than 82. Emission of an alpha particle from the nucleus of an atom results in the loss of two positive charges and a reduction of 4 in mass number; the net effect of this is transmutation to a different element. Most of the heavy elements, with atomic numbers greater than 82, are unstable with respect to alpha decay.

Beta particles are high-speed electrons and may be either positively (β^+, positron) or negatively (β^-, negatron) charged. For a beta particle to be emitted from a nucleus, which has none in its structure, an electron is created in the act of its emission. This requires that either a neutron or a proton, commonly the former, must undergo transformation to the other; a neutron thus gains a positive charge, while releasing a negatively charged electron, and becomes a proton; a proton loses its positive charge, releases a positively charged electron, and becomes a neutron. At the same time, in either case, there is released another particle, of infinitely small rest mass and without charge—the *neutrino*. When *beta decay* of a nucleus occurs, the mass number remains the same while the atomic number is either increased (β^- decay) or reduced (β^+ decay) by one. Beta decay thus results in transmutation to another element; formation of another isotope of the same element is not a possible consequence of beta decay.

Gamma rays represent electromagnetic radiation emitted from the nucleus of the atom as *photons*. Except for differences in wave length and consequently in penetrating power, gamma rays are identical with light rays; they have properties similar to those of X rays. The emission of gamma rays from the nucleus occurs as a concomitant of an excited state of the nucleus, ordinarily associated with alpha or beta decay or both; it represents an adjustment of the energy relations within the nucleus, and its terminal state is de-excitation or return to the ground state.

There are two situations in which only gamma rays are emitted from an atom; one of these has bearing on the ordinary use of isotopes. This is the phenomenon of *electron capture* (EC), by which is meant the capture by the nucleus of an electron from the outer shell of the atom; this results in the transformation of one proton to a neutron, and the reduction of the atomic number by one. An excited state of the nucleus may result, accompanied by the emission of gamma rays. Of the isotopes in common use (Table 7), those that undergo transformation to other elements, with emission of gamma rays only, are: ^{7}Be to ^{7}Li; ^{85}Sr to ^{85}Rb; and ^{133}Ba to ^{133}Ce. In addition, the transition of ^{18}F to ^{18}O and of ^{22}Na to ^{22}Ne occurs by a combination of β^+ decay and electron capture. The second phenomenon associated with gamma radiation alone is that of *isomeric transition* (IT), which represents a delay in adjusting to the ground state. Since the half-lives of isomeric states are generally short, this phenomenon is not important in the biologic application of radioisotopes.

One of the elements frequently used in physiologic experimentation is phosphorus (^{32}P), usually as orthophosphate. The physical half-life of ^{32}P is 14.2 days, and it is transformed by β^- decay to stable sulfur (^{32}S), as shown in Figure 37. There is not only a possibility of a deleterious effect on genetic material by β^- radiation from ^{32}P itself; there is also the possibility of the breakdown of nucleic acid where ^{32}P is incorporated when radiophosphorus changes to radiosulfur.

RADIOACTIVE ISOTOPES

The term *isotope*, or its synonym, *nuclide*, refers to any one of the forms an element may assume; a nuclide is characterized by the atomic number of the element and the mass number of the particular nuclide. The term isotope does not itself imply radioactivity; an isotope may be either stable or radioactive. A radioactive isotope may be designated as a *radioisotope* or *radionuclide*.

Many isotopes occur naturally; others are produced artificially. The number of known isotopes of all the elements is about 1,500. New elements, as well as new isotopes, have been formed in the laboratory. In addition to the transmutations that occur naturally, as in the decay of the heavy elements such as radium, transmutations may be induced. Of these events the most dramatic is nuclear fission, brought about in the atomic bomb, and resulting in radioisotopes of the 34 elements in the periodic system from zinc (element 30) to the rare-earth europium (element 63). In some instances several isotopes of the same element may be formed as fission products. Other radioisotopes are produced by bombardment of the nucleus with particles, commonly neutrons, which add to the mass of the nucleus that absorbs them, resulting in a new isotope of the same element, with an increase by one in the mass number. Other examples of transmutation are *deuteron-induced, alpha particle–induced,* or *proton-induced. Neutron bombardment* requires a source of *neutron flux,* commonly a *nuclear reactor.* Induction by deuterons, alpha particles, or protons requires acceleration of the particles in order that they may acquire sufficient energy to

Mass (A) Numbers

Atomic (Z) Numbers	26	27	28	29	30	31	32	33	34	35	36	37	38		
14	^{26}Si ?	^{27}Si β^+	^{28}Si 92.2%	^{29}Si 4.7%	^{30}Si 3.1%	^{31}Si β^-, γ	^{32}Si β^-								14
15			^{28}P β^+, γ	^{29}P β^+, γ	^{30}P β^+	^{31}P 100%	^{32}P β^-, γ	^{33}P β^-	^{34}P β^-, γ						15
16						^{31}S β^+	^{32}S 95.0%	^{33}S 0.75%	^{34}S 4.215%	^{35}S β^-	^{36}S 0.17%	^{37}S β^-, γ	^{38}S β^-, γ		16
	26	27	28	29	30	31	32	33	34	35	36	37	38		

Atomic (Z) Numbers	37	38	39	40	41	42	43	44	45	46	47	48	49	50	
19	^{37}K β^+	^{38}K β^+	^{39}K 93.1%	^{40}K .01% β^-, EC	^{41}K 6.9%	^{42}K β^-, γ	^{43}K β^-, γ	^{44}K β^-, γ	^{45}K ?						19
20		^{38}Ca β^+	^{39}Ca β^+	^{40}Ca 96.97%	^{41}Ca EC	^{42}Ca 0.64%	^{43}Ca 0.145%	^{44}Ca 2.06%	^{45}Ca β^-	^{46}Ca .0033%	^{47}Ca β^-, γ	^{48}Ca 0.185%	^{49}Ca β^-, γ		20
21				^{40}Sc β^+, γ	^{41}Sc β^+	^{42}Sc β^+	^{43}Sc β^+, γ	^{44}Sc β^+, γ	^{45}Sc 100%	^{46}Sc β^-, γ	^{47}Sc β^-, γ	^{48}Sc β^-, γ	^{49}Sc β^-	^{50}Sc β^-, γ	21
	37	38	39	40	41	42	43	44	45	46	47	48	49	50	

Mass (A) Numbers

FIG. 37.—Partial chart of nuclides, to show isotopes of phosphorus and of calcium with their relations to isotopes of neighboring elements. Mass (A) numbers are in vertical columns; atomic (Z) numbers are in horizontal rows. Shown are atomic numbers of isotopes, relative abundance in nature (in per cent), and type of radiation emitted. Stable isotopes are underlined. Arrows indicate pathways and direction of spontaneous decay, with nature of decay (β^-, β^+, and electron capture, EC). Alpha decay does not occur in the elements shown. (Data derived from Table of isotopes, Strominger, Hollander and Seaborg, Rev. Mod. Physics 30:585.)

enter the nucleus under bombardment. A variety of high-energy accelerators is now available for research in particle physics, as well as for the formation of new isotopes.

RADIOACTIVE DECAY

A radioactive substance disintegrates or decays in a manner characteristic of a first-order reaction; that is, decay occurs in proportion to the number of radioactive atoms present. Because radioactive decay is a random process governed by a constant probability per unit time, the fraction of atoms in a very large sample decaying in a given time interval will be constant. The *physical half-life* of a radioactive element may be defined as the time in which each atom of a radioisotope has a 50 per cent probability of decay. The net result is that during one physical half-life, a sample of radioisotope loses half of its activity.

Radiation and Bone

Of the wealth of material now available, we have chosen to limit ourselves to: (1) the metabolism of radioelements having a special affinity for the skeletal system; (2) the pathophysiologic effects upon bone of internal and external radiation; and (3) the use of radioisotopes as tracers in the study of bone.

Fixation of Radioelements by the Skeleton

Experiments with radioactive elements have firmly established the concept of the skeleton as a dynamic system. In addition to the changes in structure and in distribution of the bone mineral mediated by cellular activity, every ionic grouping in the mineral is subject to replacement. Moreover, many elements have a special affinity for the bone matrix and may remain fixed in it for long periods of time.

Replacement may occur at the surfaces and within the structure of crystals. It is appropriate to consider these phenomena as resulting from two processes: rapid ion exchange in and on the crystal surfaces and slow incorporation of the ions within the crystals by intracrystalline exchange. Both occur continuously; to them must be added the formation of new crystals during growth and reconstruction of bone; remodeling of crystals by recrystallization is also believed to occur.

Because of the manner in which bone is renewed by erosion and deposition, there is a definite pattern to which exchange conforms. In the area of growth and remodeling, where vascularity is greatest and all the crystals are of recent origin, the equilibrium between the intercellular fluids and the mineral phase is rapid and nearly complete; in such areas the uptake of administered radioisotopes is at its maximum. In the older osteons of adult compact bone and in lamellar bone, the crystals are partially isolated and less able to incorporate new ions, either physiologic or foreign, into the bone mineral. Even in such bone, however, there is diffuse deposition of radioelements, by *long-term exchange.*

The most striking sequel of administration of radioelements with an affinity for bone is their deposition in new and incompletely mineralized osteons. The result is a spotty distribution of discrete foci of intense concentration; these are the areas frequently given the designation of *hotspots.*

The concept of intracrystalline exchange has important bearing on the behavior of elements associated with the bone mineral. These elements, studied largely by the use of radioisotopes, may be divided into two groups: (1) those elements or ionic groupings that can enter into a surface reaction with the bone crystals but, because of space considerations or electric charge, cannot be incorporated within the structure; and (2) those that can substitute for the normal constituents of bone in the interior of the crystals.

An example of the first category is uranium. This element can be held at the surface as the water-soluble uranyl ion, UO_2^{2+}. Since this remains exposed to the body fluids, it is rapidly removed and excreted; it has a relatively short effective half-life. Complex ions such as citrate are also fixed at the surfaces; it is still uncertain whether carbon dioxide, as CO_3^{2-}, is held on the surface or in the crystals or both. Substitution of ions, both at the surfaces and in the interior of crystals, is taken advantage of in experimental work and in clinical investigation by administration of the radioisotopes of calcium and strontium, chiefly ^{45}Ca, ^{47}Ca, and ^{85}Sr. Radium and lead are also capable of such substitution.

In addition to the elements associated with the mineral of bone, a number of others, of which the prototype is plutonium, do not react with or substitute in the bone mineral, but do exhibit a predilection for deposition in the bone matrix. Except for ^{35}S, which substitutes in the sulfated mucopolysaccharides in the ground substance of bone and cartilage, the nature of the combinations by which elements may remain fixed for extended periods in the organic matrix is poorly understood.

Table 8 summarizes information concerning the radioactive isotopes of elements of special interest in relation to the skeleton. Those included have assumed importance either because they con-

TABLE 8

Radioisotopes of Special Interest in Relation to the Skeleton*

Z No.	Element	Isotope	Half-life†	Radiation Type and Energy, Mev‡	Decay Type and Transition Product†§	Interest for Bone
1	Hydrogen (tritium)	H^3	12.3 y	β^- 0.018	β^- to stable helium-3	H^3-amino acid to label cell constituents
4	Beryllium	Be^7	53.6 d	γ 0.478	EC to stable lithium-7	Fixed on crystal surfaces
6	Carbon	C^{14}	5,568 y	β^- 0.155	β^- to stable nitrogen-14	Fixed as CO_3^{2-}
9	Fluorine	F^{18}	109.7 m	β^+ 0.649	β^+ and EC to stable oxygen-18	Substitutes for OH^-
11	Sodium	Na^{22}	2.6 y	β^+ 0.540 γ 1.277	β^+ and EC to stable neon-22	Deposits on crystal surfaces
12	Magnesium	Mg^{28}	21.4 h	β^- 0.459 γ 0.032–1.35	β^- to 2.3-m radioaluminum-28	Fixed on crystal surfaces
15	Phosphorus	P^{32}	14.3 d	β^- 1.707	β^- to stable sulfur-32	Exchanges for P^{31} as PO_4^{3-}
16	Sulfur	S^{35}	87.1 d	β^- 0.167	β^- to stable chlorine-35	As SO_4^{2-} in ground substance
20	Calcium	Ca^{45}	164 d	β^- 0.254	β^- to stable scandium-45	Exchanges for Ca^{40}; pure beta emitter
	Calcium	Ca^{47}	4.7 d	β^- 0.69, 2.0 γ 1.3, 0.83, 0.46	β^- to 3.4-d radioscandium-47	Exchanges for Ca^{40}; gamma emitter
25	Manganese	Mn^{54}	300 d	γ 0.940	EC to stable chromium-54	Associated with bone mineral; small amount bound to matrix
30	Zinc	Zn^{65}	245 d	β^+ 0.324 γ 1.119	β^+ and EC to stable copper-65	Deposits in preosseous tissue in formation of new osteons
31	Gallium	Ga^{72}	14.2 h	β^- 0.56–3.17 γ 0.631–2.50	β^- to stable germanium-72	Deposits in regions of osteogenic activity
38	Strontium	Sr^{85}	64 d	γ 0.513	EC to stable rubidium-85	Exchanges for Ca^{40}; gamma emitter
	Strontium	Sr^{89}	51 d	β^- 1.5	β^- to stable yttrium-89	Exchanges for Ca^{40}; beta emitter
	Strontium	Sr^{90}	27.7 y	β^- 0.54	β^- to radioyttrium-90	Fallout hazard

* Physical data derived from Strominger *et al.* Table of isotopes, Rev. Mod. Physics 30:585–904, 1958.

† Half-lives: m, minutes; h, hours; d, days; y, years.

‡ Radiation type: α, alpha particles; β^-, beta particles (negatrons); β^+, beta particles (positrons); γ, gamma radiation; Mev, million electron volts.

§ Decay: β^-, β^+, α, EC (electron capture).

TABLE 8—*Continued*

Z No.	Element	Isotope	Half-life†	Radiation Type and Energy, Mev‡	Decay Type and Transition Product†§	Interest for Bone
39	Yttrium	Y^{90}	64 h	β^- 2.26	β^- to stable zirconium-90	Deposits on resorbing and quiescent surfaces
	Yttrium	Y^{91}	58.0 d	β^- 1.56	β^- to stable zirconium-91	Deposits on resorbing and quiescent surfaces
40	Zirconium	Zr^{95}	65 d	β^- 0.75 γ 0.768	β^- to 35-d radioniobium-95	Deposits on resorbing and quiescent surfaces
41	Niobium	Nb^{95}	35 d	β^- 0.158 γ 0.758	β^- to stable molybdenum-95	Deposits on resorbing and quiescent surfaces
56	Barium	Ba^{133}	7.2 y	γ 0.36	EC to stable cesium-133	Exchanges for Ca^{40} on crystal surfaces
	Barium	Ba^{140}	12.8 d	β^- 0.48 γ 0.306–0.540	β^- to 40-h radiolanthanum-140	Exchanges for Ca^{40} on crystal surfaces
57	Lanthanum	La^{140}	40 h	β^- 1.3–2.26 γ 0.093–2.9	β^- to stable cerium-140	Deposits on resorbing and quiescent surfaces
88	Radium	Ra^{226}	1,622 y	α 4.777 γ 0.186	α to radioradon-222	Exchanges for Ca^{40}; induces neoplasms
89	Actinium	Ac^{227}	21.6 y	α 4.94 β^- 0.046	1.2% α to radiofrancium-223 99.0% β^- to radiothorium-227	Deposits on resorbing and quiescent surfaces
90	Thorium	Th^{234}	24.1 d	β^- 0.192, 0.104 γ 0.090	β^- to 6.7-h radioprotactinium-234	Fixed on crystal surfaces
92	Uranium	U^{233}	162,000 y	α 4.816	α to radiothorium-229	Fixed on uranyl ion, UO_2^{2+}
94	Plutonium	Pu^{239}	24,400 y	α 4.9–5.15 γ 0.01–0.05	α to radiouranium-235	Deposits on resorbing and quiescent surfaces

stitute a hazard to man or because they are useful as tracer elements in the study of bone; others known to be bone-seekers but of only theoretical interest are omitted. The table includes the half-lives of the elements listed; the types of radiation emitted, with their energies; the types of decay and transition products; and some information concerning the interest in relation to bone.

FISSION PRODUCTS

Nuclear fission has assumed importance not only because of its destructive properties, but also because of the liberation of radioactive fission products in the testing of nuclear weapons, and because of the much greater hazard from the possible large-scale use of these weapons in war. In the detonation of a bomb, cleavage of a uranium or plutonium nucleus leads to the formation of two atomic nuclei, each of which is unstable and radioactive. The mixture of fission products emits both beta particles and penetrating gamma rays. It includes a number of elements whose half-lives vary from a fraction of a second to many years; the intensity of the radiation falls off sharply with time, owing to the rapid decay of the radioisotopes with short half-lives. Among the 34 fission-product elements, some of which are represented by more than one radioisotope, there are 14 whose rates of decay are expressed in terms of days or years, and which are produced in relatively large amounts by fission. Almost all the radioactivity remaining in a fission-product mixture after it has decayed for a week comes from the isotopes of these elements. Of these, some may be stored in bone for twenty-five to five hundred days or more, and thus constitute a potential hazard; only two are absorbed to a significant degree by the gastrointestinal tract. These are strontium and barium, both members of the alkaline-earth series. Only strontium is found in sufficient amounts among the fission products to constitute a significant hazard; for this reason, and because of the amounts of strontium liberated into the biosphere by nuclear-bomb tests, current attention is centered on the radioisotopes of this element. Of the radioisotopes of strontium liberated by nuclear fission, only ^{90}Sr has a long half-life (27.7 years); that of ^{89}Sr is fifty-one days. Thus of all the fission products, the long-term hazard to man by virtue of uptake and retention in bone narrows down to the one radioisotope, ^{90}Sr.

STRONTIUM 90

Most of the ^{90}Sr found in man and animals as a result of contamination of the atmosphere gains entrance by ingestion in foods; the pathway is from air to plants, via soil or direct uptake by leaves, and from plants to man, either directly or via the flesh or milk of animals that have eaten contaminated plants. While the behavior of strontium in plants and in the animal body is similar to that of calcium, there are significant differences in the hazard to man of ^{90}Sr. Comar (1955) and others have shown that differential behavior of calcium and strontium occurs mainly in (1) absorption from the gastrointestinal tract, (2) reabsorption in the kidney tubules, (3) transfer across the placenta, and (4) secretion into milk. In each case there is discrimination against strontium in favor of calcium, and Comar has introduced a *discrimination factor* to apply to a particular physiologic process that brings about the differential behavior. Schachter and Rosen (1959) have found that while calcium and magnesium are transported *in vitro* from the mucosal surface of the gut by a mechanism limited in capacity and dependent upon oxidative phosphorylation, this is not operative for strontium. The strontium/calcium ratio in bone is approximately equal to that in the blood. It appears that bone, *in vivo,* does not discriminate against strontium. The strontium/calcium *observed ratio,* diet to bone, has, however, been found to be low in all animals studied, owing to discrimination in intestinal net absorption and in urinary excretion. The kidneys discriminate against strontium by a preferential reabsorption of calcium; the net result is that the organism has some protection against retention of ^{90}Sr in the body.

An alternate route of entry is through the lungs. Inhalation of aerosols of fission products or of plutonium will lead to much the same distribution in the body as if the substances had been absorbed by the gastrointestinal tract. Aerosols of insoluble materials, however, are poorly absorbed through the lungs, being largely moved out of the bronchial tree by ciliary action and swallowed with the sputum. Other routes of entry, of lesser importance, are by contamination of wounds and by percutaneous absorption.

REMOVAL OF ISOTOPES FROM BONE

Many efforts have been made to find methods by which radioactive elements, once absorbed into the body, can be prevented from deposition in bone, or by which they can be removed after being deposited. Two types of approach are under consideration: (1) the use of carrier agents, such as zirconium, which form colloidal aggregates with the radioelement in the blood, from which they can then be removed by excretion through the kidney; and (2) complexing and chelating agents which form soluble, non-ionic, readily excreted complexes with the radioisotope.

Zirconium has been used successfully to remove plutonium, yttrium, and cerium; it is most effective when the blood level is highest—that is, soon after the radioelement enters the blood. It has not been useful in increasing elimination of strontium or thorium.

The chelating agents, especially polyamino acid compounds, such as ethylenediamine tetraacetic acid (EDTA) and diethylenetriamine pentaacetic acid (DTPA), have proved very useful for removing a number of radioisotopes from the body, including plutonium, thorium, yttrium, and the rare earths, such as cerium. Again, these agents have not been effective against strontium or radium.

In no case is it to be expected that removal of an element from the stable bone mineral will be practicable, since this would require virtual demineralization of the bone. The above methods may be expected to reach only the isotopes still in the blood, or at the most those in the readily exchangeable portions of the bone mineral.

Effects of Radiation upon Bone

units of radioactivity and radiation

The measure of radioactivity is the *curie*, Ci. More specifically, it is that quantity of a radionuclide in which the number of disintegrations per second (dps) is $3{,}700 \times 10^{10}$. A millicurie (mCi) corresponds to 3.7×10^7 dps, a microcurie (μCi) to 3.7×10^4 dps, and a micro-microcurie ($\mu\mu$Ci) or picocurie (pCi) to 0.037 dps. The curie unit was officially redefined in 1950 and is no longer referred to in terms of radium.

The effect of radiation in biologic systems is determined by the energy transferred to the system. The two units in common use for expressing this energy are (1) the *roentgen* (r) and (2) the *rad*. Another unit used in calculations involved in radiation protection is the *rem*, originally an abbreviation for "roentgen equivalent, man"; still another unit is the "roentgen equivalent, physical," *rep*. The roentgen unit is used for X or gamma radiation only and is based on the ionization produced in air; the rad is used for all types of radiation, internal or external, and refers to amounts of energy absorbed. The rad is the more generally useful term; it is defined as 100 ergs absorbed per gram of tissue. The roentgen is the exposure dose; the rad is the absorbed dose.

EXTERNAL RADIATION

The bones of adults have a high degree of resistance to radiation. The bones of children, however, are susceptible to injury, particularly the growth apparatus of the long bones. Such injury is not a hazard of ordinary diagnostic roentgenography, but overexposure may result from therapeutic radiation; uninformed use of fluoroscopic equipment may also have harmful effects.

In experimental animals, total body irradiation will usually result in death from doses below those necessary to cause damage to bones. Much higher doses restricted to local areas, however, may cause extensive changes in the bones. The parallel columns of cartilage cells in the epiphyseal cartilage plate become disarranged, the cartilage cells swell, and the matrix takes on a mottled and fibrillar appearance. Growth ceases, mainly as a result of interference with the ingrowth of blood vessels and with the replacement of the hypertrophic cartilage. Osteoblasts may disappear, assuming the characteristics of reticular cells. If the damage to the growth apparatus is slight, recovery will occur within a few weeks; larger doses may result in permanent impairment of growth. The changes to be expected in growing children are similar to those found in young animals.

Damage to the bones of adults is seen following very heavy and localized X-ray treatment or similar radiation from other external sources. Spontaneous fractures of the ribs, of the neck of the femur, and of the jaw have been reported under such circumstances; the lesion responsible for the fractures is necrosis. Serious marrow changes are produced at doses much lower than those approaching the threshold for damage to bone substance; damage may be done in the vascular channels of both bone and bone marrow at somewhat higher doses than those that affect the hemopoietic function and the formed elements of the marrow.

INTERNAL RADIATION

The effects of radiation from radioactive elements deposited within the skeleton are essentially similar to those of external radiation. Alpha and beta particles and gamma radiation result in similar effects; observed differences depend more upon the distribution of the element in bone and the intensity of radiation than upon differences in the type of radiation. Alpha particles, which have a very short range, do not penetrate as far as beta particles. Gamma radiation influences tissues at much greater distances from the source. On the basis of an equal amount of absorption per unit volume of tissue, alpha particles are considerably more effective than is beta or gamma radiation. For this reason, alpha emitters, such as plutonium, deposited in the endosteal surfaces of bone in close proximity to the bone marrow, are especially destructive to the marrow as well as to the bone.

BIOLOGIC EFFECTIVENESS

The biologic effectiveness of internal radiation, besides being dependent upon its quality and intensity, is determined by a combination of the *physical half-life* of the radioelement and its *biologic half-life*, which is the time required for the biologic system to eliminate one-half of the substance that has been introduced into it. The *effective half-life* of a radioisotope in a biologic system is the resultant of a combination of its physical and biologic half-lives. For those elements fixed in bone, the effective half-life may be assumed to be relatively long; in the case of the long-lived isotopes it may far exceed the life of the individual.

The *relative biologic effectiveness* (RBE) refers to a comparison between different types of radiation and different elements or isotopes. The concept has a limited usefulness, since the biologic effectiveness of any radiation depends on many factors in addition to the characteristics of the source of radiation, including biologic half-life, distribution and retention in tissues, and differences in susceptibility of tissues. Moreover, the RBE of alpha to beta radiation changes markedly with the level of dose. As a useful guide, the relative biologic effectiveness of the various types of ionizing radiations, other conditions being equal, may be approximated as follows: X rays, gamma rays, beta rays, and electrons, 1; alpha particles, 10; for tissues within the short range of alpha radiation the biologic effectiveness is some ten times as great as for other types of internal radiation.

RADIUM

There is now a great deal of information concerning the effects of radium deposited in the bones of man. Of that which remains in the bones over periods of years, it may be assumed that all is eventually incorporated within the crystals of the bone mineral, substituting therein for calcium. Since radium remains within the bone mineral, mainly within the lamellae of compact bone at some distance from the marrow cavity, and since radium and its radioactive decay products emit chiefly short-range alpha particles, the effects on the bone marrow may not be prominent. The organic matrix of bone is relatively resistant to radiation, but over a period of years considerable damage may be done (Fig. 38). In severe cases of poisoning in radium-dial painters, this has frequently been mani-

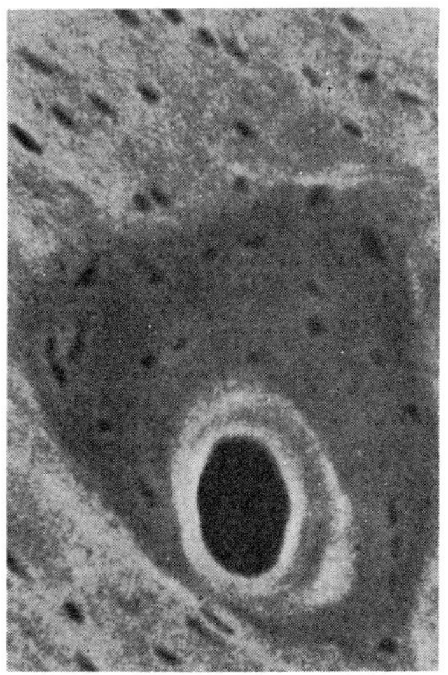

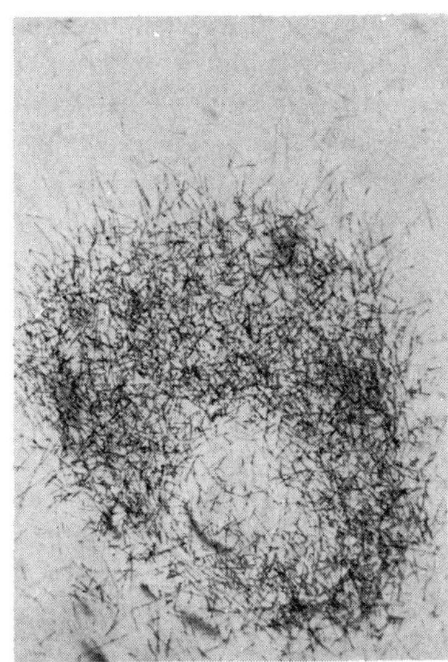

FIG. 38.—Microradiograph (*left*) and alpha-track autoradiograph (*right*) of single osteon from compact bone of a woman who received 41 weekly injections of radium chloride at age 32 and died 24 years later. Bone embedded in methyl methacrylate and sectioned at 100 μ, with high-speed rotary saw, without further treatment. Microradiograph made with 10 kv X rays on Eastman Kodak 649-0 spectroscopic plate. The osteon is labeled throughout, owing to length of period over which radium was administered. The hypercalcification around the haversian canal in the microradiograph is characteristic of radium poisoning. ×236. (From original of Fig. 2, Rowland and Marshall, Radiat. Res. 11:304. Reproduced by courtesy of the publishers.)

fested early as necrosis of the mandible, maxillae, and temporal bones. Pathologic fractures in other bones have also occurred.

RADIATION AND BONE TUMORS

A manifestation of delayed tissue damage produced by internally deposited radioisotopes, including radium, is malignancy; the induction period for appearance of the tumors following uptake of radium has varied as much as from twelve to thirty years. Of the malignant tumors of bone, the most frequent has been osteogenic sarcoma.

Information is also accumulating concerning the body burden of radium in individuals who develop bone tumors after the long latent period following exposure. So far, no case has been reported in which less than 0.4 μCi of radium, plus an undetermined amount of mesothorium, was left in the body of an individual developing an osteogenic tumor who had been exposed to radium in adult life. On the other hand, one patient with a low terminal body burden of 0.8 μCi developed a bone neoplasm. Radium had been given medically twenty-four years previously, and the total accumulated dose from mesothorium was estimated at 50 rads, with 1,100 rads from radium; these are dosage levels at which major skeletal damage has been observed in other patients.

The appearance of a bone tumor following radiation from an external source was reported in 1922; since then, many isolated cases have appeared. In a recent report of seventeen patients with bone sarcoma, sixteen of these had undergone irradiation for benign conditions. In another group of cases, osteosarcomas were observed in patients given radiation for reasons other than benign conditions of bone.

The effects of radioelements other than radium on bone have rarely been observed in man; reliance must be placed on experiments on animals. Comprehensive long-range studies on the toxicity of plutonium (^{239}Pu), radium (^{226}Ra), mesothorium (^{228}Ra), radiothorium (^{228}Th), and strontium (^{90}Sr) are under way at the Radiobiology Laboratory at the University of Utah. Osteogenic sarcomas are produced in a colony of inbred beagles following single injections of the isotopes. Radium and strontium are primarily deposited in areas where bone is being formed at the time of the injection, with some diffuse distribution; plutonium, thorium, and mesothorium localize on endosteal bone surfaces. Osteogenic sarcomas, dose-dependent and time-dependent, have been found as a consequence of all these radioelements; they are frequently multiple. The *relative biologic effectiveness* of the different isotopes depends mainly on the retained dose level of each.

Strontium, like radium, is incorporated within the crystals of the bone mineral following an initial stage of rapid uptake by exchange for calcium ions at the surface. The incidence of bone tumors in rats and rabbits is approximately proportional to the dose of the radioelement. Single and multiple tumors and extensive metastases have been observed. Radioactive yttrium and cerium also produce sarcomas in the skeletal system, especially in the long bones. Following sublethal doses of ^{32}P, a considerable proportion of the survivors develop malignant tumors, usually osteogenic sarcomas.

The pattern of bone-tumor response, as observed following introduction of ^{89}Sr or ^{90}Sr in CF_1 mice, is as follows: (1) There is a latent period, following which bone neoplasms, mostly osteogenic sarcomas, develop rapidly, and in many cases as multiple neoplasms. The latent period is not shortened by increasing the dose. (2) There is no linear relation between dose and response. (3) The data are consistent with the existence of a threshold below which sarcomas are not induced.

Radioactive Tracers in the Study of Bone

The use of radioactive elements as tracers in the study of bone dates from the observations of Chiewitz and Hevesy (1935), when they demonstrated that there was a rapid uptake of ^{32}P by bone by exchange between the phosphate ions of the bone and those of the blood. Since then the use of tracer elements has been greatly extended and has become a common procedure in many laboratories.

There are two main categories in the use of tracer elements. Either the element itself, as an ion or in an ionic grouping, may be administered and its subsequent behavior in the organism observed, usually with reference to a specific system; or a radioactive element may be combined with an organic compound that itself has specific physiologic activity, such as a vitamin or a hormone; the distribution and metabolism of the compound are followed by observing the tracer elements. A variant of this procedure is the administration of a labeled organic compound that has a specific metabolic pattern, or which may act as a building block in the synthesis of a more complex molecule; by this means complex reactions, and even cellular behavior, may be studied. Owing to the avidity of the skeleton for numerous elements, which has led to their being called bone-seekers, radioactive tracer elements have been much exploited; on the other hand, only a few labeled organic compounds have been used in studies of the metabolism of bone.

AUTORADIOGRAPHY

The principles of autoradiography are applicable to study of the distribution of radioelements in the organism in a variety of ways. The object containing radioactive material is placed in contact with a photographic emulsion, and on development an image is produced which provides visualization of the location of the radioactivity in the sample. On a gross scale, a whole bone may be cut with a saw and the cut surface placed in contact with film; thus the distribution of the radioactivity may be viewed in either sagittal or cross-sections of the bone. When desirable, serial sections may be made; in any case, studies of the deposition of radioelements in bone do not ordinarily permit decalcification.

Autoradiographs made from thin ground sections of cortical bone are easiest to interpret. The information can be expanded by histologic staining to disclose the location of the endosteum and cells, by microradiography to show the density of the mineral deposits, and by ultraviolet microscopy to reveal administered fluorescing substances incorporated in the new lamellae—all in a single section (see Fig. 16).

For study at the cellular level, high-resolution autoradiography is required, and the photographic image on the film may be enlarged to any desired size. A method in common use is to apply the photographic emulsion directly to a histologic section; by this means, the section stained by conventional methods and the photographic image of the radioactivity may be viewed together under the microscope. A variation of this method is the use of a special emulsion that records the tracks of alpha particles from heavy elements deposited in the material. Special emulsions are also available for recording tracks of beta particles.

Autoradiography may be used in conjunction with paper chromatography. The autoradiogram is made from the chromatogram, and the two methods together serve to identify the material responsible for the radioactivity.

For the most part, the information obtained by autoradiography is of a qualitative nature. Optical densities of autoradiograms have, however, been measured with a densitometer. On a microscopic scale, and with the use of high-resolution techniques, quantitative information may be obtained by counting alpha or beta tracks, or, for diffuse distribution of activity, by counting the number of darkened grains in the emulsion.

RADIOASSAY

Quantitative methods for estimation of the radioactivity in samples of biologic material require: (1) preparation of uniform samples; (2) counting of the number of disintegrations per unit of time; and (3) expression of data, with appropriate corrections. The details of radioassay are highly specialized, and are dependent upon variables that are beyond the scope of this chapter. The end result of radioassay is usually best expressed in terms of *specific activity*—the amount of radioactive element per unit weight of the element present, the weight to include both active and stable isotopes. In the fraction used to express specific activity, the denominator is the unit mass of the element, which may be in terms of weight or of moles or millimoles. The numerator may be expressed as percentage of dose; in arriving at this figure a correction is made, if necessary, for any decay that may have occurred between administration of the isotope and final count of the sample.

WHOLE-BODY COUNTING

Under certain circumstances it is desirable to obtain quantitative measurements of the radioactivity of the whole body. This has proved especially useful in the study of individuals who have ingested radioactive materials, such as radium, either accidentally or for medicinal purposes. Beginning with the use of ionization chambers in 1929 and followed by Geiger-Müller counters in 1937, the methodology has since been greatly improved, both in sensitivity and in accuracy, by the employment of large-scale scintillation assemblies.

Maximum performance of a whole-body counting facility depends upon the extent and design of the scintillation crystal array, the effectiveness of the shielding, and the use of high-capacity multichannel analyzers. An important consideration is the achievement of a high ratio of the counting rate to background radiation. These characteristics provide for high sensitivity and for the identification of gamma-emitting radioisotopes from the spectrum recorded by the analyses.

RADIOISOTOPE SCANNING OF BONE

Radioisotope scanning at the surfaces of the body has as its principal usefulness the detection, localization, and outlining of lesions in the internal organs. For these purposes there is required the administration of a suitable radioisotope that will deposit selectively and will emit gamma rays, which can be recorded by a collimated scintillation detector, moved from point to point over the area under examination. One of the early applications of the scanning method was for localization of thyroid tissue with the aid of ^{131}I.

When it is desired to determine the distribution of radioactivity in the skeleton *in vivo* by the scanning technique, there is required a radioisotope that has a special affinity for bone and emits penetrating gamma rays. If the observations are to be made on living man, it is also necessary that preference is given to a short-lived isotope. The isotopes that meet these specifications, and that have been used for clinical observation in man, are ^{47}Ca and ^{85}Sr. Calcium 47 has proved useful for detecting lesions in the skeleton, at times before X-ray evidence is conclusive. Strontium 85, which emits only gamma rays, furnishes information comparable to that obtained by the use of an isotope of calcium.

Mulry and Dudley (1951) pioneered in the localization of radioactive gallium (^{72}Ga) in bone tumors. They placed a small-bore end-window Geiger tube, jacketed by a lead shield, over the suspected area and obtained a counting rate from the gamma rays emitted by the isotope. Subsequently Dudley and his co-workers (1956) improved on the method by the use of better collimation and scintillation crystal counters. While the use of gallium has been superseded by other gamma emitters, this work was an important step in the development of skeletal scanning.

Bauer and Ray (1958) reported on the kinetics of strontium metabolism in man, having used a collimated scintillation crystal and having combined surface scanning with assay of the radioactivity of blood, urine, and feces. Their results were submitted to analysis with an electronic analog computer. Bauer and Wendeberg (1959) described the use of external counting of ^{47}Ca and ^{85}Sr in various localized bone lesions in human subjects. Corey *et al.* (1962)

reported on the application of a high-energy gamma scanner (HEG scanner) to the detection of bone metastases in patients with breast tumors, where the usual roentgenograms had not revealed the bone lesions.

Bauer and Wendeberg (1959) found that the uptake of ^{47}Ca and of ^{85}Sr in human tibial and femoral fractures was several times that in normal bone tissue. Bauer and Scoccianti (1961) reported similar findings in vertebral fractures in man. To these reports Wendeberg (1961) has added a detailed description of the observations made on patients with fractures of one tibia by using scintillation detectors over the thighs, the knees, and the tibias. The uninjured leg served as the control in each instance.

Current applications of the principles of external scanning have become progressively more refined, with increasing use of automation, including print-outs, making it possible to map skeletal lesions with a high degree of precision.

ISOTOPES AND ION TRANSFER

When ^{45}Ca or ^{32}P is administered intravenously to an animal, it is demonstrable by autoradiography within a few minutes and in specific locations. These are chiefly the new and incompletely calcified osteons incident to the remodeling of compact bone; rapid deposition also occurs subperiosteally and subendosteally in the growing bones of young animals. This occurs by *ion transfer*, a term applied to the movement of ions without specifying the mechanism. When this occurs as a one-for-one exchange, without a net change in the solid phase, it is called *ion exchange*, which may be isoionic or heteroionic. There is no essential difference between ion transfer and ion exchange in bone; both occur passively in an approach to equilibrium with the fluids with which the crystal surfaces are in contact.

Although transfer of radioisotopes has been demonstrated autoradiographically only in the direction of blood to bone, it is commonly assumed that transfer occurs in both directions, and that the areas in which deposition is demonstrable represent the labile, reactive, or exchangeable pool of calcium and phosphate in the bones. If this assumption is correct, it is these areas that are responsible for the rapid transfer of calcium from bone to intercellular fluid and blood in the homeostasis of the calcium levels in the fluids of the body; a slower transfer of ions to blood occurs as a result of osteoclastic resorption of stable bone, under regulation by parathyroid activity.

In addition to the transfer of ions from blood to areas where radioactivity is concentrated in the bones, a number of radioisotopes are deposited diffusely in association with the bone mineral; this has been called the *diffuse component* of radioisotope distribution, in contrast to the component concentrated in the new osteons and represented by the *hotspots*. The activity in the diffuse distribution of radium in bone samples from individuals who have carried radium twenty years or more has been found to be relatively uniform in cortical bone. The average magnitude of this activity is about one-half of the total body burden divided by the weight of the bones. The specific activities in the hotspots are, on the average, ninety times as great as in the diffuse component; the total amount carried in the hotspots is, however, approximately equal to that in the diffuse component, when the entire skeleton is taken into account. Similar distributions are found for ^{45}Ca; sodium, however, as ^{22}Na or ^{24}Na, is demonstrable only as diffusely deposited in short-term experiments. ^{22}Na has been found concentrated in new osteons as late as four months after it was administered.

LABELED COMPOUNDS AND BONE

The distribution and fate of hormones and vitamins in the body have been studied to a limited extent by means of labeled compounds. Examples with reference to the skeleton are estrone-16-^{14}C, tritiated estradiol (^{3}H-6,7-estradiol), ^{14}C-ergocalciferol, and tritiated amino acids.

Evidence that endosteum is a target for estrogens, characteristic for the mouse, is based on the localization of radioactivity in the skeleton when other tissues have been cleared of this activity. The patterns of distribution and metabolism of radioactive estrone are different from those of tritiated estradiol; the relation of the hormone to osteoblastic activity has not been established. When ^{14}C-labeled vitamin D was administered to rachitic rats, tissues intimately connected with the turnover of phosphate, such as bones, intestines, and kidneys, contained significant amounts of the labeled vitamin.

Tritiated thymidine has come into use as a label for cell nuclei.

Thymidine enters the structure of deoxynucleic acid (DNA) during interphase. When tritiated thymidine is administered, the nuclei of cells undergoing division are labeled, and they may subsequently be identified by microautoradiography. This procedure has been employed in the study of the life cycles and transformations of the cells of bone.

The deposition of matrix material has been studied by autoradiography after injection of various precursors, such as ^{14}C-bicarbonate, ^{14}C-glucose, ^{14}C-proline, ^{35}S-methionine, ^{14}C-methionine, ^{3}H-leucine, ^{3}H-methionine, and ^{3}H-glycine. Of these, ^{3}H-glycine has proved to be a useful tracer of newly formed matrix. In sites of bone growth in adult mice, the glycine label has been found to give a strong reaction in the cytoplasm of osteoblasts within thirty minutes after injection of the tritiated amino acid, when the preosseous tissue reacts only moderately. At four hours the radioactivity in the osteoblasts has diminished, while the preosseous tissue is heavily labeled. From these observations it has been concluded that osteoblasts elaborate a matrix precursor within their cytoplasm and release it to preosseous tissue. Direct evidence for a collagen precursor, tropocollagen, has been obtained by addition of ^{14}C-proline to a suspension of osteoblasts; this was followed almost immediately by the appearance of protein-bound ^{14}C-hydroxyproline, although collagen fibers were not detectable until a day later.

CHAPTER XIII

Postfetal Osteogenesis

Osteogenesis continues as the normal growth of bone through adolescence; it takes part in the physiologic turnover of bone throughout life. It becomes highly active in the repair of fractures and of other injuries to the skeleton. It occurs normally as extraskeletal ossification in specific genetically predetermined locations; as a pathologic process it is observed in the ectopic formation of bone. It can be brought about experimentally or in the treatment of fractures by transplantation of cells with osteogenic potencies or tissues capable of leading to formation of new bone by *induction;* bone formation may also be observed in tissue and organ cultures.

Tissue and Organ Culture

The earlier work on tissue culture of bone deals chiefly with the embryology of the skeleton. A review of the literature by Bloom (1937) describes the techniques and basic principles of the study of the behavior of cells *in vitro.* Culture techniques include tissue culture proper, cell culture, and organ culture. Proteolytic enzymes can be used to digest the extracellular matrix and isolate chondrocytes and osteocytes for analytic work with labeled amino acids and other metabolites. As a rule, however, the cells rapidly revert to an undifferentiated state; they retain their osteogenic potencies for a limited period of time.

OSTEOGENESIS FROM BONE ANLAGEN

The earliest rudiment of the skeleton is an axial condensation of the mesenchymal connective tissue in the core of the limb bud. With organ-culture methods, fragments of this tissue as small as thirty cells in volume will, when cultivated, produce the cartilage model of a bone. The cells first become enlarged, then spread apart by a homogeneous intercellular matrix, and finally are organized as bone. The shape of a bone such as the femur is predetermined in certain cells of the limb bud as early as the third day of life of the chick embryo. The cartilage model is absorbed and replaced by bone through the formation of an intermediate tissue described as *chondro-osteoid.* Under these conditions cartilage is incompletely calcified and transforms directly into bone tissue. If a chondrogenic core of the limb bud of an early chick embryo is disintegrated by enzymatic digestion of the intercellular matrix, thereby reducing isolated organs to suspensions of single cells, the suspended cells reaggregate and differentiate into masses of cartilage. Clusters formed from mixed suspensions of chondrogenic and myogenic cells produce an inner mass of cartilage and an outer sheath of muscle tissue. From this it has been concluded that the discrete limb bud of the early chick embryo is capable of reestablishing a tissue-like association and of resuming its characteristic histotypic development.

Fell (1953) demonstrated that tissue-culture and organ-culture methods permit study of the response of isolated tissues and organs to vitamins. There is a direct effect of vitamin A on skeletal tissue, specifically on the intercellular matrix of the cartilage. When a culture medium contains an excess of vitamin A, differentiation of early chick-embryo limb buds is interfered with by arrest of growth. The cellular zones of cartilage differentiate and periosteal bone develops, but the cartilage becomes soft and gelatinous and loses its characteristic basophilic and metachromatic staining reactions. In late fetal mouse limb bones, the cartilage matrix quickly disappears, leaving free chondroblasts during the rapid resorption of bone. The surrounding soft tissue grows profusely, but all that remains of the bone is a sheet of amoeboid cells containing a few fragments of bone and cartilage. Vitamin A acts only on viable cells; cartilage models heated to 45° C, just sufficient to prevent growth, lose all the effects of the vitamin.

OSTEOGENESIS FROM OUTGROWTHS OF BONE TISSUE

A fragment of bone tissue about 2 mm square, obtained from nine- to twelve-day-old rats, will produce an outgrowth in tissue culture by the coverslip method within two days. The outgrowth, representing both bone and bone marrow, consists of an inner ring of spindle-shaped cells surrounded by an outer ring of free amoeboid

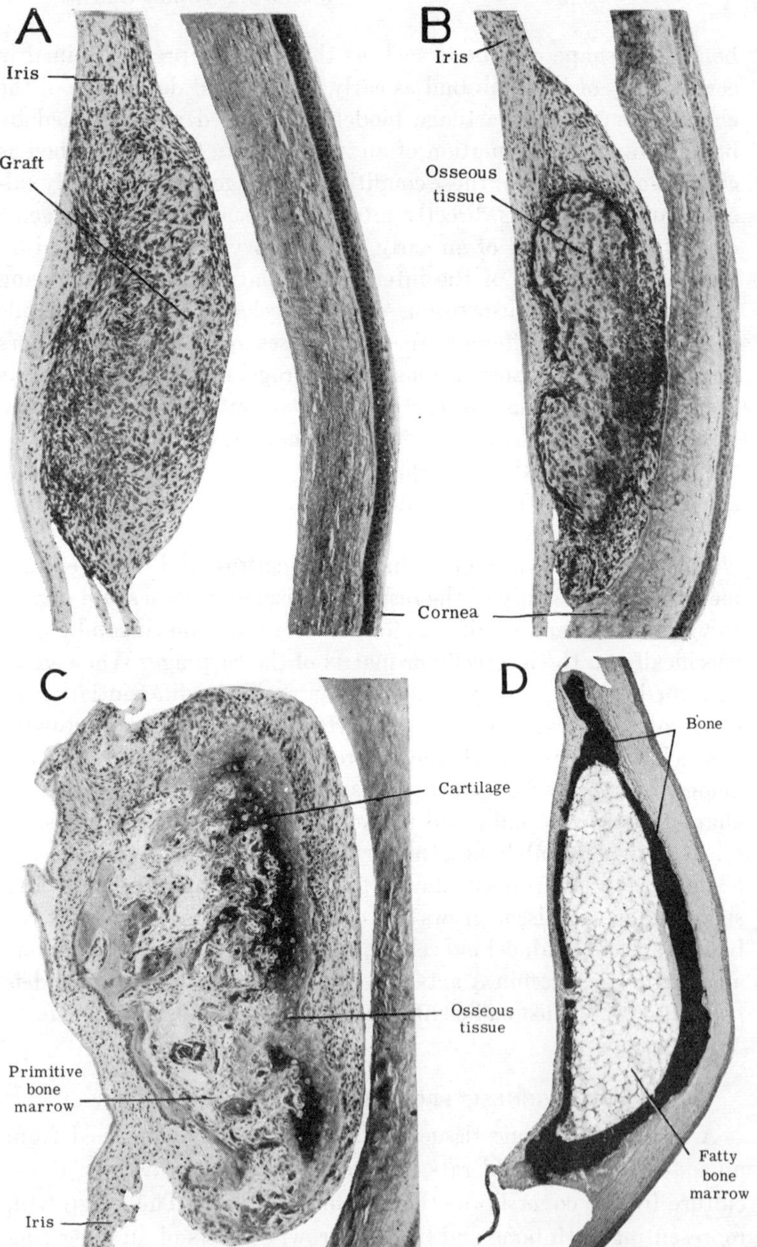

A
Iris
Graft
B
Iris
Osseous
tissue
Cornea
C
Cartilage
Osseous
tissue
Primitive
bone
marrow
Iris
D
Bone
Fatty
bone
marrow

cells, such as macrophages, eosinophil myelocytes, and heterophil myelocytes. The original explant can be excised at four days and reimplanted in other nutrient media to obtain new generations of outgrowing cells. Each outgrowth can be either subcultured or transferred as a homogenous transplant to a host site to determine its cell potencies for differentiation into bone cells.

After the cells of the outgrowth are separated from the explant of bone tissue and transplanted, a new ring of closely packed fibroblast-like cells appears in the center of the subculture. These cells are offspring of primitive mesenchyme, endothelium, reticular cells of bone marrow, or endosteum. Samples of bone and bone marrow containing all these cells produce better outgrowths and healthier cultures than do those scraped free of bone marrow.

Masses of cartilage appear by the third day; spindle-shaped cells are in the loose meshwork, where there is no bone or cartilage formation. By the sixth day the masses of bone, cartilage, or chondro-osteoid are circumscribed by a perichondrium-like layer of spindle-shaped cells. When outgrowths are transplanted to the anterior chamber of the rat's eye, cellular differentiation follows the same sequence as in a subculture, with the exception that there is less chondro-osteoid. Instead, the cartilage matrix is calcified, immediately invaded by blood vessels and perivascular connective tissue cells, and finally replaced by new bone within two weeks. The sequence is that of endochondral ossification. The process is organotypic; the cells of the transplanted outgrowth are capable of developing and becoming organized into an ossicle, filling the anterior chamber of the eye (Fig. 39).

Fig. 39.—Development of bone in the anterior chamber of the eye of the rat, from transplants of outgrowth of tissue cultures of bone from a 12-day-old rat. Fragments of bone were cultured in rat plasma and embryo extract. The outgrowths were removed after 4 days *in vitro* and transplanted to the iris of normal rats. These outgrowths contained no bone or cartilage. (*A*) After 1½ days in the eye, there was no cartilage or bone. (*B*) After 2½ days in the eye, chondro-osseous tissue developed from the culture. (*C*) After 6 days in the eye, much bone and cartilage and some marrow appeared. Zenker-formol; hematoxylin-eosin-azure II. ×70. (*D*) After 4 months, a "bone" with central fatty marrow developed. Formalin; silver nitrate–hematoxylin-eosin. ×28. (Courtesy of J. H. Heinen, Jr.) (From original photomicrographs of Fig. 120, Maximow and Bloom, Textbook of histology [6th ed.; Philadelphia: W. B. Saunders Co., 1952]. Reproduced by courtesy of the publishers.)

The osteogenic potency of the outgrowths is lost if separated from bone tissue for more than fourteen days before transfer to the anterior chamber of the eye. Nearly all samples will produce bone after eight days of cultivation, but after this time the cells revert to fibroblast-like forms and produce dense masses of fibrous connective tissue instead of bone.

CALCIFICATION OF NEW BONE IN VITRO

Chondro-osteoid and osteoid tissues appear in cultures of bone anlagen and bone outgrowths, if the amounts of calcium and phosphorus are insufficient to promote continuous deposition of bone mineral. Transplants of outgrowth in the eyes of rachitic rats do not exhibit calcification in either cartilage or bone. The same tissue can be made to calcify within a few days if the rachitic host is treated with parenteral injections of a solution of sodium phosphate or with vitamin D.

FACTORS INFLUENCING OSTEOGENESIS IN ORGAN CULTURE

Remodeling of bone and development of the internal architecture are guided by intrinsic forces present in limb buds as well as by external forces. Cartilage differentiates *in vitro* from small fragments of a limb bud by an inherited capacity of the cells for self-differentiation without the necessity for an external force. Cultures of perichondrium subjected to pressure can be stimulated to produce an excess of cartilage. Organ culture has proved a useful method for study of intrinsic and extrinsic factors in skeletal development; explants of avian sternum will form a keel in the absence of pectoral musculature, for which it normally serves as an attachment; a knee joint appears in the cartilage model of the leg from which the muscles have been removed; an explant of mouse sternal buds with rib stumps differentiates into a normal segmental structure, whereas when the rib stumps are removed before explanting, the sternum ossifies as a continuous double bar without segmentation. It is known that extrinsic factors play an important role in osteogenesis; both biochemical and mechanical influences are present. Fracture healing occurs in tissue culture just as in the normal skeleton.

The presence of enzymes in a calcifiable tissue is not necessary for calcification *in vitro;* consequently the presence of enzyme inhibitors has no effect on osteogenesis in tissue culture. Alizarin Red S added to culture media for supravital staining permits fibrous connective tissue growth and chondrogenesis but inhibits osteogenesis. Hyaluronidase causes stunting of growth of cartilage models and diminished basophilia of the cartilage matrix, without any specific effect on osteogenesis. The distribution of phosphatase in hypertrophic cartilage and osteoblasts is the same in tissue culture as in the normal skeleton.

Transplants of Bone

Progress in tissue transplantation has made it increasingly clear that several biologic principles, to some degree interrelated, are essential to the successful transfer of bone tissue, as judged by the survival of a *bone graft* or by its replacement by new bone formed by the host, with the end result, in either case, of anatomic or functional repair of a skeletal defect. Information to this effect has come from both experimental and clinical observations, the results of which may be put in a perspective of interest both to the biologist and to the surgeon.

The major principles to be taken into account are: (1) *osteogenic potency*, or the ability to form bone, expressed as *osteogenic activity* of bone-forming cells; (2) survival and proliferation of transplanted tissue or cells, giving rise to the formation of new bone originating from the transplant; (3) the *immune response* of the host to the transplanted tissue or cells, which may be the major factor in determining whether the transplant will survive; (4) *induction* of new bone formation, under the influence of specific properties residing in the implant, conferring osteogenic potency on the tissues of the host; and (5) a nonspecific affinity of the host for the interstices of an implant of devitalized bone or of an inert material, leading to its removal and replacement by bone.

The work of Medawar (1957) and Burnet (1961) for which the Nobel prize in medicine was awarded in 1960, has firmly established the thesis that the immunologic defenses of the organism against foreign proteins are responsible for rejection of homogenous transplants of skin. This mechanism is doubtless operative with respect to homografts of bone, although the fate of transplants of homogenous bone is determined in part by factors not applicable to skin grafts, in which the success of the procedure depends entirely upon the survival of the donor cells. Such survival may, in fact, lessen the probability of acceptance of a bone graft. For reconstructive surgery of the skeleton, when viability is not essential and only an absorbable framework may be required, it is often possible to use implants of bone derivatives or even of inert substitutes for bone.

OSTEOGENIC POTENCY

A connective tissue having the capacity to form bone has *osteogenic potency;* when this characteristic becomes manifest, the cell exhibits *osteogenic activity.* Osteogenic potency may be inferred and osteogenic activity observed in many situations in the organism, most prominently in embryonic and postfetal formation and growth of bone and in the healing of fractures. We are here concerned with the ability of transplanted cells to survive, proliferate, and exhibit osteogenic activity, and with the means by which osteogenic potency may be conferred on cells and osteogenic activity elicited and observed.

IMMUNE RESPONSE

Of the factors entering into the problems of tissue transfers, that of the greatest interest, both experimental and clinical, is the immune response of the host to the transplant; upon this depends the interpretation of many of the results obtained from experimental transfers of bone, as well as the feasibility of surgical transfers undertaken for the repair of defects in the skeleton. There is an increasing body of evidence that the general principles arrived at by transfer of soft tissues, including skin, are applicable also to bone.

In recent years the terminology of the field of tissue transplantation has been revised by Russell and Monaco (1965). *Orthotopic* is the term employed to denote a graft of any genetic origin that is placed in an anatomic position normally occupied by the same kind of tissue; for example, a fragment of bone in a bone defect. *Heterotopic* bone grafts are those placed in unusual locations, such as the belly of a muscle or the anterior chamber of the eye. Table 9 lists terms and definitions receiving general approval to describe the genetic characteristics of a graft. Two other terms, contributed by Longmire *et al.* (1964), are also useful: *homovital* for functional and *homostatic or nonviable* but functional grafts. These terms are particularly applicable in the field of bone physiology because, when

bone tissue is transplanted into an orthotopic site, osteocytes lose viability and the bulk of the tissue is a relatively inert, unresorbed mass. Since it can perform a mechanical function just as normal living bone, regardless of implant type, the tissue is simply an interstructural implant.

With the exception of *autologous* or *isogeneic transfers*—that is, transfers within the body of the same individual or between identical twins—foreign antigens are introduced into the body of the host whenever bone is transferred from one individual to another, or when extracts of bone are administered to experimental animals;

TABLE 9

TERMINOLOGY OF TISSUE TRANSPLANTATION

Old Terminology	New Terminology	New Adjective	Definition
Autograft	Autograft	Autologous	Graft in which donor is also recipient
Isograft	Isograft	Isogeneic	Graft between individuals identical in histocompatibility antigens
Homograft	Allograft	Allogeneic	Graft between genetically dissimilar members of same species
Heterograft	Xenograft	Xenogeneic	Graft between species

Reprinted with permission from P. S. Russell and A. P. Monaco, The biology of tissue transplantation. Boston: Little, Brown & Co., 1965.

the antigens are proteins foreign to the host. The sequelae of such transfers are influenced also by the choice of *allogeneic* or *xenogeneic* bone and by the state of the transplanted tissue; antigenic activity is much greater in bone with living cells than in derivatives of bone. The current concept is that when fresh living allogeneic tissues are transferred, antigens pass directly via the host lymphatics to the regional lymph nodes, where antibodies are formed; the spleen also reacts to antigens reaching it through the blood, but this response is quantitatively of lesser importance. The antigens in allogeneic bone that lead to the production of antibodies have not been accurately identified; they are formed by and reside in or on cells; their formation is under the genetic control of the nucleic acids of the cell. For as long as transferred allogeneic bone proliferates, it continues to form antigens, and hence to invoke the immune response of the host. For this reason the usefulness of fresh, living allogeneic bone grafts is limited, and such transfers are rarely made.

Clinically, transfers of tissue may be made without immune response within the same individual or between identical twins; experimentally this condition may be simulated by transfers between animals of the same inbred strain; such inbred strains of mice are generally available. Inoculation of newborn mice or embryos *in utero* with cells or tissue from a different strain of mice leads later to their ability to tolerate skin grafts from mice of the donor strain.

The antibodies produced by the host in the presence of an allogeneic transplant of tissue are mainly carried by cells; these are probably the lymphocytes produced by the regional lymph nodes and released into the circulation. This has not been demonstrated for transplants of bone. An allograft enclosed within a porous membrane will survive if the pores of the membrane are small enough to prevent the passage of whole cells but large enough to permit the diffusion of substances dissolved in the plasma, including humoral antibodies. There is evidence that the cells of living implants of xenogeneic tissue are killed by circulating cytotoxins, produced by the host in response to the foreign proteins of the implant; the participation of humoral antibodies in the immune response to allogeneic transplants is not excluded, although their effects on grafts are negligible.

The mechanism of the reaction of the host to allogeneic transplants of bone is not clear. In the case of skin transplants, Medawar (1957) has characterized the delayed reactions as fundamentally cellular as opposed to humoral, and has stated that they depend upon the activation, deployment, and peripheral engagement of the lymphoid cells. There is no doubt that allografts of solid tissues lead to inflammatory reactions, in which round cells and histiocytes predominate. Descriptions of the histologic features of the inflammatory reactions to homotransplants of bone in rabbits are reported by Bonfiglio and his collaborators (1955).

Enneking (1957) has reported histologic studies of the response of rats to autologous and allogeneic transplants of bone. Until the fifteenth day after transplantation there was no difference in the response of the host. After the fifteenth day only the proliferations of autologous transplants consistently survived and aided in repair. The majority of allogeneic transplants (34/52) invoked a major inflammatory host response, which obliterated the periosteal proliferations and prevented repair or replacement of the transplants. A smaller number (11/52) brought about a minor inflammatory response, which did not prevent the reactive bone of the host from crossing the transplant-host junction and repairing and replacing the transplant. A still smaller number (7/52) were accepted as though they were autogenous. The difference in the reactions of the host are probably attributable to the degree of inbreeding of the Sprague-Dawley rats used in the experiments. Enneking has also investigated the effect of whole-body X-irradiation on one of the partners of parabiotic rats, the other being shielded. This brought about, as a rule, a temporary immunoparalysis of the irradiated rat, permitting it to accept a fresh transplant from the other partner as though it were autologous; the nonirradiated rat, on the other hand, had a reduced rate of rejection of transplants from the irradiated partner, but still exhibited a characteristic immune response.

A group at the University of Otago, New Zealand (Heslop, Zeiss, Nisbet, 1957) has published a series of studies on autografts and homografts of cortical bone in rats, when all implants were made into the subdermal tissue. They have reported on survival of osteocytes, osteogenesis, the reaction of the host, vascularization of the grafts, and the production of immunologic tolerance to allografts. They found that many osteocytes survived up to 250 days near the outer surface of both autografts and allografts, and they propose an ingenious explanation for the survival of osteocytes in homografts. This is that lymphocytes of the host, carrying antibodies, are unable to penetrate into the compact bone of the graft, which thus protects the osteocytes from destruction. They observed the usual differences between autografts and allografts with respect to osteogenesis and vascularization. They produced a high degree of tolerance to homografts in rats by subcutaneous injection of spleen cells within twenty-four hours after birth; when the recipients were adult they were grafted with implants from the donors of the spleen cells. In the animals with induced tolerance, the reaction of the host to allografts was modified, approximating the reaction to autografts; the degree of approximation corresponded to the degree of tolerance conferred. In general, the results of these investigators support the application to allografts of bone of the principles derived by Medawar and others from homografts of skin and other tissues.

While the response of the host to transplants of fresh allogeneic bone is of great interest, and will be made use of in the interpretations in this chapter, such transplants are now made only rarely in man. The fate of experimental allografts or xenografts has limited bearing on the success or failure of incorporation of tissue that has been devitalized and treated in such a way as to reduce its antigenicity and preserve it for storage in bone banks. Dead bone, especially in the form of a massive implant of cortical bone, is absorbed so slowly that it liberates only very small amounts of antigen. The denser the deposit of mineral, the more inaccessible the antigenic proteins of the matrix (Fig. 40, *a* and *b*).

INDUCTION

Induction is the influence that one tissue may have upon another in close contact with it, as a result of which the second tissue is induced to exhibit activities not previously in evidence. An example relevant to this chapter is the formation of bone following implantation of bone from another individual. In such instances the implant does not itself proliferate and form new bone, but it may cause the cells of the host to differentiate into osteoblasts and to organize in the form of a bone. The study of induction is aided by the use of biologic systems that are not complicated by an immune response on the part of the host. For this reason autologous implants are favorable for observation of induction phenomena; the anterior chamber of the eye also provides a favorable environment, even for allogeneic transplants, since interference by cell-borne antibodies is reduced.

Induction systems for bone formation generally obey laws governing cellular differentiation. The inductor is transmitted by a specific tissue, such as growing cartilage or urinary bladder epithelium, for a specific period of time. This may require a long exposure or latent period and may have a relatively short period of action. Normally the inductor is produced by proliferating cells, but it can emanate from resting, degenerating, or devitalized tissue. Recent observations demonstrate more conclusively than ever before that the proteins of the matrix of bone and dentin contain the precursor of the inducing substance. When bone or dentin is decalcified, lyophilized, and implanted in the belly of a muscle, a bone-induction system is set up over a period of three weeks. All the available

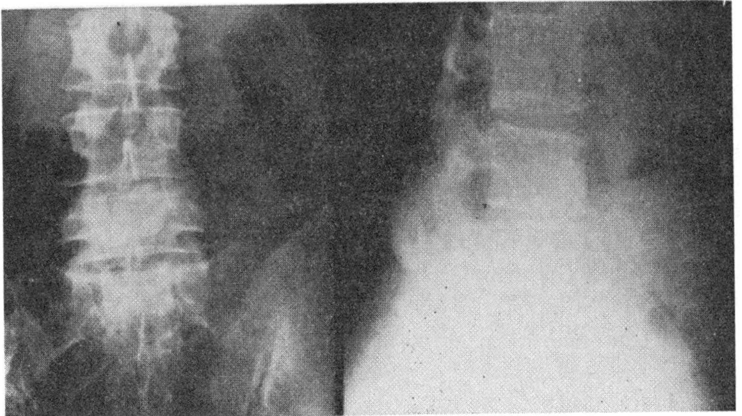

A

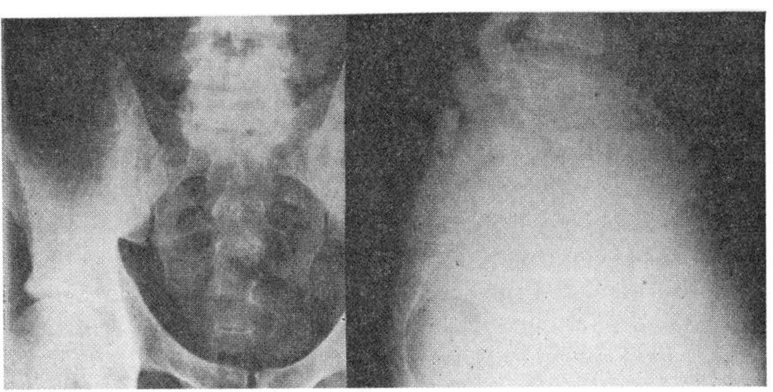

B

FIG. 40.—Roentgenograms of processed xenogeneic bovine implants employed as H-block for internal fixation. (*A*) Fixation of the 4th and 5th lumbar spinous processes, 7 years after the operation for degenerative joint and disk disease in a 58-year-old woman. Autologous bone is employed for a graft across the interlaminar spaces. There is no immune response to the xenogeneic bone proteins, in approximately 60 per cent of the cases. In 40 per cent, the immune response is expressed in the form of an envelope of inflammatory tissue and scar around the H-block as shown in *B*, in the lumbosacral region in a 20-year-old man. Note the area of radiolucent tissue around the implant. Some, but not all, of these individuals display a positive cross-species immune response to horse serum proteins.

interstitial spaces, old vascular channels, or osteocyte canaliculi or dentinal tubules are repopulated with lymphocytes, plasma cells, wandering histiocytes, and mesenchymal cells derived from migratory cells of the circulating blood. Later the surfaces are covered with ingrowing capillary sprouts, fibrous connective tissue, and giant cells. The interaction of mesodermal cells and mesodermal derivatives in excavation chambers in old matrix during the process of resorption induces differentiation of preosteoblasts, osteoblasts, and new bone. Urist (1965) has termed the process *autoinduction* because, while the protein matrix has the geneic characteristics of another individual, both the inducing and the induced cells are derived from the same individual. Immune responses, other than those associated with autologous or allogeneic tissues, interfere considerably with bone induction. When decalcified, lyophilized xenogeneic bone matrix is transplanted into muscle, the yield of new bone is always very scanty and the incidence of positive results may be only 1 or 2 per cent (Fig. 41).

The bone inductor is believed to be transmissible over a short distance and not diffusible or extractable in synthetic solutions *in vitro*. The cells being induced to form bone are always connective tissue cells at a receptive stage of development; resting or adult cells can be induced to form bone only rarely, if at all. Lash *et al.* (1957) have observed induction of cartilage by embryonic spinal cord in tissue culture even after interposition of a millipore membrane. Büring and Urist (1967) described both intrachamber and transfilter bone induction. In the bone induction systems in the living animal the evidence is that contact between the extracellular secretions of interacting cells is important and that the inductor is transmissible only across channels between adjacent cells.

There are many theories concerning the mechanism of induction. We prefer to follow Weiss (1950) who postulates progressive recruiting of cells for a given type or differentiation, spreading from a focal area like an infectious wave; cells that have attained a certain differentiated character can communicate their state to their neighbors, which then pass it on further, and so on down the line. This should require physical factors as well as chemical agents, participating in many sorts of combinations; there must be many degrees of specificity and complexity, employing a great variety of mechanisms.

CRITICAL CONDITIONS FOR TISSUE TRANSFERS

Many tissues, both of skeletal and of nonskeletal origin, have been tested for osteogenic activity or for the ability to produce new bone by induction, by transfer of samples to isolated soft parts of the body or to defects in bone. The results are conditioned by: (1) the density of the tissue transferred; (2) whether the donor tissue comes from embryonic, young, or adult animals; (3) whether it comes from a tissue in which latent potencies have been reactivated by injury; (4) whether the transplant is autologous, allogeneic, or xenogeneic; (5) whether fresh or preserved tissue is used, and the state of the tissue when transferred; and (6) the nature and state of the host bed. The reaction produced by preserved tissues depends upon the method of preservation and the period of storage; whether the tissue has been simply frozen, or frozen at very low tempera-

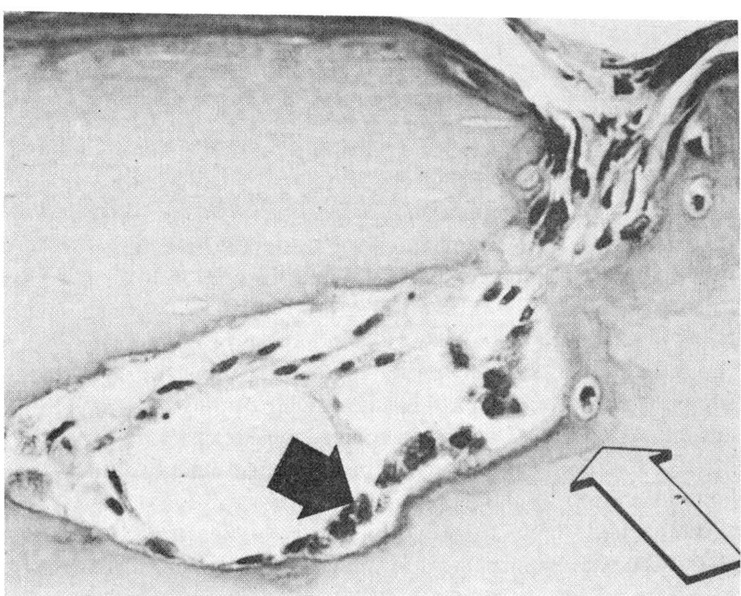

FIG. 41.—Photomicrograph showing bone induction in excavation chamber in decalcified bone matrix. The transparent arrow points to a cement line between dead old matrix and live new bone. The black arrow points to proliferating osteoblasts. Note empty enlarged lacunae in old matrix. (Reproduced from Science 150: 893, 1965, by courtesy of the publishers.) © 1965 by the Am. Assoc. Advan. Sci.

tures; whether the tissue has been coagulated by heating, boiling, or chemical solutions, or dehydrated before transplantation; and whether the donor tissue or its cells, if living, provoke an immune response from the host.

Allografts of bone will vascularize, proliferate, and survive for a limited time only, owing to the immune response of the host. Cornea, fascia, cartilage, and undifferentiated connective tissue cells will survive autologous transfer, and at times even allogeneic transplantation; either they are nonantigenic, inaccessible to cell-borne antibodies, or they resist their effects; acceptance of allogeneic transfers must in some cases be related to the quantitative as well as qualitative immune response on the part of the host. In the case of bone, clinically the bulk of the transplant is unaltered, unaffected, and inaccessible to the host, but like cornea, it performs a structural function and is chiefly responsible for the success of such procedures.

TRANSPLANTS OF OSTEOGENIC TISSUE TO EXTRASKELETAL SOFT PARTS

Many kinds of host beds can be used to study osteogenesis under conditions in which there is no possibility of contact with pre-existing osteoblasts. Transparent chambers may be placed in a rabbit's ear or under the skin of a mouse as receptacles for transplants. As in the case of the anterior chamber of the eye, the degree to which they will accept homogenous tissue may be related to their ability to exclude cell-borne antibodies. A favorite site for transplants of bone, or of tissue to be tested for induction of bone formation, is the subcapsular space of the kidney. Autogenous transfers to this site may survive and lead to results similar to those observed in the anterior chamber of the eye; homogenous transfers, unless from litter mates or from inbred strains, more commonly lead to new bone formation by induction.

Transplants have also been made to muscle, brain, mesentery, testis, synovial membrane, and subcutaneous tissue; the success of such transplants depends upon the same factors as in the case of the subcapsular space of the kidney. The universal requirements of any transplant for the production of new bone are: (1) that the host tissues establish contact with the donor cells; (2) that the transplant leads to a proliferative response of new capillaries and undifferentiated connective tissue cells from the host bed, in addition to such proliferations as may be produced by the transplant itself; and (3) that it does not lead to an immune response capable of destroying the implant; this requirement is best met by autogenous transplants, more rarely by allogeneic implants, and virtually never by xenogeneic transfers except when devitalized, processed, and used as a massive implant.

Tissues that will not produce new bone following fresh autogenous transplantation are: fascia, ligaments, muscle, tendon, elastic cartilage of the external ear, and semilunar cartilage of the knee. The formation of bone follows autologous transplants of periosteum; bone marrow, with or without cancellous bone; epiphyseal and articular cartilage; compact bone; and fibrocartilaginous callus after an injury to the bone of the donor.

The nature of the bone formed following an autologous transplant differs with the tissue transferred to the new location. Periosteum from young growing animals includes an active osteoblastic layer and will produce new bone consistently after transfer to the anterior chamber of the eye. Periosteum from an adult animal will produce either no new bone at all or very little following transplantation. The same tissue removed several days after a fracture contains proliferating osteoblasts and has osteogenic activity. A transplant of osteogenically active periosteum to the anterior chamber of the eye produces a mass of compact bone, without an intermediate stage of cartilage and without the appearance of bone marrow. Such a reaction is histotypic; it forms only one kind of tissue.

Survival and proliferation of autologous tissues, themselves capable of forming bone, may also be observed when bone marrow or cancellous bone, or a mixture of the two, is transplanted to the anterior chamber of the eye of the rat. Transplantation of the fibrocartilaginous callus leads to differentiation of mesenchymal cells into osteoblasts (Fig. 42). The fibrocartilaginous mass is replaced by bone and bone marrow; such a reaction is organotypic, since it forms a complete ossicle. The anterior chamber of the eye is slow to differentiate between autogenous and homogenous tissue; transplants from other animals of the same species may be equally well accepted. Implants of the outgrowth from tissue cultures from bone of the same species also lead to the formation of bone in the anterior chamber of the eye; again the reaction is organotypic, and a complete ossicle results before the tissue is destroyed by the immune response.

The behavior of transplants of epiphyseal cartilage is of particular interest. This tissue consists chiefly of hyaline cartilage, and is a remnant of the cartilage model of embryonic bone, engaged in endochondral growth. Following autologous or allogeneic transplantation in the eye of the rat, it continues to produce new bone by endochondral ossification; new bone arises, however, not from transplanted cells, but from ingrowing cells of the host. Bone induction similarly follows transplantation of the germinal epiphyseal layer of articular cartilage of a young growing animal. A thin split-

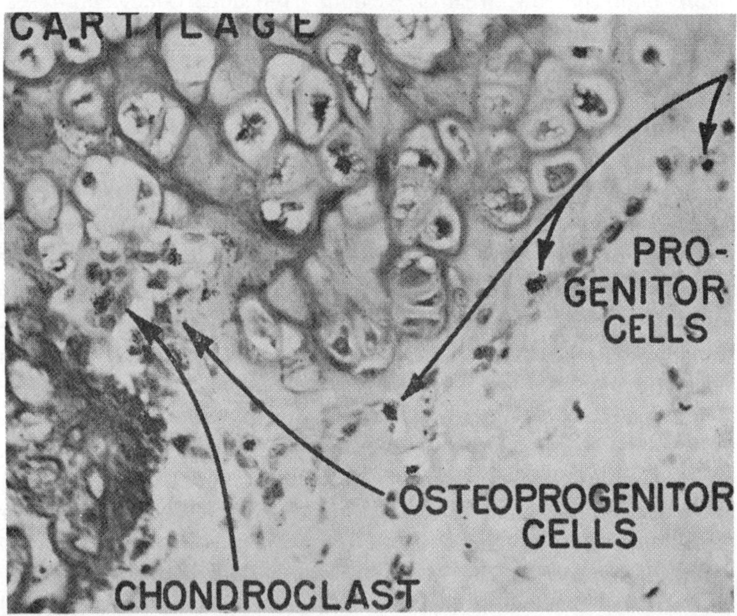

Fig. 42.—Autoradiograph showing excavation chamber in isogeneic fibrocartilaginous callus in the anterior chamber of the eye of a rat, 48 hours after an injection of ^{3}H-thymidine (1 μc per gram of body weight). Note high percentage of labeled nuclei in the osteoprogenitor cells in an excavation chamber containing capillary sprouts. Irrespective of whether the progenitor cells arise from the cells of the donor or the host bed, proliferation and differentiation into osteoblasts follow transplantation. Cartilage does not metabolize ^{3}H-thymidine or proliferate in the eye following transplantation but undergoes histolysis and resorption, and induces ingrowth of perivascular connective tissue cells of the host.

thickness graft that contains only germinal cells of the gliding surface induces formation of cartilage. Following transplantation of autologous and isogeneic articular cartilage labeled with ^{3}H-thymidine, Urist *et al.* (1965) noted histolysis with mobilization and activation of chondrocytes. In excavation chambers produced by sprouting capillaries and chondroclasts, activated chondrocytes are inducing cells. Perivascular connective tissue cells are responding cells. Interaction of inducing and responding cells leads to differentiation of precursor cells, osteoblasts, osteocytes, and new bone.

Transplants of autologous compact bone subcutaneously or to the eye exhibit little ability to form new bone; usually a new layer of bone is formed on the surface of the transplant, by apposition. Transfer of autologous compact bone to any new location in the body leads to death of all or most of the osteocytes; survival and proliferation of osteoblasts, together with induction, account for the success of such transplants. Fresh allografts in higher mammals do not ordinarily survive, owing to the immune response of the host; early death of a homograft, with consequent reduction in its antigenic potency, is conducive to success of the graft; formation of bone under these circumstances is prima facie evidence of operation of the induction process, as it is also in the case of bone derivatives.

TRANSPLANTS TO HOST BED OF BONE TISSUE

The most favorable conditions for survival of transplants of osteogenic tissue are afforded by a fresh autologous graft of cancellous bone, including bone marrow, to a well-prepared host bed of bone. Such transplants are commonly used in clinical surgery for fusion of joints, internal fixation to produce union of fractures, and filling of surgical defects. These conditions offer a high degree of probability that some of the transplanted tissue or of its cells will survive, proliferate, and produce bone; to this is added the probability that the transplant may cause the cells of the host to become engaged in osteogenesis by induction. Burwell (1964) contends that a special group of cells of the bone marrow is the main source of osteogenic and inducing cells. While conditions responsible for new bone formation by induction are unknown, except that both physical and chemical factors are involved, tissues other than fresh autologous bone are considered less active and less desirable for reconstructive surgery. Experimental and clinical observations, however, leave no doubt that nonviable materials are effective regardless of limited knowledge of how or why they accomplish their purpose. In Table 10 materials currently under investigation have been classified as bone implants, derivatives, and substitutes, and distinguished from transplants, because they exhibit either very little or no viability and an unknown capacity for induction.

Recent experimental observations suggest that inert materials, with neither viability nor capacity for induction, can assume the appearance of a bone transplant. Various parts of the skeleton of young individuals are able to incorporate inert materials in an in-

TABLE 10

MATERIALS USED FOR EXPERIMENTAL BONE SURGERY

TRANSPLANTS
- Fresh autologous bone
- Fresh isogeneic bone (from identical twin)
- Embryonic bone (for temporary survival)

IMPLANTS—Allogeneic or xenogeneic bone
- *Pretreatment*
  - Refrigerated in plasma
  - Frozen (−30° C)
  - Freeze-dried
  - Boiled in physiologic salt solution
  - Autoclaved
  - Preserved in:
    - Aqueous glycol
    - β-propiolactone
    - Merthiolate
  - Irradiated by:
    - Cathode ray
    - Cobalt 60

DERIVATIVES—from allogeneic or xenogeneic bone
- Decalcified bone
  - Extracted with EDTA
- Anorganic bone
  - Extracted with ethylene diamine
- Os purum
  - Extracted with potassium hydroxide
- Collapatite
  - Extracted with urea, saline, and ether or detergents
- Extracted with hydrogen peroxide

SUBSTITUTES
- Metal
- Methyl methacrylate
- Polyurethane
- Calcium sulfate
- Hydroxyapatite

volucrum and thereby bridge large gaps and restore the continuity of a bone. The skeleton of a nongrowing or adult individual is not able to produce the same amount of new bone and generally requires bone transplants to bridge a gap. When there is no gap and only internal fixation is required, derivatives of bone, or bone substitutes may often be used with good results.

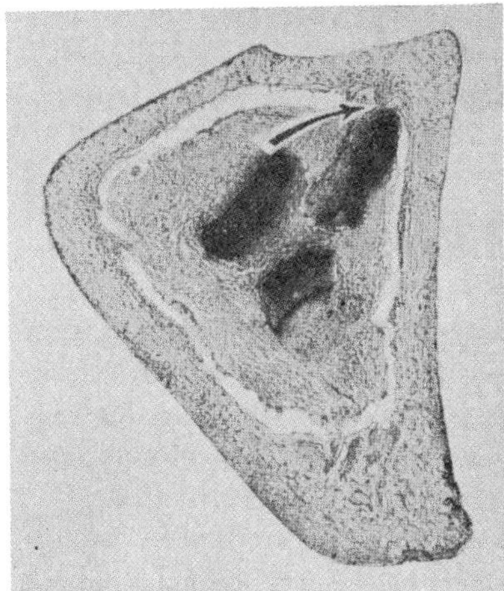
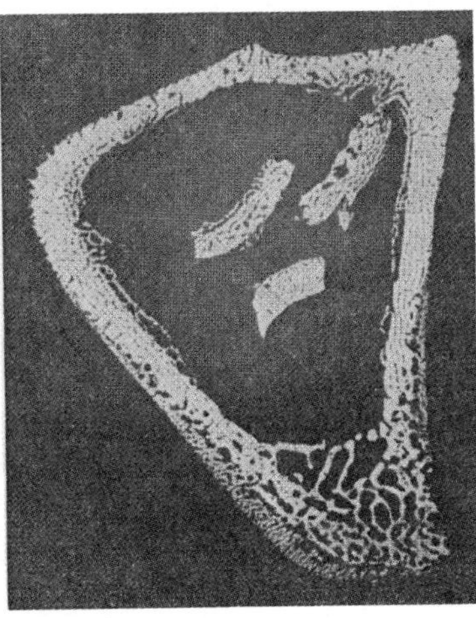

Fig. 43.—Microradiograph (*left*) and autoradiograph (*right*) of a cross-section through tibia of a rabbit, with homologous graft of bone inside the marrow cavity. The donor was a 6-week-old rabbit injected with 1 mCi of ^{90}Sr 5 days before the transplant into a host of the same age. The tibia was excised 4 weeks later. The microautoradiograph made with stripping film records the radioactivity in the bone of the donor while the bone of the host shows only low level of diffuse radioactivity. The arrow points to contact of the homograft with the bone of the host, where new bone is growing out from the endosteum. ×7. (From originals of Figs. 4A and 4C, Urist, MacDonald, and Jowsey, Ann. Surg. 147:137 and 138. Reproduced by courtesy of the publishers.)

Radioisotope studies reveal little about induction after the first layer of bone is deposited on the donor tissue. Allogeneic bone, either fresh or frozen, labeled with ^{45}Ca, ^{90}Sr, ^{90}Y, or ^{91}Y and implanted into bone defects in clean hosts, becomes joined to new bone produced by the host through a cement layer or line (Fig. 43). The mineral constituents of the donor tissue are in solution in the tissue fluids of the host, but are not able to diffuse across the cement line. Correlated histologic sections, microradiograms, and radiochemical analyses of the whole skeleton reveal that the donor tissue is reabsorbed in some places and covered with new bone in others; a large part of the radioisotope is excreted and a small part is redeposited systemically throughout the entire skeleton. There is no local transfer of bone mineral from the donor to the new bone of the host. The donor tissue accomplishes its purpose to enable the host to fill a defect, fuse a joint, or unite a fracture when only a small fraction of its surface area has been resorbed. There is a definite affinity of the new bone of the host for interstices of an implant, whether it be transplanted dead or living bone, or a bone derivative or substitute.

Extraskeletal Bone

When osteogenesis occurs in a part of the body where bone formation does not normally occur in a particular species, it is termed *ectopic* or *heterotopic* bone formation. Ectopic bone formation is an abnormality and is to be distinguished from *extraskeletal bone* in various locations in many animals, examples of which are leg tendons and fascia in the turkey, the laryngeal cartilages of man, and the penis of almost all mammals except the higher primates.

The number of organs and the many different kinds of pathologic lesions in which ectopic bone formation has been described seem not so important as that connective tissue elements, rather than the specialized tissues, give rise to the osteoblasts associated with the appearance of bone. Nearly all the organs and tissues in the body—eye, brain, tongue, lung, heart, blood vessels, breast, testes, and anterior abdominal wall—are capable of harboring bone. Ectopic bone formation is also very well known in connection with wound healing, infectious processes, degenerative diseases, and aging. The unanswered question is what is the source of the inducing matrix or inducing cells in such systems.

ECTOPIC OSSIFICATION IN MUSCLE

Ossification of muscle arises from disease or following injury. *Myositis ossificans traumatica* is a localized form developing rapidly in the deep muscles of the thigh or arm within a period of three weeks after a contusion and subsiding within six months. *Myositis ossificans progressiva* is a rare congenital or familial disorder, sometimes associated with microdactyly, continuing throughout the life of the individual, generally involving the muscles of the neck, back, and hips. It is associated with inflammation, loss of striations of muscle cells, atrophy or reduction in the amount of cytoplasm, and proliferation of sarcolemmal sheath cells; later, after mitotic division, spindle-shaped connective tissue cells between the muscle fibers differentiate into new bone or cartilage or both. Smith and associates (1966) observe electromyographic changes and various intrinsic alterations in muscle fibers prior to invasion by connective tissue or bone. After six months, in nearly all cases, the bone deposit fuses with the cortex of the nearest bone. The new bone matures or becomes compact bone, and persists for years as an exostosis. Surgical excision frequently is followed by recurrence and involvement of a large segment of the muscle. The local conditions generating myositis ossificans are unknown.

Calcification of necrotic soft parts and muscle fibers closely adjacent to areas of osteogenesis has been regarded as evidence that calcification is a precursor of ossification. It is now clear, however, that ossification and calcification can be entirely separate and that calcium salts are not required for the initiation of osteogenesis, although calcified necrotic tissues are frequently areas in which ectopic ossification may ensue. Osteogenesis occurs in the healing of a mechanical injury or a pathologic lesion, but it always begins from newly proliferated connective tissue. Ectopic ossification is therefore not to be regarded as metaplasia of connective tissue elements previously in existence in the lesion; not as a simple sequel to deposition of calcium salts in dead tissue; but as a reaction of perivascular connective tissue cells, growing into injured tissue from surrounding areas.

EXPERIMENTAL OSSIFICATION IN MUSCLE

Chemical injury to muscle tissue by injections of 40 per cent alcohol or acid alcohol in rabbits leads to the formation of fibrous scar, amorphous deposits of calcium salts, and in some instances new cartilage or bone or both. Injections of 2 per cent calcium chloride produce calcification in bundles of collagen fibers, amorphous deposits of calcium salts, and calcified plaques of hyaline between the adventitia and the lamina elastica externa of the arteries outside the area of the damaged muscle. Some of these blood vessels exhibit lamellar bone formation associated with erosion of the calcium deposits. In the center of the lesion where there is liquefaction, caseation, necrosis, or disintegration of the structure of the tissue, the conditions are not favorable for bone formation. Osteogenesis appears where muscle cells atrophy, sarcolemmal sheath cells proliferate, and young fibrous connective tissue cells differentiate into chondroblasts and osteoblasts and form islands of new cartilage and bone.

Saline, alcoholic, and calcium chloride extracts of bone produce results not much different from those obtained with the extracting solution alone. When bone formation occurs, the results may be attributed to physicochemical factors arising *in situ* rather than to an exogenous osteogenic substance. It is common to find amorphous deposits of calcium salt, patches of hyalinized scar, and bizarre cells resembling preosseous, precartilaginous, or osteoid tissue. Unabsorbed injured muscle tissue, however, has the capacity to produce new bone formation, but the occurrence rate is very low and the source of the inducing cells is obscure; Bridges and Pritchard (1958) were able to produce formation of cartilage, which eventually was replaced by bone, by implanting small pieces of alcohol-devitalized smooth cardiac or skeletal muscle beneath the capsule of the kidney in rabbits. This is interpreted as induction of cartilage formation by the implant of dead muscle in a host bed that is conducive to osteogenesis; it suggests that new bone formation by autoinduction occurs when muscle is devitalized by injections of alcohol, with or without substances extracted from bone.

OSSIFICATION OF TENDON

Bone formation normally occurs in modified tendinous tissue at the point of bony insertions. Tendons also ossify following injury, but such deposits are generally small and not so extensive as those developing spontaneously in birds. The process has recently been described in detail in the turkey. In these birds, during the first fifteen to twenty weeks of life a new matrix, rich in acid mucopolysaccharide, accumulates between the collagen bundles of the tendons; the original tendon collagen bundles undergo changes in their chemical constitution; and osteons, similar to those in skeletal bone, appear as the result of formation of absorption cavities, which are then filled in with concentric lamellae of bone. All three of these tissues mineralize and persist, with the result that the tendon eventually consists of mineralized collagen bundles interspersed with calcified haversian bone. The origin of the bone-inducing cells in ossifying tendon is not known.

ECTOPIC PERIARTICULAR OSSIFICATION

Patients with anterior poliomyelitis and other paralytic conditions frequently develop multiple foci of ectopic bone. This is usually preceded by extensive atrophy of bone, mobilization of large amounts of bone mineral, excessive excretion of calcium and phosphorus in the urine, and formation of kidney stones. There is thus a sequence of events that seems to relate ectopic bone formation to the *atrophy of disuse* of skeletal bone; this sequence is not necessarily associated with any change in the levels of serum calcium, phosphorus, or phosphatase. The localization of formation of bone is determined by degeneration of muscles, tendons, and the soft-tissue elements of the joints; the result is a periarticular distribution of the deposits of new bone.

OSSIFICATION IN THE URINARY TRACT

In circumstances created by disease and following surgical operations, the urinary tract has a tendency to ectopic bone formation greater than that of any other tissue; this seems to be related to the transitional epithelium of the calyces and pelvis of the kidney, the ureter, and the mucosa of the urinary bladder. Ossification occurs in the kidney of man within a fibrous capsule formed around old renal calculi. Deposits of bone can often be found after surgical incisions in the pelvis of the kidney or in the ureters. Bone has been produced experimentally by ligation of the renal artery in rabbits. It begins independently of any calcification and develops in the loose vascular connective tissue under the epithelium of the calyces.

When urinary bladder is transplanted to the fascia of the anterior abdominal wall, the transitional epithelium proliferates and spreads in all directions to form a fluid-filled cyst. The roof of the cyst consists of the original implant and appears inert; the walls consist of spreading epithelium and induce formation of *lamellar bone* all along the line of contact with the host bed. This is to be regarded as an example of induction in which the bone arises from growing connective tissue cells of the host under the influence of the proliferating cells derived from urinary bladder. The nature of the inductor that is transmitted from one cell to another is unknown. It appears, however, that this induction system for bone is highly specific and dependent upon a factor transmitted from dividing cells of transitional epithelium. Transplants of columnar epithelium from other viscera proliferate and produce fluid-filled cysts but not new bone. The yield of new bone is high in the dog and cat, low in the guinea pig, and almost nil in the rat. The spleen is unfavorable as a host bed for osteogenesis for autologous as well as allogeneic transplants of urinary bladder. The fascia of the anterior abdominal wall and the capsule of the kidney are relatively favorable sites. With allografts of urinary bladder in dogs a reticulocyte-lymphocyte-plasma-cell response surrounds the spreading epithelium but never the new bone; this indicates that the bone cells are derived mainly from the body of the host.

CHAPTER XIV

Healing of Fractures

Mammals have inherited from lower vertebrates an extraordinary capacity to repair injury and replace missing parts of the skeleton. The proliferative reaction is equally vigorous in experimental and clinical healing of fractures. A bone is not simply patched together by scar tissue, as in the healing of most other organs. Bone repair is ordinarily so complete that it is impossible to find the area of a fracture or of a large defect one year after injury. New-bone formation is an automatic reaction to any form of injury of bone tissue. The injury and the reaction are so much a part of each other that the damaged tissue seems to introduce local factors that produce osteogenesis. The site of an otherwise unrecognizable bone injury can be located by the appearance of new-bone formation. The important unsolved problem of the physiology of fracture repair is the nature of the stimulus released by injury that incites connective tissue cells to differentiate into bone cells.

The injured bone tissue immediately shows inflammation, then revascularization, and finally substitution by new bone that grows into it from adjacent endosteum and periosteum. In membrane bones the process is proliferation and direct extension of new bone from old bone. In long bones this involves preliminary formation of a model of fibrous connective tissue and cartilage through which osteogenesis is drawn into and across the fracture gap from each side. The fibrous connective tissue, cartilage, and bone are organized in the form of a complex structure termed *callus*. The interaction of cells and tissue resulting in healing of a fracture is an example of organization of diverse means to a common end.

Organizing Hematoma

As in wound healing in every other part of the body, fracture healing begins with the clotting of extravasated blood. The hemorrhages flow into the fracture gap and flood the soft parts, the bone marrow, periosteum, endosteum, and haversian canals. The organization of the blood clot begins within twenty-four hours on all surfaces, and fibrin is replaced by granulation tissue, in part of hematogenic origin, within a few days. Stinchfield and his associates (1956) observed that anticoagulants administered to rabbits at the time of a fracture caused delayed union. Both heparin and dicumarol have the same effect and prevent the formation of the fibrin clot between the bone ends. Adverse influences upon induction, cellular proliferation, and chondroitin sulfate synthesis are also possible, but the most important information gained from such experiments is that a trellis of fibrin is a mechanical necessity for ingrowth of cells capable of differentiating into fibrocartilaginous callus. It is by this means that a preliminary structure can form to bridge the gap whenever there is displacement of a fracture.

Dedifferentiation

Immediately after the formation of the blood clot and the manifold general physiologic alarm and adaptation reactions, bone regeneration begins. In the bone ends there is hyperplasia and hypertrophy of previously existing osteogenic cells. Between the bone ends in and around the surface of the hematoma, there is cell dedifferentiation, cell migration, proliferation, differentiation, and morphogenesis. Dedifferentiation heralds all tissue reparative processes because it activates cells. It causes nuclei to swell and develop vesicles. It increases the ratio of the volume of nucleus to cytoplasm and accelerates the rate of mitosis. Immune reactions to the products of histolysis may initiate dedifferentiation. Enzymes of the acid protease group increase in the tissue during cell differentiation. As soon as cell dedifferentiation gives way to cell multiplication, growth, and differentiation, there is a rise in tissue dipeptidases. These changes characterize the process of repair of all mammalian organs. What distinguishes bone from tissues that have lost regenerative ability in the course of vertebrate evolution, such as spinal cord, muscle, and skin, is the exceptional ability to set up an embryonic induction system involving mesodermal derivatives in postfetal life. Bone induction is discussed at length in Chapter XIII.

Necrosis of Bone

In a large bone of adult man, with a closed noncomminuted fracture, at least 0.5 cm of the shaft is damaged above and below the fracture line. If the fracture is comminuted and displaced, small and large bits of dead bone are found floating in the fibrinous clot. The necrotic bone is distinguished by pyknotic nuclei, autolyzing osteocytes, and empty lacunae. Increasing acidophilia distinguishes the devitalized matrix of bone from the undamaged tissue at the site of a fracture.

Fibrocartilaginous Callus

The torn ends of periosteum, endosteum, and bone marrow adjoining the fracture line supply cells of histogenic origin; these proliferate and differentiate into fibrous connective tissue, fibrocartilage, and hyaline cartilage. This growth of new tissue is contributed to also by cells of hematogenic origin—monocytes and possibly lymphocytes—that have responded to the stimulus of the inflammation and have participated in the organization of the hematoma. The interaction of mesodermal cells of hematogenic and histogenic origin leads to new bone formation by induction.

The appearance of cartilage in the callus is most prominent in fractures of long bones with displacement or large defects; here the cartilage is a temporary filling material for later replacement and bridging of the defect by new bone. Small drill holes and thin saw cuts produce relatively little cartilage and are repaired chiefly by growth of connective tissue cells and osteoblasts from one surface to another. Although fibrocartilaginous callus is an inseparable part of the healing of fractures of long bones, it is very thin, more fibrous, and less cartilaginous when the bone ends are compressed together between transfixation pins and turnbuckle clamps.

When the defect is large, a model of connective tissue and fibrocartilage is formed, similar to the cartilage model of embryonic osteogenesis. The conditions giving rise to cartilage, instead of bone, in the fracture callus are not known. Age, regional factors, and species differences, however, influence the capacity of the individual to produce cartilage. Growing animals produce more cartilage than adults; they frequently form islands of cartilage concurrently with formation of trabeculae of new bone. Long bones formed as cartilage models in fetal life invariably produce cartilage in a fracture callus. Flat bones formed by intramembranous ossification heal without the appearance of cartilage; surgical defects in the calvarium heal along the edges of the bone, but osteogenesis in this area of the skeleton in adult life is indolent and fails to produce complete filling.

Rats and rabbits have a greater capacity to form cartilage than do guinea pigs, dogs, and men; motion and function cause an increase in the amount of cartilage. Low oxygen tension and low blood supply in the fracture gap are said to promote chondrogenesis; the evidence is scanty.

The significance of cartilage in fracture callus merits further study. While chondrogenesis in mammals is relegated to an accessory or nonessential part of bone repair, it plays a dominant role in lower animals. In reptiles, if the metabolic processes are slowed by low body temperatures, cartilage transforms directly into bone. Similar phenomena can be seen in chondro-osteoid in rachitic mammals and in various pathologic lesions in man. Lacroix (1953) believes that cartilage acts as an organizer, and that it not only elaborates the skeletal tissues, but also arranges them in their normal order.

Osteogenesis

New-bone formation begins in young individuals on the inner and outer surfaces of the damaged bone as early as 48 hours after injury. It arises from periosteum and endosteum, at some distance from the fracture line, and grows toward the fracture gap, enveloping and replacing the fibrocartilaginous callus. This bone originates from cells with inherited osteogenic potency; as it advances into the fibrocartilaginous callus, perivascular connective tissue cells are drawn into osteogenesis and are transformed into osteoblasts (see Fig. 8).

Bone does not form at random within the fibrocartilaginous callus, but grows by extension of periosteal and endosteal new bone. The tendency has been to regard the fibrous connective tissue and cartilage of the callus only as a model or scaffold for osteogenesis, to be invaded and replaced by bone. As in the case of embryonic cartilage models of bone, however, it is reasonable to regard the cartilage as playing an active rather than a passive role in osteogenesis and to assume that the cartilage exerts its influence through the mechanism of *induction.* This concept is strengthened by the observation that when autogenous, homogenous, and even devitalized transplants of fibrocartilaginous callus are made to the anterior chamber of the rat's eye, they lead to production of new bone.

In both the embryonic cartilage model and the fibrocartilaginous callus, connective tissue cells that otherwise would not have exhibited osteogenic potencies are induced to do so by the proximity of bone or cartilage. The formation of new bone may thus require the participation both of cells predisposed to exhibit osteogenic activity and of others that do so less readily, but enter into the process under the influence of induction. The end result is replacement of the fibrocartilaginous callus by bone, bony union of the fracture fragments, and reorganization of the callus with removal of excess bone.

When a polyethylene tube is implanted across a gap in the shaft of the fibula of a young animal, the plastic prevents sealing of the bone ends. The events of repair are separated in time and space as the cells migrate into the tube. Osteogenesis is prepared for and initiated during a preliminary stage of migration and mitotic division of reticular cells. Cartilage and to some extent bone develop in a fluid- and fibrin-filled space. The conditions for survival of the cells in this environment are limited and temporary. Resorption of calcified cartilage or bone, however, provides the conditions for continuation of osteogenesis; resorption can occur with or without the action of osteoclasts. The sequence of events within the walls of the polyethylene tube is: (1) outgrowth of capillaries and mitotic division of reticular or endosteal cells; (2) differentiation of chondroblasts and osteoblasts; and (3) alternating phases of resorption and reconstruction of bone. Guided by the plastic tube, osteogenesis occurs across a gap that could otherwise not become bridged by new bone.

Role of Periosteum

The external callus of the healing fracture develops from periosteum. In adults this membrane is morphologically indistinguishable from ordinary dense connective tissue. In young growing individuals and in adults after a fracture, the periosteum consists of an inner layer of proliferating osteoblasts and an outer layer of fibrous connective tissue, including fibroblasts. After an injection of ^{3}H-thymidine, periosteal connective tissue cells display a higher percentage of labeled nuclei and mitotic figures than the fibroblasts or osteoblasts. The layer of connective tissue cells is activated by the injury to the underlying bone, and it differentiates into osteoblasts and new bone until the outer layer is separated from the cortex as a spindle-shaped mass, enveloping the ends of the bone and forming the external bony callus.

The contribution of the periosteum to the repair of bone is of major importance. An intact periosteal tube is capable of regenerating a large segment of a rib or the entire diaphysis of a long bone. In very young individuals this regeneration is complete. In adults with less active periosteum, the end result is imperfect and inadequate.

These observations indicate that the osteogenic potency of the periosteum is derived from and somewhat dependent upon a close and continuous association with bone. If the periosteum is excised, the body can replace it with a new connective tissue membrane. This applies itself closely to the shaft and can function as well as the original periosteum in producing an external callus for repair of a fracture. Some parts of the skeleton, such as the proximal portion of the neck of the femur, the patella, and other locations from which the periosteum disappears after growth is complete, must depend entirely upon endosteal bone formation for repair.

The extremes can be seen in the healing of fractures when the marrow cavity is obliterated by a steel rod for intramedullary fixation and the repair of bone occurs almost entirely by periosteal activity. The regeneration of bone is rapid and efficient where the periosteum is well developed and can re-form when damaged. The repair of bone is slow in the neck of the femur, where the periosteum is vestigial, inactive, absent, or not regenerated.

Species Differences

The organization of fracture healing is the same in all vertebrates. Some differences from the repair described in mammals can be seen in birds, reptiles, and amphibia. Bone repair has been little studied in fishes. Removal of fibrocartilaginous callus is extremely slow in cold-blooded animals; some of the cartilage that is uneroded by blood vessels appears to transform directly into bone. Pritchard and Ruzicka (1950) described removal of cartilage by chondroclasts in the lizard. There was virtually no calcification of fibrocartilaginous callus, and alkaline phosphatase activity of the tissue was always extremely low in the frog. The chief source of new bone in all species, however, is periosteum and endosteum.

Blood Supply

The vascular network of the callus is an entirely new growth of small arteries, capillaries, and veins, arising as branches of blood vessels of surrounding muscles, periosteum, and bone marrow. As is the case in the granulation tissue of any healing wound, the new blood vessels, including the smooth muscle of the arteriolar walls, originate, at least in part, from differentiation of perivascular connective tissue cells. The magnitude and complexity of the system correspond to the size of the callus. In specimens injected with dyes or radiopaque solutions it may be demonstrated that callus is abundant and healing is rapid in areas with large collateral circulation, such as the metaphyses of the long bones. It is slow in areas such as the head of the femur, where the blood supply is limited to terminal arteries.

The circulation in the midshafts of long bones is reduced in adult life to a volume barely adequate for compact bone and insufficient for rapid regeneration of large areas of damaged bone. Since callus is new growth with a new system of vessels, the vascular bed develops in proportion to the proliferative response of the bone tissue and is usually adequate to accomplish the healing of a fracture. After the fracture is united, there are regression of connective tissue, absorption of excess cartilage and bone, and disappearance of the entire vascular system of the callus. This is a characteristic of the healing of fractures that distinguishes callus from neoplasms of bone and from such conditions as myositis ossificans.

Uniting of Fracture

The bridging of a fracture by new bone, as seen in a sagittal section, follows a plan resembling that of a fixed-arch bridge. The principle is that of cantilevering, and is frequently seen in contemporary architecture. The new bone grows out upon the surface of the model and envelops the fibrocartilaginous callus to form an arch of new bone over the fracture gap. Like ribs and spandrels let down from the arch of a bridge to suspend the deck, the new bone grows through and replaces the cartilage centripetally toward the fracture gap. Finally the deck is laid down between the fracture ends and provides for permanent union. When the fracture is healed, the superstructure disappears, leaving only the bone required for union of the fracture ends (Figs. 44, 45, 46).

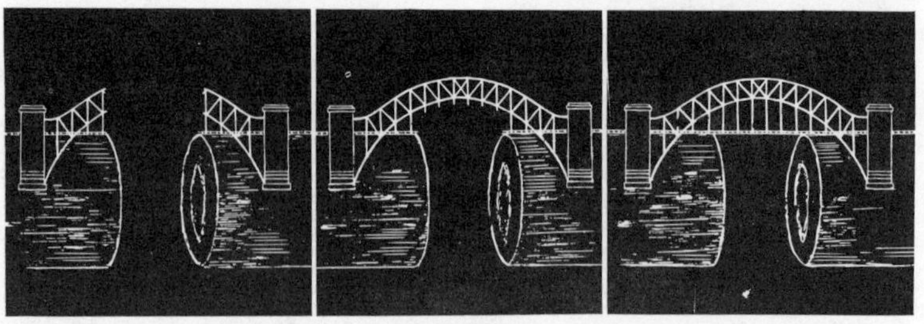

Fig. 44.—Comparison of the union of a fracture of a long bone with the construction of a fixed-arch bridge. Schematic drawing of the Hell Gate Bridge, New York City, 1917.

Left—Stage 1: Bridge, a tower or elevated abutment is constructed on each embankment of the gap to be spanned. *Fracture,* new bone is deposited on the cortex on each side of the fracture line.

Center—Stage 2: Bridge, by the method of cantilevering out, an arch is constructed over the gap. *Fracture* (see also Figs. 45 and 46), new bone from both fragments grows over the fracture line and not between the main fragments.

Right—Stage 3: Bridge, the deck of the bridge is laid down between ribs and spandrels suspended from the arch. *Fracture,* new bone, showing the formative structure of the haversian systems of the compacta, appears between the arch of spongiosa and the cortex and continues to develop directly from the new bone, replacing the last remnants of the fibrocartilaginous callus between the cortical ends. There are no isolated areas of bone formation which appear to be spontaneous or metaplastic in origin. (From Fig. 28, *A, B, C,* Urist and Johnson, J. Bone Jt. Surg. 25:36. Reproduced by courtesy of the publisher.)

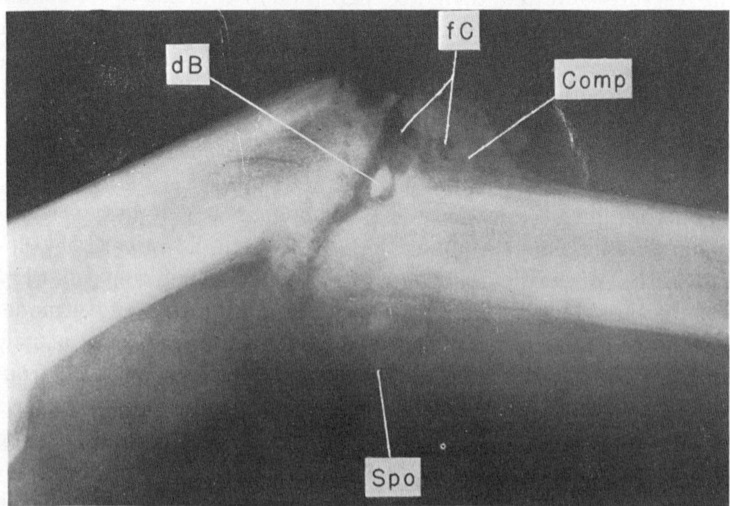

Fig. 45.—Roentgenogram of a fracture of the femur after 85 days of healing, showing a spindle of bony callus inclosing the fracture site but not yet joining the cortical ends, which are still separated by fibrocartilaginous callus (*fC*). *Spo* indicates spongiosa; *Comp,* compact bone; and *dB,* an isolated fragment of dead cortical bone. (From Fig. 25, Urist and Johnson, J. Bone Jt. Surg. 25:32. Reproduced by courtesy of the publisher.)

The shape of the callus and the volume of tissue required to bridge a fracture depend upon the amount of bone damage and displacement. The healing time is directly proportional to the total volume of damaged bone and the breadth of the fracture defect. In impacted fractures a microscopic plate of fibrocartilage is formed at the line of the injury and is replaced by new bone within a few weeks. In displaced fractures the defect becomes filled with a great mass of fibrocartilaginous callus and fibrous tissue, requiring months or years to be replaced by new bone.

The healing time of each bone in the body is predetermined and related to regional conditions. Accurate estimates are available for fractures in the skeletons of the rat and of man. In general, the bones of the upper extremity heal more rapidly than those of the lower extremity. In man, in fractures with the bone ends in contact,

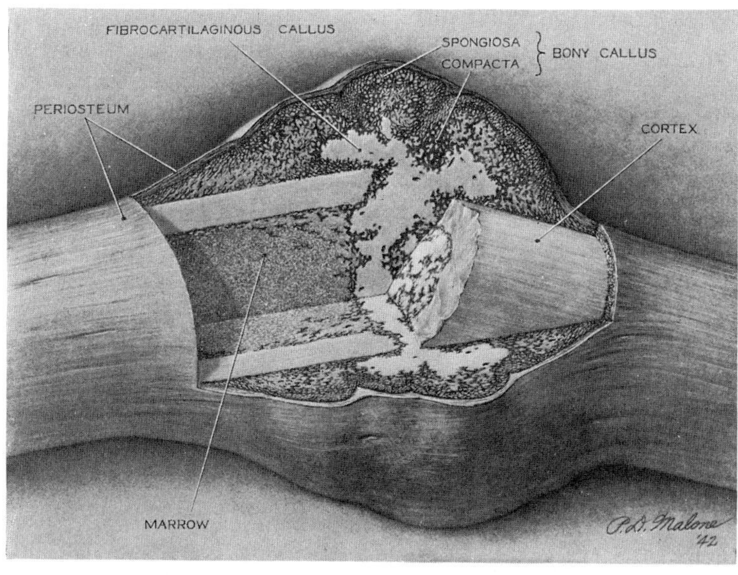

FIG. 46.—Artist's reconstruction of the fracture site, drawn from a clay model of the roentgenogram in Fig. 45. Histologic sections of various parts of the callus were placed on the appropriate plane of the sectioned surfaces and reproduced as magnified. The cartilage, fibrocartilage, and dense fibrous tissue of the fibrocartilaginous callus are seen as a homogeneous, glistening, white scar between and about the fracture ends. (From Fig. 27, Urist and Johnson, J. Bone Jt. Surg. 25:35. Reproduced by courtesy of the publisher.)

humerus and forearm bones unite in three months. The femur and tibia usually require six months. In rats the same fractures heal in four and eight weeks. Spiral fractures heal more rapidly than transverse fractures. Separation of the fragments, even when slight, will greatly increase the healing time in fractures through dense compact bone in adults. Young individuals produce more callus and heal fractures faster. Double fractures of the midshaft require sequences of healing following the direction of flow of the nutrient arteries. In the femur the distal fracture line unites first and the proximal later. In the tibia the proximal fracture line unites first and the distal later; it may even fail to unite at all if the period of immobilization is insufficient.

Systemic Factors

The local and the systemic factors in bone repair are interdependent. The minimum subsistence level of nutritional factors essential for life is apparently all that is required to heal a fracture. The callus appears to hold the highest priority on all tissue-building materials in transport. Multiple fractures in rats heal without delay. The animal loses a large part of its body weight, owing to loss of muscle tissue. Metabolic-balance studies with nitrogen, phosphorus, potassium, and sulfur indicate that muscle-tissue catabolism supplies all the materials needed for building bone matrix. The body elects to catabolize muscle to meet the exigency of the moment when there is need for rapid construction of new bone.

Calcification of Callus

The growing callus is calcified in the same way as cartilage and bone in other parts of the skeleton. Calcification occurs only in a specially prepared matrix. New bone ordinarily calcifies in the callus as soon as it is formed, provided sufficient concentrations of calcium and phosphate ions are present in the blood plasma. In healing fractures in rickets, calcification and ossification can be entirely separate phenomena. In the early stages of fracture healing in rickets, the new bone is laid down as osteoid tissue without any calcium salts. The fibrocartilaginous callus also fails to calcify and leads to the formation of chondro-osteoid rather than bone. The sequence is the same as in the rachitic metaphysis, and it results in a disorganized mass of callus and a measurable delay in union of the fracture.

New-bone formation advances into the callus along a broad front from each side and replaces fibrous connective tissue, fibrocartilage, and hyaline cartilage alike as it moves across the fracture gap. Wherever a calcifiable tissue is encountered, calcium is deposited at the line of contact with the osteogenic tissue or bone. In the early stages of healing, particularly in young individuals, the rate of calcification may lag behind the rate of new-bone formation. The bone trabeculae formed under these conditions have thin osteoid borders. Such small areas of uncalcified cartilage and bone in the callus are encountered in patients on standard or average hospital diets and do not indicate rickets. The levels of serum calcium, inorganic phosphorus, and alkaline phosphatase are not appreciably altered during fracture healing.

X-ray diffraction patterns of the mineral in callus are typical of hydroxyapatite. The orientation of the crystals as observed by X-ray diffraction and by polarization microscopy is in the long axes of the collagen fibers. Densitometric measurements reveal a relatively slight increase in deposition of bone mineral after the initial calcification is complete. The content of organic material, as observed by microinterferometry upon decalcified sections of bone, is the same in partially mineralized and fully mineralized bone.

Tracer Studies of Fractures

Radioisotopes of calcium, strontium, phosphorus, and sulfur are avidly removed from the circulation by growing callus. Uptake of ^{35}S occurs with synthesis of chondroitin sulfate and other mucopolysaccharides in the matrix of fibrocartilage and hyaline cartilage 4 to 21 days after the injury. ^{45}Ca or ^{90}Sr is deposited in the calcifying new-bone matrix and in the zone of provisional calcification during endochondral ossification at from 4 to 120 days of healing. The areas of uptake of ^{32}P correspond closely to those of ^{45}Ca; it is deposited in a more concentrated form as hydroxyapatite than as organic phosphorus. Because of the relatively low concentration of sulfated mucopolysaccharides in bone tissue, less ^{35}S can be found in bone matrix than in cartilage matrix; the ^{35}S content of the callus is accordingly markedly reduced in the course of the replacement of the fibrocartilaginous callus by bone.

The time relationships and sequence of events in bone repair may be observed by administration of tracer doses of ^{45}Ca. Preliminary repair, with callus formation and calcification, occurs within a few weeks after trauma, while resorption, reconstruction, and redistribution of the bone tissue continue for months and sometimes years. For the most part, however, increase in mineral density, hardness, and weight-bearing capacity develop together. In this respect the bone tissue forming in the callus is similar to that in the skeleton as a whole.

Minerals, Vitamins, and Hormones

The search for a substance that might stimulate healing of fractures has motivated study of the effects of minerals, vitamins, and hormones upon callus formation. Thus far nothing specific has been found either to suppress or to stimulate bone repair. The situation is much the same as with the present state of knowledge of the physiology of wound healing in general. Certain phases of the formation of fibrous connective tissue are affected by systemic factors, such as vitamin C or cortisone. By subjecting experimental animals to deprivation of vitamin C or overdosage of cortisone, it is possible to produce a poor quality of callus, but eventually the fracture will heal.

Delayed Union or Nonunion of Fractures

A large part of the literature on bone regeneration has been written by physicians who hoped to find an answer to the problem of slow-healing fractures in man. The emphasis of textbook dogma on the subject has been upon mechanical causes and mechanical treatment. Observations on callus formation, using histochemical techniques, suggest that nonunion is not the absence of healing per se, but the failure to set up an induction system for new-bone formation in the area between the bone ends. The adult human tibia, the bone that offers one of the great challenges to fracture treatment, provides the material most suitable for study of slow-healing fractures.

When bone repair is observed in a consecutive series of control cases compared with matched cases of ununited fractures, the healing time is always proportional to the total length of the damaged area of bone and the breadth of the fracture gap. The adult human tibia produces about 1 cm of bone per year—0.5 cm from each bone end. After eighteen months the rate of proliferation subsides to the normal slow rate of turnover of tibial bone tissue. If the area of bone damage and fracture gap exceeds 1 cm and if the fracture does not unite within eighteen months, the interior of the callus may develop an amorphous center, with fibrinoid and hyaline degeneration of connective tissue (Fig. 47).

Fibrinoid

Fibrinoid forms in the interior of the callus if the fracture is extensive, complicated by infection, or difficult to immobilize. The occurrence is similar to that in chronic adventitious bursitis, except that the lesion develops in the space between the bone ends rather than in the subcutaneous region over a bony prominence. The formation and composition of fibrinoid indicate that it is a by-product of trauma and repair.

Morphologically, fibrinoid is a mass of collagen and ground substance in all stages of degradation. It is like fibrin, as its name implies, but it is not fibrin. It is acellular, homogeneous, highly refractile, and acidophilic. It has the staining reactions of mucopolysaccharides—that is, it stains metachromatically with toluidine blue, pink with PAS reagents, and a mixture of orange, brown, yellow, and blue with phosphotungstic acid and hematoxylin. X-ray diffraction and the electron microscope reveal disoriented collagen fibers in the early stages and only amorphous material remaining in the later stages of fibrinoid degeneration.

After any mechanical disturbance of the fracture site, if it contains fibrinoid, the amorphous material may split apart and produce a cavity filled with mucinous fluid in the center of the callus. Fibrinoid imbibes water, and the internal pressure created by osmosis may be sufficient to break metallic appliances used for internal fixation and to refracture necrotic bone. If motion and friction are not controlled, fibrinoid degeneration continues indefinitely, and a permanent pseudarthrosis may develop. All the new bone formed in the area then becomes converted into compact bone inside and around the cortical ends, but not across the fracture site, and this forms articulating false-joint surfaces.

Immobilization acts as a deterrent to the formation of fibrinoid and permits refilling of the defect with new fibrocartilaginous callus. By this means the degradation can be reversed up to eighteen months after injury, and bone repair can progress simply by pro-

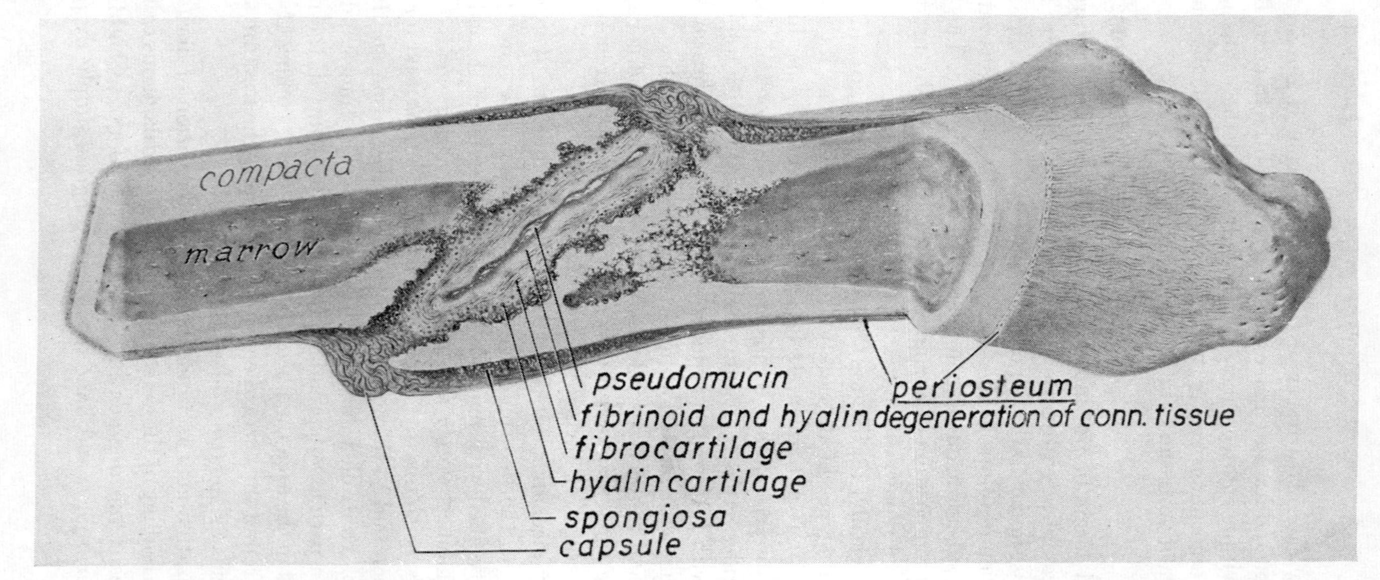

FIG. 47.—Artist's drawing to illustrate the gross and microscopic anatomy of the callus of an ununited fracture at 2 years and 9 months of healing, reconstructed from small samples of tissue obtained from all parts of the fracture site and the bone ends of the tibia of a man thirty-five years of age. (From original drawing of Fig. 7-*G*, Urist, Mazet, and McLean, J. Bone Jt. Surg. 36-A:949. Reproduced by courtesy of the publisher.)

longed immobilization. After eighteen months, excision of the fracture site and close coaptation of the bone ends is more likely to produce union.

Injury to blood supply has been regarded by many writers of many years past as the main cause of failure of bone repair. This generally occurs in adult life in parts of the skeleton where there is inadequate collateral circulation, dense avascular compact bone, arteriosclerosis, or excessive splintering of cortex due to osteoporosis.

A bone graft of any kind produces a new proliferative response from the bone ends and new-bone formation by induction across the fracture gap. Homogenous and autogenous bone appear to be equally effective in most cases. Inlay, onlay, and intramedullary grafts are all capable of producing union in the majority of cases. The success of the operation depends upon the proliferative response of the bone ends rather than upon the technique or the material employed. These observations suggest that the mechanical treatment of fractures can be overemphasized and that early open operations and metallic internal fixation should be used only in unusual circumstances. More reliance should be placed upon the primordial power of the human skeleton to regenerate injured and missing substance.

CHAPTER XV

Pathologic Physiology of Bone

We shall restrict our consideration of pathologic conditions to a few of those illustrating the effects of disturbances of the normal physiology of bone. These will include abnormalities in the formation of bone matrix, defective calcification of matrix, and the effects upon bone of hypersecretion of the parathyroid glands. They will exclude all new growths and infections of bone, a variety of polyglandular syndromes, and both systemic and localized affections whose genesis is not clearly understood.

Atrophy, Osteoporosis, and Rarefaction of Bone

Strictly speaking, *atrophy* of bone should refer to loss of substance or of volume; *osteoporosis* to an increased porosity—that is, to a decrease in the hard portions of bone substance in favor of a relative increase in the soft portions; and *rarefaction* to decreased density—that is, to a decrease in the weight per unit of volume. Since roentgenograms do not distinguish clearly between conditions resulting in a decrease in the density of the shadows cast by bones, and since the nature of the condition is often obscure, both in the clinic and at autopsy, the tendency is to use the three terms interchangeably. Excluded from these terms, however, are rickets and osteomalacia, both of which are differentiated from osteoporosis or rarefaction by failure of calcification of the matrix, production of which is not changed. Also excluded is softening of bone by the increased resorption of hyperparathyroidism. *Demineralization* or removal of bone mineral without alteration in the underlying organic matrix does not occur in the living animal, and as a descriptive term it serves no useful purpose. The same objections can be raised to the term *remineralization*. Atrophy is a word commonly used to describe deficient formation of new-bone matrix, and we have used this as a general designation. Occasionally it is useful to apply these terms in connection with descriptions of a specific condition, such as the osteoporosis of Cushing's syndrome.

Atrophy of bone is unlike atrophy of soft tissues. In soft tissues, such as skin, muscle, or liver, atrophy produces a reduction in the size as well as in the number of cells, and results in shrinkage of volume. Atrophy of bone occurs without change in volume or external dimensions, but mass may be reduced as much as 75 per cent. Internal architecture gradually becomes attenuated and almost disappears. This is seen in its most typical form in the bones of paralyzed limbs or parts immobilized in casts for long periods of time; these exhibit the *atrophy of disuse*, and a diminished mass of bone tissue per unit volume of the bone. An atrophied bone is everywhere brittle and of a more spongy consistency than normal. In cross-section the cortex is paper thin; the periosteal surface is smooth and relatively unaltered; the intramedullary surface is composed of a yellow, fatty, fibrous tissue. In roentgenograms the bone tissue casts a homogeneous diffuse shadow with the individual trabeculae widely separated, thin, and difficult to outline. A loss of 23–30 per cent of the bone mineral is necessary to produce an appreciable change in roentgenograms of the bone; in severe cases of atrophy, with extreme roentgenographic changes, more than 50 per cent of the mineral of the skeleton may be lost. The microscopic structure of atrophied cancellous bone consists of very thin trabeculae, branching, deficient in length, and with smooth surfaces completely devoid of osteoblasts. The bone marrow is uniformly fatty, fibrous, and hypoplastic.

Bone atrophy may be systemic, regional, or local. The use of the term *osteoporosis* usually refers to a systemic condition, in contrast to the local atrophy of disuse. The terms *senile osteoporosis* and *postmenopausal osteoporosis* add to the confusion in the literature on this subject. Radiographically and microscopically, physiologic atrophy of the bone tissue in old age resembles the atrophy of disuse or osteoporosis. Atrophy generally develops from simultaneous decrease in the rate of bone formation and increase in the rate of resorption. The rapidity with which the atrophy of disuse develops in an immobilized limb has suggested that an increased rate of destruction may also be an important factor. This view is supported by the observation of calcium balance and urinary ex-

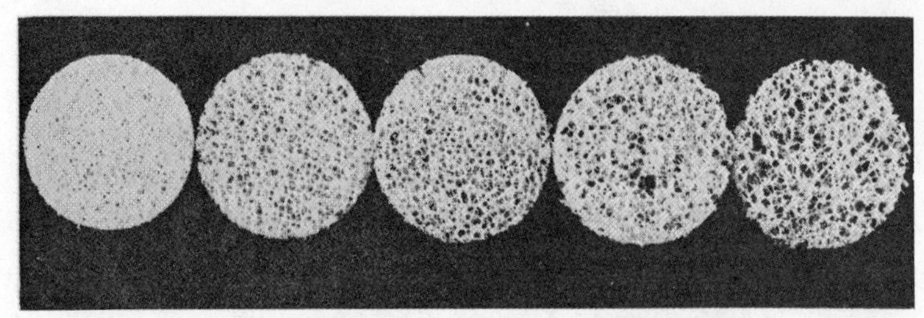

A

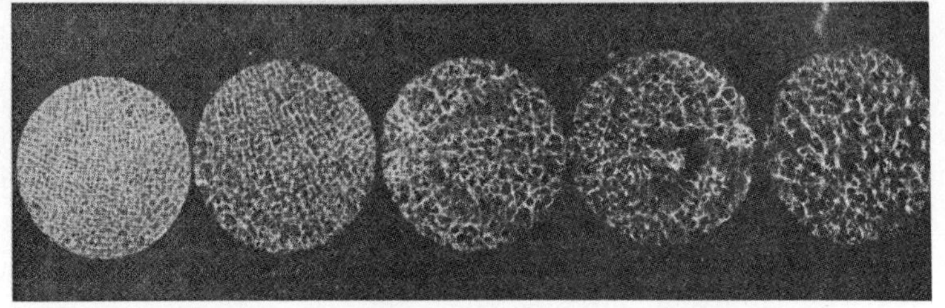

B

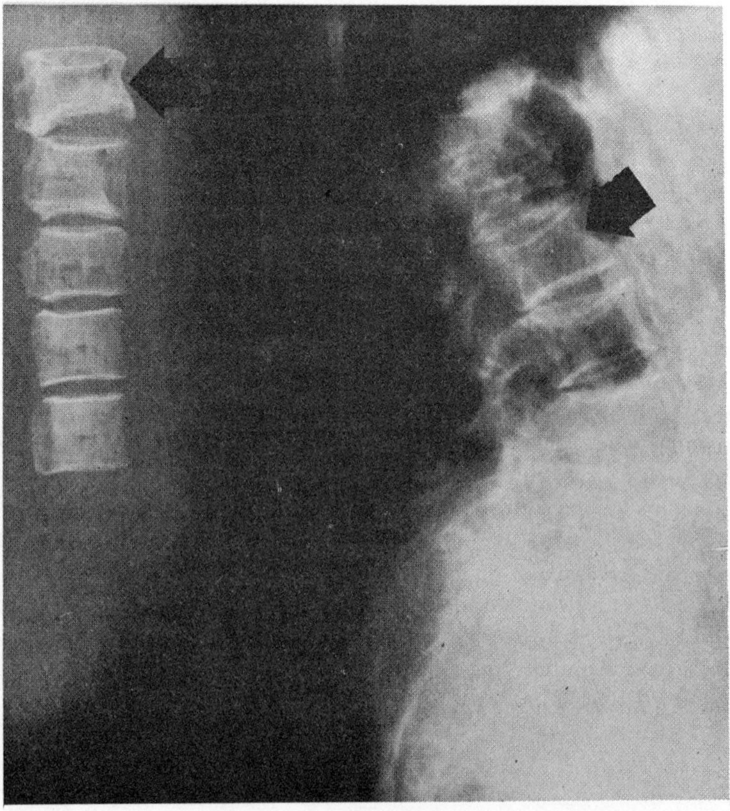

C

Fig. 48

cretion during immobilization. Normal young men immobilized in plaster casts lose 1–2 per cent of their total body calcium within six to seven weeks. A growing boy placed in a partial body cast for a fracture of the neck of the femur suffered extreme atrophy of the immobilized parts of the skeleton, with hypercalcemia and increased excretion of calcium in the urine. The occurrence of kidney stones in patients immobilized in casts is frequently observed; this is a complication derived from prolonged hypercalcemia and hypercalcuria.

The Problem of Osteoporosis

The most common systemic bone disease and the most important unsolved problem in the biology and medicine of the skeletal system is osteoporosis. The condition develops from simultaneous reduction in cortical and spongy bone in ribs, vertebrae, pelvis, and necks of the femurs; loss of spongiosa is most rapid, but slow decrease in cortical bone mass is critical because this leads to mechanical failure, or spontaneous or pathologic fractures. The roentgenographic appearance in the spinal column in osteoporosis, osteitis fibrosa, and osteomalacia sometimes can be surprisingly alike. Multiple myeloma and various widespread malignant tumors in middle-aged individuals can also produce these bone changes, and can deceive inexperienced or unwary observers, especially during early stages of the disease. Only a thorough hospital investigation to exclude other bone disease can establish a diagnosis of osteoporosis.

Urist and his associates (1963; 1964) divide patients with osteoporosis into two groups: physiologic and pathologic. Physiologic osteoporosis is the time-dependent, slow process of aging, atrophy, or failure of retention of bone mass that occurs in proportion to reduction in muscle mass after age fifty. Figure 48 illustrates a degree of change that is characteristic of physiologic osteoporosis. Pathologic osteoporosis causes a disproportionate, rapid loss in

---

Fig. 48.—(*A*) Photographs of disks of cancellous bone removed from the center of the first lumbar vertebra with the use of a cork borer, illustrating five degrees of vertebral bone density. The maximum bone density in a young man is shown on the left. The minimum bone density is in an osteoporotic individual as shown on the far right. (*B*) Roentgenograms of the five samples of cancellous bone shown in *A*. (*C*) Roentgenograms of lumbar spine of a patient with severe osteoporosis with minimal bone density (*right arrow*) and spondylometer readings including a specimen with comparable low bone density (*left arrow*).

bone mass, generally in the age interval between fifty-five and seventy years, and is characterized by *spontaneous collapse of vertebral bodies in the dorsal spine* (Fig. 48 *A* to *C*). In the lumbar spine there is concurrent resorption and remodeling of the cortical end plates and ballooning of the intervertebral disks. This is associated with a compensatory increase in the thickness of hypertrophy of the vertical trabeculae. Using a method of *spondylography*, it is possible to demonstrate five stages of the process of reduction in bone mass per unit volume with compensatory increase in vertical trabecular markings (Fig. 48 *A* to *C*).

Some observers hold that pathologic and physiologic osteoporosis are similar in almost every respect except a quantitatively greater reduction in bone mass. We are inclined to search for some differences. In physiologic osteoporosis, the bones of the axial and appendicular skeletons are reduced in density in definite although unequal proportion, and are subject to fracture only from accidental falls or external forces. In pathologic osteoporosis, the bones of the axial skeleton are always much more severely affected than the appendicular skeleton, and multiple fractures occur spontaneously and without any significant external force. Histologically, there is often an abnormally large number of empty osteocyte lacunae, and both trabecular and haversian bone are enveloped in fibrous and lipoid connective tissue. The cortex becomes porous, light in weight, hard in substance, and very brittle. Microradiographs show fully calcified new and old lamellar bone, but the vascular channels contain plugs of amorphous calcium deposits. Bone accretion, as determined by tracer studies, is frequently normal, but may be either low or high, depending upon the age of the patient and the stage of the disease.

Urist and Fareed (unpublished) observed that subjects with pathologic osteoporosis are only infrequently found at autopsy—that is, those with spinal columns showing generalized decrease in bone mass, thickening of the vertical trabeculae, ballooning of the lumbar disks, and collapsed thoracic vertebral bodies throughout. Only 1 per cent of males and less than 5 per cent of females in their series of over 200 autopsies had clinically significant osteoporosis. Unlike living patients with osteoporosis, autopsy populations have relatively little reduction in bone mass and no pathologic fractures or ballooned disks, but they do exhibit other conditions, such as spondylosis, metastatic bone disease, and single traumatic lesions. An autopsy survey by Caldwell and Collins (1961) reveals no point at which an osteoporotic can be distinguished from the nonosteoporotic in measurements of bone density or bone calcium. Thus, bone density as determined by total calcium is only one index, and not a typical feature, in either the incidence or the development of pathologic osteoporosis. Villanueva *et al.* (1966) measured bone mass in cross-sections of ribs and demonstrated lower values in some patients without severe pathologic osteoporosis than in others with the disease. The problem remains, therefore, to explain the fact that the incidence of pathologic osteoporosis is higher in relatively healthy subjects observed in old people's homes than in autopsy populations. In homes for the aged, it is as high as one-fourth of the female and one-tenth of all healthy males of average age seventy-five. Undoubtedly, advanced age is a factor, but it is not the critical one, because the majority of people develop spondylosis, not osteoporosis.

Trotter and her colleagues (1960) measured bone mass in still another sample of the population of the United States—the bodies found in a medical-school anatomical dissecting room. If their samples were comparable to those found in a hospital autopsy room, they would be a mixture of a very few cases of pathologic osteoporosis and a great many cases of physiologic osteoporosis, but they do not distinguish between the two. They note instead that bones of both white males and American Negro females are normally denser than those of white females. Urist (1960) selected a sample of white males with severe debilitating disease; not only was the incidence of osteoporosis lower in males than in females, but the bone changes were relatively slight and more like physiologic than pathologic osteoporosis. In a hospital population of subjects severely disabled with pathologic osteoporosis there was a ratio of seven females to one male. Sex, race, and aging, or involutional changes in the skeleton, are underlying factors in both physiologic and pathologic osteoporosis, but in the latter there is a precipitous fall in the amount of vertebral cortical bone, rather than a gradual decline. This is associated with failure to repair the trabeculae or replace lost bone tissue with new bone. The question whether the incidence of fractures in the aged is a manifestation of a fracture factor of unknown nature is difficult to answer. Microfractures in the interstitial lamellae are a common finding in the bones of the aged, especially in the neck of the femur, but neither their causation nor their relationship to vertebral collapse is clear. Bauer (1960), investigating the epidemiology of fractures in adult individuals in Sweden, postulates the existence of an endogenous fragility factor, exclusive of aging or osteoporosis, predictable and constant for populations and for special sites of predilection in the human skeleton. In the United States, the epidemiology of fractures has been investigated chiefly in the Negro population; for some unknown reason, possibly genetic, the 9 per cent of the population that is derived from African Negro ancestry infrequently shows pathologic osteoporosis and very rarely has fractures of the hip. In Puerto Rico, investigated by Smith and Rizek (1966), and in other populations of the world sampled by Nordin (1966), the relationship between race and pathologic osteoporosis was similar but not always so clear-cut.

A satisfactory experimental laboratory mammal for study of osteoporosis is yet to be found. Mice and cats fed on all-meat diets, supplemented with vitamin D during the period of rapid growth or during lactation, develop a physiologic form of osteoporosis. Deer found in areas where the grass is poor develop a hunger-osteopathy form of osteoporosis. Canadian geese lose bone mass and suffer from pathologic fractures in the far north at the conclusion of the egg-laying cycle. A spontaneous form of osteoporosis, related to genetic factors but in some respects resembling the disorder in man, is found in the white leghorn hen bred for heavy egg production. This condition is known in the poultry industry as *cage layer fatigue;* it is aggravated by confinement in close quarters and improved by exercise. Osteoporosis, experimental as well as clinical, is characterized by normal levels of serum calcium, phosphorus, and alkaline phosphatase. Mineral, vitamin, and general nutritional status are usually within normal limits. Metabolic-balance studies upon young subjects with rapidly progressive osteoporosis reveal daily losses in calcium, phosphorus, and nitrogen in the urine and feces in excess of the amounts in the dietary intake. Aged individuals with slowly progressive osteoporosis, commonly seen with fracture of the neck of the femur as the presenting symptom, are usually not in negative calcium, phosphorus, or nitrogen balance. The pathogenesis appears to be a depressed or very low rate of accretion, associated with high or normal rate of resorption.

The etiology of osteoporosis is rarely demonstrable in man. Patients with Cushing's syndrome are exceptional; the effects of exogenous hypercortisonism are seen more frequently, both in man and in experimental animals, and are not uncommon in children. Proliferation of connective tissue cells, including osteoblasts, is inhibited by corticosteroids; large amounts of calcium are unabsorbed. On correction of hypercortisonism, young individuals may regain bone structure by appositional new-bone formation, but recovery of the original mass of skeletal tissue has not been observed in adults. Neither has it been possible to prove that middle-aged individuals can regain bone mass from either physiologic or pathologic osteoporosis treated by various methods for periods as long as twenty years. For over thirty years, physicians in the United States have prescribed sex hormones, following the rationale of Albright and Reifenstein (1948 see Chapter X) that the condition is related to postmenopausal imbalance between gonadal and adrenocortical hormones. In the absence of quantitative data on the output of metabolites of these hormones, and failure to prevent further fractures by replacement therapy, sex hormones are used more for supportive than specific treatment.

Fluoride ion deficiency is now being looked upon as a factor in the occurrence of osteoporosis in man. Bernstein and his associates (1966) made a survey of the density of the lumbar spine in 11,015 subjects over age forty-five residing in areas of North Dakota where the water fluoride was over 4 parts per million (ppm), compared with areas where it was under 0.15 ppm, and conclude that the incidence of osteoporosis and vertebral fractures was higher in persons with low intake of fluoride. The incidence was 5–10 per cent in females and 50 per cent in males over age fifty living in high-fluoride areas. Previously, Leone and his associates (1954) made a similar survey in Bartlett and Cameron counties in Texas, and found some patients with osteoporosis living in areas of high concentrations of fluoride in water. Rich *et al.* (1964) employ fluoride ion for treatment of osteoporosis, and note slight positive calcium balances. Our experience with some thirty-five cases treated over a period of five years shows no improvement in the roentgenographic picture of the vertebrae and no prevention of further fractures.

Longer experience with a larger number of cases is necessary to substantiate the basis of F^- therapy for either prevention or cure of osteoporosis. It is conceivable that lifelong intake of 1 ppm of F^- in the water supply may promote bone retention in aging and lower the degree of physiologic osteoporosis, but whether it can be expected to alter the progress of pathologic osteoporosis materially can be determined only by careful scientific studies on future generations.

An older view is that osteoporosis results from a deficient calcium intake. Nordin (1960), supporting this concept, holds that osteoporosis may be associated with either low intake, insufficient absorption, or high excretion of calcium. Whedon and his associates (1959) have observed the influence of accompanying debilitating disease, immobilization, inadequate intake of minerals, and treatment with an intake of 2 g or more of calcium daily; they report retention of as much as 200 mg per day in osteoporotics sixty years of age, as well as in normal control adults. Rose (1964) claims that high calcium intake magnifies the errors inherent in the balance method, and that when patients are brought back for a second study, positive calcium balance usually is no longer present. It seems that it has sometimes been possible to arrest negative calcium balance by very high calcium intake, but never possible to establish a positive calcium balance in an adult patient for a very long period of time. This applies to high intake of sex hormone and fluoride ion, as well as to high calcium intake.

A protein-starvation theory, citing the effects of protein-deficient diets or gastrointestinal disorders, is based upon the similarity of bone changes in hunger osteopathy and in osteoporosis. Except for the osteoporosis of hypercortisonism, endogenous or exogenous, there is generally no abnormality of protein metabolism. One may generalize by saying that calcium-deficient diets, castration, hypercortisonism, hyperthyroidism, weight loss from starvation or debilitating disease—all may accelerate the progress of the disorder in individuals predisposed to it. This supports the view of a nonspecific aging suggested by the higher incidence of the condition in the aged population. Young patients with osteoporosis have the external appearance of individuals ten to twenty years older than their chronological age. Urist and Vincent (1961) have observed a decline in the excretion of 11-deoxy-17-ketosteroids in young women with osteoporosis; this was observed also after age seventy in women without osteoporosis, and was attributed to the nonspecific effects of aging upon the adrenal cortex.

As has been noted, osteoporosis in adult life is refractory to treatment and irreversible with respect to recovery of normal density of the bone. Until the etiology is known, or an antiosteoporosis factor is isolated, or a specific stimulant for osteogenesis is found, treatment with high-calcium diets or sex hormones, or with combinations of the two, or with fluoride ion, will continue to be of limited value.

Rickets and Osteomalacia

RICKETS

Rickets may be defined as a failure of calcification to keep pace with the growth of bones. This implies that rickets is a disease of the growing child; a somewhat similar pathologic condition seen in the adult, under extreme deprivation of vitamin D and minerals, is known as osteomalacia.

One of the most constant and most characteristic sequelae of what may be called a functional deficiency of phosphate—generally as the result of a low intake of vitamin D—is the lowering of the concentration of inorganic phosphate in the blood plasma. The simplest conception of rickets is that which attributes all the symptoms and findings in this disease to the lowered plasma phosphate.

In experimental animals fed with rachitogenic diets, the earliest evidence of rickets is failure of calcification at the epiphyseal-metaphyseal junction and the appearance of uncalcified osteoid tissue on the surfaces of growing trabeculae of bone. The failure of calcification, particularly in the epiphyseal cartilage, is responsible for the subsequent pathologic changes, all of which result from the growth and accumulation of cartilage and osteoid tissue.

VITAMIN D–RESISTANT RICKETS

There is a series of disorders characterized by the skeletal manifestations of rickets or osteomalacia but resistant to therapy with vitamin D. Various forms have been described; for the most part they have in common a disturbed function of the renal tubules, resulting in a relative phosphaturia with a lowering of the serum phosphate level, conducive to a failure of calcification. At the other end of the scale there is a condition known as *idiopathic hypercalcemia*, believed to be a manifestation of hypersensitivity to vitamin D. Fanconi (1955) has described the variations in sensitivity to vitamin D, and his name is prominently associated with the clinical manifestations of these variations. Harrison (1957) has also described the varieties of rickets and osteomalacia associated with hypophosphatemia, including the Fanconi syndrome. Engfeldt *et al.* (1956), who have reported microradiographic studies of the bones in refractory rickets, have observed that the structural features differ from those in ordinary rickets, and have concluded that the condition is genetically determined. Treatment with massive doses of vitamin D is commonly employed, with variable success. Any improvement so obtained has been attributed to the calcemic effects of the large doses of vitamin D; this treatment does not influence the morphology and does not cure the disease.

OSTEOMALACIA

Osteomalacia is the adult form of rickets. Since it involves only the bones of adults, in the absence of the growth apparatus of infancy and childhood, it is characterized pathologically by failure of newly formed bone matrix to calcify. In borderline cases osteoid margins on otherwise calcified trabeculae of bone may be demonstrated; advanced cases are notable for softening of all the bones and consequent deformities.

Osteomalacia has been known for centuries in India and the Middle East. It is now rare in Europe and America, but it occurred in combination with osteoporosis in some of the European countries during World War I, associated with pregnancy and dietary privations. Classic osteomalacia was carefully studied in China, where it had assumed endemic proportions, resulting from lack of vitamin D, combined with a very low intake of calories, protein, calcium, and phosphorus. Even under these extreme conditions it is rare except as a sequel to pregnancy, with its drain on the skeletal system of the mother. It also occurs, but very rarely, in males.

Several conditions occur, also rarely, in which the bones have the roentgenographic and microscopic characteristics of osteomalacia, but without the usual etiologic factors. The most common form accompanies an excess of fat in the stools, with failure to absorb vitamin D. Renal *tubular acidosis* may also be accompanied by softening of the bones; this condition is distinct from *renal rickets*, which is commonly a manifestation of secondary hyperparathyroidism.

In both rickets and osteomalacia the serum calcium is usually maintained at a normal level; the inorganic phosphate of the serum is low; the alkaline phosphatase is high. Secondary enlargement of the parathyroid glands is common in both disorders.

Hyperparathyroidism

Primary Hyperparathyroidism

Primary hyperparathyroidism is the idiopathic form of hyperparathyroidism. In most instances there is a single adenoma; more rarely there are multiple adenomata; carcinoma is still less common. Idiopathic hypertrophy, in which the increase in the size of the glands is in part attributable to enlargement of the cells, also occurs.

The manifestations of primary hyperparathyroidism are the result of hypersecretion of the parathyroid hormone; they are independent of the nature of the disorder of the gland. The most common and almost pathognomonic finding is elevation of the serum calcium level. The increase in concentration of the total calcium is divided between calcium ions and undissociated calcium proteinate, distributed in accordance with the law of mass action. With few exceptions, increase in the calcium ion concentration of the serum is diagnostic of primary hyperparathyroidism, especially if it is accompanied by a normal protein and low phosphate level. Any finding of a serum calcium level above 11 mg per 100 ml (2.75 mmoles per liter) or a calcium ion concentration above 5.5 mg per 100 ml as estimated from serum calcium and serum protein (Fig. 34) should arouse suspicion. Serum calcium values above 15 mg/100 ml are rare, but they may occur.

Although hyperparathyroidism first made itself known by its production of skeletal disease, skeletal changes are by no means an essential part of the findings. Hypercalcemia leads to increased excretion of calcium in the urine; this in turn leads to the formation of kidney stones. The possibility of hyperparathyroidism is brought to the attention of the physician as often by kidney stones as by symptoms and signs originating from the skeleton.

The gross skeletal changes in advanced cases are characterized by softening of the bones, with consequent deformities and fractures. The diagnosis is often suggested by the roentgenographic findings of generalized decrease in density of the bones, often accompanied by cysts and tumors. The microscopic findings are those of greatly increased resorption of bone, with numerous osteoclasts. These are accompanied by increased osteoblastic activity, indicative of attempts to repair the damaged trabeculae of bone. Attempts at repair also result in an excess of fibrous connective tissue; this has led to the use of the term *osteitis fibrosa* to describe the pathologic changes in the bones. Such bone matrix as is present, old and new, is calcified; it is not correct to refer to the changes in the bone as *decalcification.*

In many cases of hyperparathyroidism, certainly in borderline cases, no bone changes can be found. They may also be prevented by providing a liberal intake of calcium. When bone changes are present, the serum phosphatase level is elevated; when they are absent or are prevented by increased calcium intake, the serum phosphatase is within the normal range.

SECONDARY HYPERPARATHYROIDISM

Hyperplasia of the parathyroid glands, accompanied by increased secretory activity, occurs under the following conditions: rickets or osteomalacia; pregnancy; renal insufficiency, associated with retention of phosphate; and calcium deprivation. All these conditions predispose toward low serum calcium; hyperplasia of the parathyroid glands is compensatory; hypersecretion rarely leads to elevation of the serum calcium above normal values. Erdheim's description of enlargement of the parathyroid glands in osteomalacia (1907) led to some later confusion between primary and secondary hyperparathyroidism. This was not entirely clarified until after Mandl (1925) had performed the first parathyroidectomy, for adenoma of the gland.

Of the foregoing conditions, only renal insufficiency leads to enough increased activity of the parathyroids to bring about skeletal changes. These changes, because of their association with glomerular nephritis, have become known as *renal rickets.* The sequence of events, each stage being dependent upon the one just before, is: (1) renal insufficiency; (2) diminished excretion of phosphate; (3) elevation of serum phosphate level; (4) depression of serum calcium level; (5) hyperplasia of parathyroid glands with hypersecretion; and (6) resorption of bone.

In adults the pathologic changes in the bones are indistinguishable from those of primary hyperparathyroidism. In children there are, in addition, changes in the epiphyses that closely resemble those seen in true rickets. The blood findings in both adults and children usually include normal or slightly low calcium levels, high phosphate levels, high serum phosphatase, and severe acidosis with low carbon dioxide combining power. Calcium deposits are frequently found in blood vessel walls and soft tissues around joints.

Pathologic Calcification

One of the most serious manifestations of bone disease is pathologic calcification in vital soft-tissue organs. It is less serious and less likely to be associated with bone disease when it is classifiable as *dystrophic* calcification and limited to one locality, such as a shoulder tendon or an adventitious bursa. It is very serious when it is classified as *metastatic* calcification and associated with hypercalcemia based upon bone disease. In metastatic calcification, the deposits form in the kidneys (nephrocalcinosis), arterial walls, dura, heart muscle, stomach wall, lungs, and the subcutaneous tissues over the bony prominences of elbows, hands, knees, or other parts exposed to minor traumata. Metastatic calcification follows any disturbance of calcium homeostasis, either kidney disease with failure of renal excretion or failure of tubular reabsorption of calcium and phosphate ions. Some of the more common disorders of calcium homeostasis are hyperparathyroidism and extensive bone destruction from multiple myeloma, metastatic carcinoma, vitamin D intoxication, Paget's disease with atrophy of disuse, acute posttraumatic metabolic syndrome, and immobilization. The calcium deposits are prominent in the cytoplasm of the cells of organs that excrete acidic products of metabolism and thereby become more alkaline: for example, lungs, which secrete carbonic acid; the stomach, which secretes hydrochloric acid; and the kidneys, which secrete phosphoric acid. The calcium deposits develop in the cytoplasm of the cells. To some extent the metastatic calcification is reversible and the deposits disappear when the hypercalcemia is corrected by therapeutic measures, Extensive calcium deposits have also been observed in arterial walls in patients treated with the artificial kidney for acute renal disease.

Hypoparathyroidism

Insufficiency of secretion of the parathyroid glands occurs from accidental removal or injury of parathyroid glands in surgical operations on the thyroid gland. In most instances, fortunately, the condition is transient, simply a manifestation of interference with the blood supply or partial ischemic necrosis of parathyroid glands. When the condition is permanent, it is necessary to treat the patient with daily supplements of readily available calcium in the form of drops of a 30 per cent solution of calcium chloride and dietary supplements of vitamin D.

Idiopathic or spontaneous hypoparathyroidism is an *uncommon disorder*, but it is possible to find some cases among persons said to have epilepsy. Albright and Reifenstein (1948) reviewed the literature, including autopsy findings in twelve cases. The gland cells were atrophied and replaced with fat cells. In addition to tetany, most of the patients had numbness of the extremities, cramps, carpopedal spasms, laryngeal stridor, and convulsions. Cataracts, calcification of the basal ganglia, atrophied fingernails, and moniliasis are common complications. Aplasia and hypoplasia of the teeth occur in children. Defective calcification of the dentin is seen in young adults. The bones may be denser than normal, owing to a low rate of osteoclastic resorption, but this is difficult to demonstrate by clinical roentgenography alone. The laboratory findings are pathognomonic: high serum inorganic phosphorus, low serum calcium, and low alkaline phosphatase; excretion of calcium in the urine is almost nil, but periods of remission with transient hypercalcuria may occur. Granstrom and Hed (1966) note that patients with idiopathic hypocalcemia are so sensitive to vitamin D that a sunbath can produce a period of hypercalcuria. A suggestion of Moore (personal communication) that patients with idiopathic hypoparathyroidism may suffer from excess secretion of calcitonin deserves investigation by biopsy, extracts of tissue, and trials of treatment with radioiodine.

Albright and Reifenstein (1948) also describe pseudohypoparathyroidism, a syndrome characterized by epileptiform seizures in individuals with short stature, brachydactyly (mainly short metacarpal bones), early closure of epiphyseal plates, and pathologic calcification of ligaments and tendons of the extremities. These patients have active or hyperactive parathyroid glands, but do not respond to injections of bovine or porcine parathyroid extract; they respond to vitamin D, however, as do normal individuals. Pseudopseudohypoparathyroidism is now also established in the literature as a clinical entity and should be mentioned briefly. The skeletal deformities are similar but the patients have subcutaneous ectopic bone rather than calcinosis; the serum calcium and phosphorus concentrations are normal; the responses to both parathyroid extract and vitamin D are also normal. We may assume that many combinations of skeletal, parathyroid gland, and metabolic anomalies are possible, presumably from aberrations of genetic elements.

Paget's Disease

Osteitis deformans or Paget's disease, a disorder of unknown etiology, is characterized by a succession of osteolytic and osteoblastic changes in the structure of bones during adult life. It is an affliction of the skeleton of man and animals, found in prehistoric fossil bones as well as in modern times. The condition may be widespread in the skeleton, but it is a localized rather than generalized condition. It advances either up or down the structure of each bone along a wedgelike front and leaves it broadened, deformed, and decreased in density. In the typical roentgenogram of Paget's disease, the cortex becomes thick and the trabecular pattern coarsened and interwoven. Microscopically, along the moving surface of the osteolytic wedge osteons are resorbed by means of the appearance of large numbers of osteoclasts, and the haversian canals remain enlarged and distorted; in another nearby area, osteoblasts may deposit lamellae of new bone between irregular thick cement lines and transform the cortical bone into a mosaic pattern.

The laboratory findings are of special interest in advanced cases with involvement of the entire skeleton. In such patients the serum alkaline phosphatase may rise to levels above 100 King-Armstrong units. Hypercalcemia occurs if such patients are immobilized in bed because of a pathologic fracture. Recent investigations reveal the strong possibility that the bone reaction in Paget's disease may arise from an aneurysmal alteration of the capillary circulation of bone. Specimens of blood obtained by cardiac catheterization reveal increased oxygen tension of the venous blood from a region of extensive Paget's disease. Venous congestion, high pulse pressure, increased cardiac output, enlargement of the heart, hypertension, severe arteriosclerosis, and local heat over the involved bones suggest that multiple arteriovenous shunts may be present inside the skeleton. However, nothing abnormal has been demonstrated by arteriography.

Osteopetrosis

Abnormalities of bone causing an increase in the amount of hard tissue at the expense of the soft tissue, with relatively little alteration of the external volume, are generally classified as osteopetrosis or marble bones. This disorder is uncommon in man, occurring chiefly in infants with fatal anemia; it is found occasionally by coincidence in asymptomatic or abortive form in roentgenographic examinations of adults. It is sometimes inherited as an autosomal recessive trait. The original patient, twenty-six years old, was described by Albers-Schönberg (1907), but nothing about the etiology has been found by study of hundreds of cases since then. Histologic sections reveal a dense spongiosa and thick cortex with bands of osteoid tissue and densely calcified cartilage. The bone tissue may be woven rather than lamellar in structure. Microradiographs show thick cement lines and active but distorted remodeling processes. Owing to the brittleness of the bones, pathologic fractures are common. The blood is generally normal with respect to calcium, phosphate, and alkaline phosphatase.

Storey (1960) has produced a condition simulating osteopetrosis in rats by intermittent administration of large doses of vitamin D. Alternate cycles of hypervitaminosis D rickets and of recovery result in the association of hypercalcification and osteoid tissue in the same bones at the same time; the bone changes in some respects resemble those seen in osteopetrosis. The conclusion is that the important mechanism in the pathogenesis of osteopetrosis is an accentuated rhythm of bone changes similar to those produced experimentally.

There are two living aquatic mammals of the order *Sirenia*, the manatee and the dugong, that have dense and massive bones, variously characterized as osteosclerosis, pachyostosis, and osteopetrosis. The bones of the axial skeleton, as well as of the upper extremities, consist almost entirely of compact bone and dense cancellous bone of a fetal type, with no medullary cavities and virtually no hemopoiesis. The thyroid gland is large and contains large follicles filled with colloid. With the aid of fossil material, representing extinct species, and because of a low basal metabolic rate, together with histologic evidence of low thyroid activity, there have been attempts to account for the skeletal peculiarities on an endocrine basis and to relate them to osteopetrosis as it occurs in man.

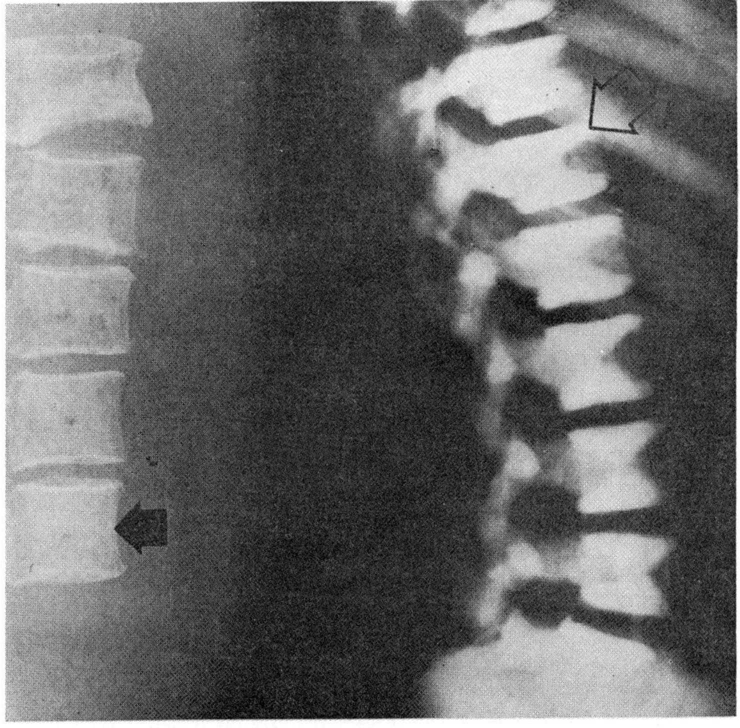

FIG. 49.—Roentgenograms of the lower spinal column of a 12-year-old girl with osteopetrosis and the spondylometer readings of five levels of density of cancellous bone. The most dense specimen of nonosteopetrotic vertebra (*left*) is relatively radiolucent compared with osteopetrotic bone. Owing to the inclusion of calcified cartilage, the osteopetrotic vertebral bodies are chalk-white (*right arrow*) with maximum radioopacity.

We have confirmed the findings of Fawcett (1942) that the entire skeleton of the Florida manatee, *Trichechus latirostis*, has some features in common with osteopetrosis. Osteoclasts are scarce, bone resorption is scanty, and periosteal bone formation continues in certain locations with relatively little internal remodeling throughout the life of the animal. There are, however, resorption cavities and other evidences of bone resorption, albeit at a slow rate. Moreover, we do not see large amounts of unabsorbed cartilage matrix. Pachyostosis may be a better name for the dense bones of the Sirenias. While the bones of the manatee resemble those in patients with marble-bone disease, and while they are suggestive of the changes associated with the anoxia of hypothyroidism, there is no real reason for equating osteopetrosis and pachyostosis.

Genetic Disorders of Connective Tissue

There is a group of skeletal disorders that are inheritable and represent inborn errors of metabolism, usually affecting both the collagen and the ground substance of bone. Their manifestations may not be confined to the skeleton, but since the mucopolysaccharides are highly concentrated in cartilage matrix and collagen is so densely packed in bone, the disorders may be brought into sharpest focus in the skeleton.

Hypophosphatasia, described as rickets with a deficiency of alkaline phosphatase, is a relatively rare metabolic disorder. It is believed to be inherited through an autosomal recessive gene. The bone lesions result from inability of osteoblasts to elaborate calcifiable organic matrix. The presence of phosphorylethanolamine in the blood and urine results from the inability of the insufficient phosphatase in the body to hydrolyze the ester phosphate linkage.

The *Hurler-Pfaundler syndrome*, also known as *gargoylism* or *lipochondrodystrophy*, an inborn error of connective tissue metabolism, presents an enzymatic defect in which there is accumulation and urinary excretion of large amounts of chondroitin sulfate B and heparin sulfate. It is characterized by grotesque facies and defects involving the entire skeleton. Genetically, two types are recognized: (1) a form transmitted by an autosomal recessive gene, affecting both males and females; and (2) a form transmitted as a sex-linked recessive, affecting only males.

The *Morquio syndrome*, or *chondro-osteodysplasia*, is a condition in which the chondrocytes fail to mature, ossification centers are disorganized, and there are extensive deformities of all the joints. It is characterized by small stature and short midphalanges of the hands and feet. There are deficiencies in matrix formation and diminished alkaline phosphatase activity in the epiphyseal plate.

Osteogenesis imperfecta is a connective tissue disease, transmitted as an autosomal dominant, in which the brittle and soft bones are usually the most prominent feature. The organic matrix of the bone is defective; collagen is mainly affected, and it has been suggested that the collagen is anomalous in its amino acid sequence.

The *Marfan syndrome*, in addition to having a predilection for the eye and aorta, is also manifest in the skeleton by excessive length of the round bones of the extremities and by defects in the ligaments and tendons, resulting in loose-jointedness. It is attributed to transmission as an autosomal dominant.

Alkaptonuria, recognized by characteristic changes in color in the urine, owing to the presence of large quantities of homogentisic acid, results from a lack of homogentisic acid oxidase. *Ochronosis*, or a dark pigmentation of cartilage, tendons, ligaments, and the sclera, is the most notable clinical feature. At autopsy, cartilage and fibrocartilage are deeply pigmented; pigmentation may also be observed in tendons and, in advanced cases, in the bones. According to Milch (1960), who has studied the condition in interrelated families, what has appeared to be a dominant form is probably a recessive form appearing in successive generations through the mating of homozygous affected persons with heterozygous carriers; consanguinous matings increase the likelihood of its occurrence.

CHAPTER XVI

Evolution of Bone

Looking back over four hundred million years in the fossil record, we see that teeth and bones are responsible for nearly all our present knowledge of the evolution of vertebrates. Rainwater and dissolved fluoride ion of the soil, filtering through the bones of buried animals, transform the apatite into fluorapatite. Because apatites and fluorapatites are among the most durable of minerals, they preserve the shape of the hard parts of the countless animals that have lived since the Cambrian period of the Paleozoic era. They preserve the skeletons of vast populations of millions of species of invertebrates and vertebrates that have become extinct since the beginning of geologic history. Some fossils are only a case or impression of the external form of a shell or bony skeleton; these are generally less informative than remnants of the original hard parts. The fossil record of the boneless vertebrates is almost unknown and must be supplemented with studies in comparative physiology if we are to learn about the origin and evolution of the skeleton. In this chapter, the vertebrate-fossil record will be discussed in the light of recent knowledge of calcium, phosphorus, and bone physiology in living vertebrates. It emphasizes the oneness of the fundamental problems of evolution, biology, and health sciences, gives a broad perspective of the past and present, and completes our introduction to the physiology of bone.

The relationships between the structure of the skeleton and the chemical composition of the blood of lower and higher living vertebrates suggest that the skeleton and the fluids of the body are parts of a single chemical system and constitute indivisible parts of a continuum. And as a corollary to that statement, it may be said that evolutionary changes in the structure of the endoskeleton and in the composition of body fluids are concurrent events. This is plain to see in the three great classes of fishes alive today: the hagfishes and lampreys, which possess no calcified tissues; the elasmobranchs—such as the shark, skate, and ray—which have a great deal of hard tissue in the form of calcified cartilage; and the teleost fishes, such as tuna and trout, which possess a skeleton of true bone tissue. The concentration of salts in the blood of the hagfishes is about 4 per cent (1,200 mmoles/liter), in the elasmobranchs about 3 per cent (900 mmoles/liter), and in the bony fishes only 1 per cent (300 mmoles/liter). The lower the total ion and total calcium content of the body fluids, the more active is the metabolism of the skeleton. As vertebrates develop a calcified internal skeleton, the body fluids also become more viscous and better aerated, and the concentrations of divalent ions, particularly calcium, become independent of the concentration of calcium in the external environment. Consequently, ionic and osmotic independence is achieved after the vertebrates have efficient mechanisms for calcium homeostasis. Homeostasis of calcium, phosphate, sodium, and other ions reaches a high degree of perfection with the appearance of the mammalian bone cell. Vertebrate evolution depends upon the homeostatic ability of the organism. Fitness in the neo-Darwinian sense is more than reproductive capacity and physical vigor; it is a complex expression of homeostatic ability. Homeostasis, therefore, is the arcanum of life.

Origin of Bone

When we observe the evolution of the skeleton from the Agnatha up the scale of the higher vertebrates, we see striking changes in the character of the bone tissue. In the terrestrial vertebrates the bone tissue is cellular and plays a very active part in metabolism. It is continually being remodeled, as old bone cells die and are replaced by new ones. The hard tissues of the lower vertebrates, by contrast, have more similarity to teeth; for the most part they are acellular, and they do not undergo internal remodeling.

Tarlo and Tarlo (1965) present the interesting suggestion that the elements of teeth and bone evolved at the same time in the form of armor in an ancient order of extinct vertebrates known as the Heterostraci. The Heterostraci belonged to the class Agnatha, also known as the ostracoderms. One example is the species *Pycnosteus tuberculatus*, which had a carapace made of three layers; a thin inner layer of laminated bonelike tissue called aspidin; a thick middle nonlaminated spongy layer of highly vascular modified aspidin; and an even thicker outer layer of tubulated dentin-like tissue arranged in ornate tubercles. There was no enamel in the Heterostraci.

A glossy hard outer covering of laminated tissue with a superficial appearance of enamel can be seen in the carapace of the Osteostraci, an order of ostracoderms that were contemporaries of the Heterostraci. A typical osteostracian is *Trematapsis mammillata*, described by Denison (1963). The middle and deep layers of its body armor consisted not of aspidin, but of hard tissue containing stellate cells resembling the osteocytes of the true bone of modern teleost fishes.

Nothing comparable to these mixtures of dental and bone tissues is found in the skeletons of any of the living vertebrates. Such relationships as exist between the highly active form of bone tissue found in modern higher vertebrates and the various forms of hard tissue found in fossil vertebrates are neither continuous nor interdependent. A fossil vertebrate with one form of bone appears in one stratum and vanishes completely in the next, presumably because some parts of the record are unpreserved. Another, with a different hard tissue, appears in the next era and may or may not have a relationship with the previous one. Only the overall plan seems to call for hard tissue first as armor, later as both teeth and armor, and still later as armor, teeth, and an endoskeleton, random or nonrandom in occurrence, in the various species of fossil fishes. Schaeffer (1961) summarizes the fossil record to show: (1) extinct jawless ostracoderms (benthonic cephalaspids) with an exoskeleton of bony armor from the Ordovician to the Devonian era; (2) extinct heavy-jawed placoderms with an endoskeleton of uncalcified or calcified cartilage and some perichondrial deposits of bone, but with most of the bone in dermal elements of the exoskeleton, in the period from the Silurian to the Permian; chondrichthyes (sharks, rays, skates, and ratfishes) with only cartilage, mostly calcified, but no bone in the endoskeleton, and an exoskeleton of teeth and placoid toothlike scales, from the Devonian to recent eras; osteichthyes (lungfishes, coelecanths, and typical recent bony fishes) with endoskeleton generally well ossified, although believed to show phyletic reduction or persistence of a fetus-like cartilaginous state in some groups, from the Devonian to recent eras.

Unlike cellular elements, the mineral composition of vertebrate hard tissues has not changed in over four hundred million years. It is an apatitic calcium phosphate in the extinct Agnatha as in the living mammals. The calcium stored in apatite serves manifold physiologic functions: it promotes growth, acts as cofactor for clotting of blood, controls permeability of membranes to water, reduces neuromuscular irritability, and triggers the contraction of muscle. Phosphorus stored in apatite is equally vital and is clearly responsible for the superiority of the vertebrates over all other living things. Phosphorus enters into complex chemical combinations with lipids, carbohydrates, and proteins to form the very basis of the chemistry of living cells. Phosphorus is essential for both synthesis and breakdown of glycogen for the release of energy. The organism is enabled to obtain a continuous supply of phosphorus as inorganic phosphate by the equilibrium between readily available stores of phosphate ion and phosphate in solution in the body fluids. This makes a virtually inexhaustible, self-replenishing source of supply. The system possesses incredible efficiency, even buffers the body fluid and acts to excrete excess acids in the urine. Thus the skeletal system both dispenses and conserves phosphorus, the one element that is more difficult than any other for plants and animals to acquire in open competition in nature.

A physiologist's interpretation of the fossil record is that the fish that possessed hard tissue only in the form of acellular armor and teeth had a skeletal system inadequate for the metabolic needs of higher organisms. Possibly this inadequacy contributed to their extinction. All the fast-moving living vertebrates, on the other hand, possess an internal skeleton that provides a reservoir of calcium and phosphorus in a readily available and utilizable ionic form. Slower moving elasmobranchs and the chimaeras have cartilage, rather than bone, in the internal skeleton, and have contrived, as we shall see, a peculiar body-fluid chemistry to accompany it.

Recent investigations of the biochemistry of the body fluids suggest that bone is an organ of adaptation of marine vertebrates and is active during migration into fresh water. To survive in fresh water, a marine animal must be able to maintain the level of 2.5 mmoles/liter of calcium in its body fluids, irrespective of the low concentration of this element (only 0.75 mmoles/liter) in the surrounding environment. Radioisotope kinetic studies are few, but they suffice to indicate that skeletal tissues, whether cellular or acellular, are relatively inactive in marine environments and clearly active in fresh-water habitats. Living vertebrates achieve ionic independence of their external environment through four separate but interrelated mechanisms: (1) membrane phenomena, including protein binding of metal ions; (2) ion exchange in calcified tissues; (3) vitamin D metabolism; and (4) action of parathyroid hormone upon the kidney and bone cells. From a study of these four mechanisms, we are not able to answer the question of the habitat of the extinct earliest bony vertebrates, but we should be able to trace some important pathways of the evolution of skeletal tissues of higher animals.

Membrane Phenomena

The archaic mechanism for maintaining calcium homeostasis is seen in the cyclostomes—the hagfishes and lampreys. These animals have no hard tissue in the skeleton and must regulate calcium concentration solely by controlling ion transfer across membranes of the gills, intestines, skin, and kidneys. In addition, calcium can also be removed from or returned to the circulating fluids by reactions with proteins, mucoproteins, and lipoproteins of various intra- and extracellular membranes. Compared with that of higher vertebrates, the capacity of these animals for adaptation is limited. The hagfishes live at the bottom of the sea and maintain a level of total ions in the blood that is the same as the ion level of the surrounding water, more than four times higher than the level found in higher vertebrates. Their level of calcium is 5–5.5 mmoles/liter, over twice that of any bony vertebrate.

The late Homer Smith (1936), celebrated American philosopher and physiologist, correlated the body chemistry of the hagfish with the low capacity of its kidney to filter blood. He noted that the lamprey evolved a more efficient and elaborate kidney than the hagfish, and regarded this step as the parting of the ways between the invertebrates and the vertebrates. Urist and van de Putte (1967) contend that that historic moment occurred earlier and possibly in a marine habitat, because a very fundamental distinguishing feature of vertebrate body chemistry is the reduction in the concentration of calcium in the extracellular fluid. Marine invertebrates have levels of calcium the same as or higher than that of sea water, while the marine vertebrates *always* have calcium levels only one-half to one-fourth that of the environment, depending upon whether homeostasis is sustained by only soft tissue or also by various hard tissues and associated hormonal factors.

Gill membranes, for example, may act as a calcium pump, transferring the calcium from fresh-water streams with concentrations of 0.7 mmoles/liter to the circulating fluids of the body with ion concentrations of over 1.25 mmoles/liter. In this way the animal must absorb calcium against a concentration gradient. The mechanism is inefficient in that it requires a lower vertebrate like the lamprey to circulate enormous volumes of water through its gill chambers and kidneys. Supplemented by microscopic deposits of calcium phosphate in the inner ear, in *statoliths*, the lamprey is able to obtain enough phosphate ions to thrive and reproduce in inland lakes. In fact, one species, *Petromyzon marinus*, is so abundant in the Great Lakes region of the United States that it has all but destroyed the trout and whitefish industry. Instead of migrating out to sea, the adult lamprey remains in the freshwater lakes, preys upon various species of large fish, and thereby completes the parasitic phase of its life cycle. Carlström (1963) observed that the cyclostomes are the only vertebrates with statoliths of calcium phosphate in their inner ears. All vertebrates having a calcified endoskeleton, including man, have statoliths composed of calcium carbonate. It is as though lampreys and hagfishes, having no tissue inside the skeleton to store mineral, located an incredibly small amount of matrix to hold a precious supply of phosphorus.

According to Romer (1946), sometime before the end of the Devonian era the Ostracodermi dispensed with their protective armor and gave rise to the ancestors of the present-day lampreys. Since soft-bodied animals leave little or no trace of themselves in the fossil record, there is no way to prove or disprove this point of view. Only the vascular or dermal layer of the armor of the fossil vertebrates can be regarded as the forerunner of bone tissue. Judging from the structure of Ordovician fossils, armor had a physiologic activity comparable to that of the teeth of modern vertebrates—that is, it could have entered into ion exchange processes. Mineralized tissue comparable to the bones of living animals, with the capacity to turn over large volumes of calcium, phosphorus, and protein, appears in the Devonian era with the evolution of actinopterygian ancestors of modern teleost fishes.

Physiology: Exoskeletal and Endoskeletal

Lower vertebrates like the elasmobranchs, which do not possess bone tissue, store apatite in an endoskeleton of calcified cartilage and in an exoskeleton of teeth and denticles. Present-day sharks, skates, and rays are covered with dental armor or placoid scales and possess well-developed jaws equipped with many rows of teeth. Each tooth is covered with a dense transparent layer of vitrodentin (durodentin). Controversy exists as to whether the vitrodentin of fishes is fundamentally the same as tetrapod enamel. Unit-cell dimensions of shark and bony-fish apatites in both *c* and *a* axes are shorter than in apatites obtained from the teeth of land-dwelling vertebrates. Electron micrographs of the crystal structure and amino acid analysis of the organic matrix reveal other significant differences. Thus the process of evolution involves alterations or modifications at all levels of structure, chemical, molecular, and morphologic, simultaneously. Evolution culminates in the Mammalia with hard dental enamel that has beautiful prismatic crystals secreted by ameloblasts; some fossil amphibians and only a few reptiles have achieved it in a modified form.

The combination of teeth, scales, and calcified cartilage represents a large amount of hard tissue but does not have the characteristic of bone. The endoskeleton of the shark is composed entirely of cartilage, only partly calcified. The calcium deposits are highly reactive with tetracycline, alizarin, fluoride, radioisotopes, and other mineral-seeking ions. In sharks, the calcium deposits are arranged in the interior of the vertebral centra in elaborate designs that are frequently representative of the genus (Fig. 50). According to the fossil record, elasmobranchs are over a hundred million years more recent than the Osteostraci, and are therefore not truly primitive vertebrates. Some writers trace the ancestry of the elasmobranchs and the holocephalans back to a branch of vertebrates called the Placodermi, a class of armored fishes that became extinct about 350 million years ago. The placoderms had dermal armor, with some calcified cartilage but little or no bone in the endoskeleton. They were contemporaries of both the ostracoderms and the early Devonian higher bony fishes. Because the endoskeleton had large amounts of calcified cartilage, the placoderms' body-fluid ion concentrations in all probability were comparable with those of modern elasmobranchs.

The chemistry of the body fluids of the elasmobranchs and holocephalans is so different from that of other fishes that it can be

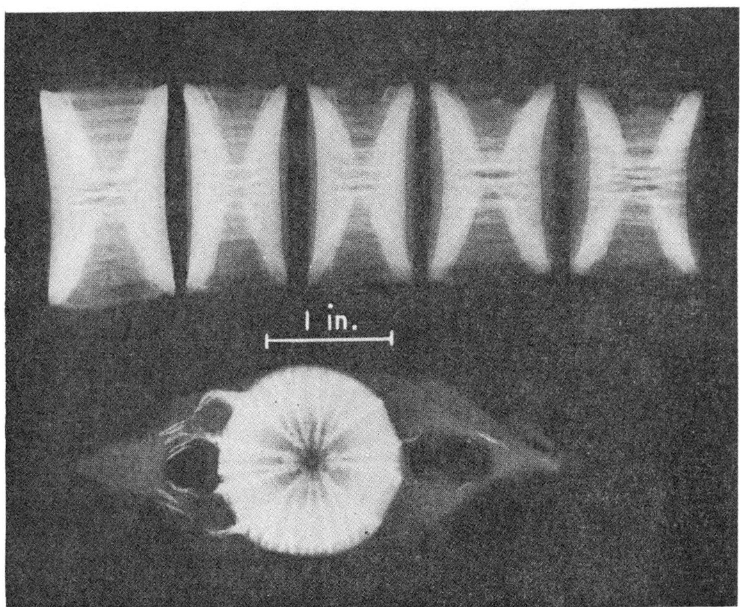

FIG. 50.—Roentgenograms of a segment from the lumbar region of a large shark. The radioopaque areas represent deposits of calcified cartilage. An end-view of one vertebral body (*bottom*) from the shark Eulamia obscura (*top*) reveals the pattern of the calcified cartilage characteristic of the genus.

used for classification or broad identification (Table 11). The total ion and total calcium concentrations are approximately half that of sea water, and approximately twice that of the blood plasma of bony vertebrates. In addition, urea and trimethylamine oxide are retained in the body fluids to raise the osmotic pressure of the blood to that of sea water. The gill membranes and kidney tubules have a relatively *low* permeability to urea, and all the tissues and organs of elasmobranchs are adapted to concentrations that are twenty to thirty times higher than those found in other animals. Strangely enough, this same process of urea retention is used by estivating lungfish and by an amphibian, the crab-eating frog, *Rana cancrivora*, when it migrates to the sea. The frog skin, relatively permeable to salts and water, becomes more impermeable to urea, and has independently reorganized this specialized process of osmoregulation.

The elasmobranchs clearly represent a group of vertebrates that have retained old biochemical mechanisms—such as urea retention—while instituting a new one, storage of calcium and phos-

TABLE 11

KEY TO CHEMICAL IDENTIFICATION OF THE SERUMS OF MAJOR GROUPS OF SOME LOWER VERTEBRATES

(Range of Values in mmoles/l)

Group	Na	Ca	Urea	Total Ion Concentration
Marine-Cyclostome	500–600	5–6 *	0.05–0.1	1,000–1,200
Holocephali	260–270	4.5–5.5	300–350	500–550†
Marine Elasmobranch	225–250	4.0–5.0	250–330	480–490
Fresh-Water Elasmobranch	175–200	3.0–3.5	100–150	350–400
Coelacanthini	166–170	3.0–3.5	350–400	325–375
Marine Teleosts	165–175	2.5–3.5	0.1–0.2	300–350
Fresh-Water Teleosts, or Potamodromous Lampreys	130–140	2.3–2.5	0.1–0.2	250–275
Lampreys, Migrating; Potamodromous	90–100	2.2–2.5	0.1–0.2	175–200
Spawning King Salmon, only during spawning	K=0.1–0.5 Na=150–140	2.2–2.5	0.1–0.2	275–285
Sturgeon, either Marine or Fresh Water	130–140	1.8–2.0	0.1–0.2	275

* Crustaceans, either marine or fresh water, display as high or even higher values of hemolymph calcium, but, to a large extent, this is bound to protein and may be in transport from gastroliths to shell during intermolt.

† Marine reptiles, i.e., turtle, *Caretta caretta*, may present also a serum total ion concentration of over 500 mmoles/l. (Potts, W. T. W., and Parry, G.: Osmotic and ionic regulation in animals. New York, Macmillan Co., 1964.)

phorus in calcified cartilage. The deposits are more readily accessible for ion exchange reaction than those in teeth, scales, or exoskeletal bone. A highly reactive reservoir of calcium and phosphorus in calcified cartilage in the interior of the body probably aids the fish during migration from the sea into fresh-water rivers and lakes. One species, *Carcharhinus leucas*, can thrive in a low-calcium environment in inland lakes in many parts of the world, such as Nicaragua, New Guinea, and India.

Bone Tissue and Vitamin D Metabolism

Osteichthyes, both extinct and living bony fishes, consist of actinopterygians (typical bony fishes), dipnoans (lungfishes), and crossopterygians (lobe-finned fishes); they generally have had, or still have, a well-ossified endoskeleton. Although the fossil evidence may not be well documented, and although recent forms have gone back and forth between fresh-water and marine habitats in geologic history, Romer (1946) proposes that true bony fishes evolved in fresh water. If fresh-water origin, a reduced exoskeleton, and a well-ossified endoskeleton can be correlated, they would seem to point to the importance of cellular bones as organs of adaptation and calcium homeostasis in evolution.

Endoskeletal bone appears to replace cartilage by means of perichondrial and endochondral ossification, and exoskeletal or dermal bone regresses or assumes the form of intramembranous ossification of various parts—for example, the vault of the cranium of most mammals. Dipnoan and crossopterygian fishes show reduced amounts of exoskeletal bone and retention or increase of endoskeletal bone. The relatively large actinopterygian assemblage consisting of chondrosteans (sturgeon), holosteans (gar, pike), and teleosteans (recent true bony fishes) exhibits extraordinary variability. Some chondrosteans have mostly cartilage and very little bone in the endoskeleton; others have the reverse. In general, the teleosts, which are the most advanced forms of actinopterygians, have the most marked reduction in exoskeleton and striking increase in endoskeleton, particularly bone containing viable true osteocytes. Acellular bone, found mostly in recent marine teleost fishes, often contains degenerate or calcified bone cells, and accordingly displays physiologically inactive osteocytes.

Osteichthyes have highly active cellular bone when found in

fresh-water habitats. In marine fishes in which the skeleton is acellular or relatively inactive, morphogenesis assumes two patterns. The bone cells may secrete a calcifiable matrix but remain outside the tissue, or the cells may become embedded in the tissue, die, and calcify within the matrix. Acellular bone, however, does not undergo internal remodeling in the lifetime of the fish and contributes relatively little to the turnover of calcium in the metabolic processes of the body. Marine species have calcium readily available in solution in the external environment in concentrations about four times higher than in the blood. In fresh-water streams and rivers, bone tissue is absolutely essential for instantaneous turnover and regulation of calcium, phosphate, and other electrolytes found in the blood.

Bone tissue performs the function of a closed-cycle storage unit or servo system for calcium, phosphorus, and sodium homeostasis. In the bony fishes, vitamin D metabolism evolved to increase the rate of turnover of calcium, and thereby also other ions. Because vitamin D increases the rate of absorption of calcium and phosphorus, it is metabolized in larger quantities by bony fishes in fresh water. In sea water, where the concentration of calcium is so high that the exogenous sources can take over the physiologic functions of the skeleton, vitamin D is not necessary. For this reason, perhaps, teleosts that do not migrate into fresh water, such as cod and tuna, accumulate large concentrations of vitamin D in the liver. Until relatively recently, cod-liver oil was of great importance to man for prevention of rickets and osteomalacia. Now vitamin D is synthesized by irradiation of ergosterol, and fish-liver oil is rarely prescribed by physicians.

Parathyroid glands seem not to exist in teleost fishes, or at least have not yet been definitely identified. Ultimobranchial bodies, however, from which the parathyroids are derived, are found to become hyperplastic in the cave-dwelling fish *Astyanax mexicanus*. Whether the response is to ultraviolet radiation and vitamin D metabolism of skin, or to pituitary gland response to visual light perception, or to some other reactions, remains to be determined. Urist and van de Putte (1967) recently reported that in the sturgeon, a specialized survivor of a primitive actinopterygian (believed by paleontologists to have lost much endochondral bone), the level of the serum calcium is low, only 2–2.2 mmoles/liter. The sturgeon also is virtually devoid of vitamin D in the liver, even when it is taken in a marine habitat. In contrast to the sturgeon, migratory teleosts, even from the same waters, have more than ample endoskeletal bone and store vitamin D in large quantities. In fishes that have ample vitamin D and endoskeletal bone, calcium and phosphorus metabolism is so efficient that teleosts like the salmon can migrate hundreds of miles upstream and support high-energy metabolism for fast swimming without feeding for many weeks. The role of the thyroid gland in calcium metabolism of fishes, including the phylogenetic history of the newly discovered hormone calcitonin, is a fertile field for investigation.

Terrestrial Life, Parathyroids, and Bone Remodeling

Amphibians, reptiles, birds, and mammals not only have a well-developed internal bony framework for mechanical purposes, but also have a cycle of cellular elements, osteoblasts, osteocytes, and osteoclasts to deposit new minerals and mobilize inaccessible or remote parts of the mineral stores. The bone is arranged in two forms: (1) dermal or exoskeletal, and (2) nondermal or endoskeletal. Dermal bone is intramembranous bone formed in skin for protection or support of vital soft parts. All dermal bone is intramembranous, but not all intramembranous bone is dermal bone. In man, for example, the cranium is membrane bone, but it has no relation to the dermis. It is intramembranous bone nevertheless, and may not have evolved from the dermal head plates of the ancient vertebrates. The carapace of the turtle is a striking example of true dermal bone.

Three events were interrelated in the rise of the amphibia: (1) the differentiation of highly active cellular elements of endoskeletal and exoskeletal bones; (2) the evolution of the crossopterygians, which migrated from an aquatic habitat onto land; and (3) the evolution of the parathyroid glands. Vitamin D metabolism appears earlier in the teleost fishes. Inasmuch as parathyroid hormone is ineffectual in mammals in the absence of vitamin D, it is reasonable to assume that the evolution of the parathyroid glands was dependent upon the development of enzyme systems for vitamin D metabolism. Additional evidence for this sequence of events comes from the fact that injections of bovine parathyroid extract are ineffective in teleosts and elasmobranchs, but can elevate the extracellular fluid calcium within three hours in amphibians and all other higher vertebrates. Thus a vitamin D–parathyroid hormone synergism evolved to regulate osteoblastic, osteocytic, and osteoclastic activity, and to maintain a high degree of precision of calcium and phosphorus homeostasis. This was achieved by earliest cartilaginous vertebrates first through binding reactions of membrane and protein calcium, then by the bony fishes by deposition of apatite in an endoskeleton, then by the fresh-water fishes by supplementation with vitamin D metabolism to increase the rate of calcium and phosphate turnover, and ultimately by the crossopterygian fishes amphibians, and reptiles through fine regulation by a negative feedback control by the action of the parathyroid hormone on renal tubules and bone cells.

Bibliography

CHAPTER II

Bone as a Tissue

Bélanger, L. 1965. Osteolysis: An outlook on its mechanism and its causation. *In:* P. J. Gaillard, R. V. Talmage, and A. M. Budy (eds.), The parathyroid glands, pp. 137–43. Chicago: The University of Chicago Press.

Bloom, W., and Fawcett, D. W. 1968. A textbook of histology. 9th ed. Philadelphia: W. B. Saunders Co.

Bourne, G. H. (ed.). 1956. The biochemistry and physiology of bone. New York: Academic Press, Inc.

Cooper, R. H., Milgrim, J. W., and Robinson, R. A. 1966. Morphology of the osteon. An electron microscopic study, J. Bone Jt. Surg. 48-A: 1239–71.

Fawcett, D. W. 1966. The cell: Its organelles and inclusions. An atlas of fine structure. Philadelphia: W. B. Saunders Co.

Frost, H. M. (ed.). 1964. Bone biodynamics. Boston: Little, Brown and Co.

Hancox, N. M. and Boothroyd, B. 1965. Electron microscopy of the early stages of osteogenesis, Clin. Orthop. 40:153–61.

Heller-Steinberg, M. 1951. Ground substance, bone salts, and cellular activity in bone formation and destruction, Am. J. Anat. 89:347–79.

Lipp, W. 1954. Neuuntersuchungen des Knochengewebes. II. Histologisch erfassbare Lebensäusserungen der Knochenzellen, Acta Anat. 22:151–201.

McLean, F. C., and Budy, A. M. 1959. Connective and supporting tissues: Bone, Ann. Rev. Physiol. 21:69–90.

Nelson, G. E., Jr., Kelly, P. J., Peterson, L. F. A., and Janes, J. M. 1960. Blood supply of the human tibia, J. Bone Jt. Surg. 42-A:625–36.

Owen, M. 1967. Uptake of ^{3}H-uridine into precursor pools and RNA in osteogenic cells, J. Cell. Sci. 2:39–56.

Robinson, R. A., and Cameron, D. A. 1958. Electron microscopy of the primary spongiosa of the metaphysis at the distal end of the femur in the newborn infant, J. Bone Jt. Surg. 40-A:687–97.

———. 1964. Bone. *In:* S. M. Kurtz (ed.), Electron microscopic anatomy, pp. 315–40. New York: Academic Press, Inc.

Rodahl, K., Nicholson, J. T., and Brown, E. M., Jr. (eds.). 1960. Bone as a tissue. New York: McGraw-Hill Book Co., Inc.

Sledge, C. B. 1966. Some morphologic and experimental aspects of limb development, Clin. Orthop. 44:241–64.

Urist, M. R., and McLean, F. C. 1957. Accumulation of mast cells in endosteum of bone of calcium-deficient rats, A.M.A. Arch. Path. 63:239–51.

Wassermann, F., and Yaeger, J. A. 1965. Fine structure of the osteocyte capsule and of the wall of the lacunae in bone. Z. Zellforsch. 67:636–52.

Weidenreich, F. 1930. Das Knochengewebe. *In:* W. von Möllendorff (ed.), Handbuch der mikroskopischen Anatomie des Menschen, 2, Part II, 391–520. Berlin: J. Springer.

Weinmann, J. P., and Sicher, H. 1955. Bone and bones: Fundamentals of bone biology. 2d ed. St. Louis: C. V. Mosby Co.

Young, R. W. 1964. Specialization of bone cells. *In:* H. M. Frost (ed.), Bone biodynamics, pp. 117–39. Boston: Little, Brown and Co.

CHAPTER III

Histogenesis and Organization of Bone

Amprino, R. 1965. Bone structure and function. *In:* W. Bargman (ed.), Aus der Werkstaat der Anatomen, pp. 1–16. Stuttgart: Georg Thieme Verlag.

Bassett, C. A. L. 1965. Electrical effects in bone. Scient. Amer. 213:18–25.

Bassett, C. A. L., Pawluk, R. J., and Becker, R. C. 1964. Effects of electric currents on bone *in vivo*, Nature 204:652–54.

Becker, R. O., and Bachman, C. H. 1965. Bioelectric effects in tissue, Clin. Orthop. 43:251–53.

Bloom, W., and Bloom, M. A. 1940. Calcification and ossification. Calcification of developing bone in embryonic and newborn rats, Anat. Rec. 78:497–523.

Bridges, J. B., and Pritchard, J. J. 1958. Bone and cartilage induction in the rabbit, J. Anat. 92:28–38.

Dhem, A. 1967. Le remaniement de l'os adulte. Brussels: Editions Arscia.

DHEM, A., and VINCENT, A. 1965. Analyse microradiographique du squelette, Recipe 10:515–36.

ENGSTRÖM, A., and FINEAN, J. B. 1967. Biological ultrastructure, 2d ed. New York: Academic Press, Inc.

FROST, H. M. 1963. Bone remodelling dynamics. Springfield, Ill.: Charles C Thomas.

FROST, H. M., and VILLANUEVA, A. R. 1960. Observations on osteoid seams, Henry Ford Hosp. Med. Bull. 8:212–19.

FROST, H. M., VILLANUEVA, A. R., and ROTH, H. 1960. Measurement of bone formation in a 57-year-old man by means of tetracyclines, Henry Ford Hosp. Med. Bull. 8:239–54.

HAUMONT, S. 1963. Le zinc dans le tissu osseux. Brussels: Editions Arscia.

HAUMONT, S., and MCLEAN, F. C. 1966. Zinc and the physiology of bone. *In:* A. S. PRASAD (ed.), Zinc metabolism, pp. 169–86. Springfield, Ill.: Charles C Thomas.

KNESE, K.-H. 1963. Zell- und Faserstruktur des Knochengewebes, Acta Anat. 53:369–94.

———. 1966. Zytogenese und topochemische Reaktion der frühen und späten epitheloiden Osteoblasten, Z. Zellforsch. 69:93–128.

LACROIX, P. 1951. The organization of bones. Philadelphia: Blakiston Co.

LEBLOND, C. P., and LACROIX, P. 1959. Réactions de la zone de calcification dans les ostéones en formation, C.R. Acad. Sci. 249:934–36.

LÖE, H. 1959. Bone tissue formation. A morphological and histochemical study, Acta Odontol. Scandinav. *Suppl.* 27, 17:311–427.

MCLEAN, F. C. 1958. The ultrastructure and function of bone, Science 127:451–56.

———. 1965. Internal remodeling of compact bone. *In:* L. J. RICHELLE and M. J. DALLEMAGNE (eds.), Calcified tissues, pp. 1–9. Liège: University of Liège.

MCLEAN, F. C., and BLOOM, W. 1940. Calcification and ossification. Calcification in normal growing bone, Anat. Rec. 78:333–59.

MCLEAN, F. C., and ROWLAND, R. E. 1963. Internal remodeling of compact bone. *In:* R. F. SOGNNAES (ed.), Mechanisms of hard tissue destruction, pp. 371–83. Washington, D.C.: Am. Assn. Adv. Science.

MURRAY, P. D. F. 1936. Bones. Cambridge: The University Press.

NEUMAN, W. F., and MULRYAN, B. J. 1967. Synthetic hydroxyapatite crystals. III. The carbonate system, Calcified Tissue Res. 1:94–104.

POMMER, G. 1885. Untersuchungen über Osteomalacie und Rachitis, nebst Beiträgen zur Kenntnis der Knochenresorption und -apposition in verschiedenen Altersperioden und der durchbohrenden Gefässe. Leipzig: F. C. W. Vogel.

SHAMOS, M. H., and LAVINE, L. S. 1964. Physical bases for bioelectric effects in mineralized tissue, Clin. Orthop. 35:177–88.

———. 1965. Bioelectric effects in tissue, Clin. Orthop. 43:254–56.

SOGNNAES, R. F. (ed.). 1960. Calcification in biological systems. Washington, D.C.: Am. Assn. Adv. Science.

———. 1963. Mechanisms of hard tissue destruction. Washington, D.C.: Am. Assn. Adv. Science.

STRANDH, J. 1961. Microchemical studies on single haversian systems, Biochim. Biol. Sper. 1:60–65.

TOMES, J., and DE MORGAN, C. 1853. Observations on the structure and development of bone, Phil. Trans. Roy. Soc. London 143:109–39.

TONNA, E. A., and PILLSBURY, N. 1959. Mitochondrial changes associated with aging of periosteal osteoblasts, Anat. Rec. 134:739–60.

TRUETA, J. 1963. The role of the vessels in osteogenesis, J. Bone Jt. Surg. 45-B:402–18.

TRUETA, J., and AMATO, V. P. 1960. The vascular contribution to osteogenesis. III. Changes in the growth cartilage caused by experimentally induced ischaemia, J. Bone Jt. Surg. 42-B:571–87.

VERNINO, D. M., and LASKIN, D. M. 1960. Sex chromatin in mammalian bone, Science 132:675–76.

VINCENT, J. 1957. Les remaniements de l'os compact marqué à l'aide de plomb, Rev. Belg. Path. 26:161–68.

VINCENT, J., and HAUMONT, S. 1960. Identification autoradiographique des ostéones métaboliques après administration de Ca 45, Rev. Franç. Étud. Clin. Biol. 5:348–53.

WALLGREN, G. 1957. Biophysical analyses of the formation and structure of human fetal bone. A microradiographic study, Acta Paediat., *Suppl.* 113:1–80.

WOLFF, J. 1892. Das Gesetz der Transformation der Knochen, Berlin.

CHAPTER IV

STRUCTURE AND CHEMICAL COMPOSITION OF BONE MATRIX

BELCHIER, J. 1736*a*. An account of the bones of animals being changed to a red colour by aliment only, Phil. Trans. 39:287–88.

———. 1736*b*. A further account of the bones of animals being made red by aliment only, Phil. Trans. 39:299–300.

BERGSMA, D., and MILCH, R. A. (eds.). 1966. Structural organization of the skeleton: A symposium. Birth Defects Orig. Art. Ser. 2.

DORFMAN, A. 1959. The biochemistry of connective tissue, J. Chron. Dis. 10:403–17.

EASTOE, J. E., and EASTOE, B. 1954. The organic constituents of mammalian compact bone, Biochem. J. 57:453–59.

ENGFELDT, B., and STRANDH, J. 1960. Microchemical and biophysical studies of normal human compact bone tissue, with special reference to the organic component, Clin. Orthop. 17:63–68.

GERSH, I., and CATCHPOLE, H. R. 1960. The nature of ground substance of connective tissue, Perspectives Biol. Med. 3:282–319.

GLIMCHER, M. J., and KATZ, E. P. 1965. The organization of collagen in bone: The role of non-covalent bonds in the relative insolubility of bone collagen, J. Ultrastruct. Res. 12:705–29.

GLIMCHER, M. J., KATZ, E. P., and TRAVIS, D. F. 1965. The solubilization and reconstitution of bone collagen, J. Ultrastruct. Res. 13:261–74.

GROSS, J. 1964. Studies on the biology of connective tissues: Remodeling of collagen in metamorphosis, Medicine 43:291–303.

HERRING, G. M. 1964. Chemistry of the bone matrix, Clin. Orthop. 36: 169–83.

IRVING, J. T. 1960. Histochemical changes in the early stages of calcification, Clin. Orthop. 17:92–102.

JACKSON, S. FITTON, HARKNESS, R. D., PARTRIDGE, S. M., and TRISTRAM, G. H. (eds.). 1965. Structure and function of connective and skeletal tissue. London: Butterworth.

KAUFMAN, E. J., GLIMCHER, M. J., MECHANIC, G. L., and GOLDHABER, P. 1965. Collagenolytic activity during active bone resorption in tissue culture, Proc. Soc. Exptl. Biol. (N.Y.) 120:632–37.

MCCLUSKEY, R. T., and THOMAS, L. 1958. The removal of cartilage matrix, *in vivo*, by papain. Identification of crystalline papain protease as the cause of the phenomenon, J. Exptl. Med. 108:371–84.

MATHEWS, M. B., and GLAGOV, S. 1966. Acid mucopolysaccharide patterns in aging human cartilage, J. Clin. Invest. 45:1103–11.

MILCH, R. A., RALL, D. P., and TOBIE, J. E. 1958. Fluorescence of tetracycline antibiotics in bone, J. Bone Jt. Surg. 40-A:897–910.

PETRUSKA, J. A., and HODGE, A. J. 1963. Recent studies with the electron microscope on ordered aggregates of the tropocollagen molecule. *In:* G. N. RAMACHANDRAN (ed.), Aspects of protein structure; Proceedings of a symposium. New York: Academic Press, Inc.

PONSETI, I. V. 1957. Skeletal lesions produced by aminonitriles, Clin. Orthop. 9:131–44.

ROBINSON, R. A., and ELLIOTT, S. R. 1957. The water content of bone. I. The mass of water, inorganic crystals, organic matrix, and "CO_2 space" components in a unit volume of dog bone, J. Bone Jt. Surg. 39-A: 167–88.

ROGERS, H. J. 1949. Concentration and distribution of polysaccharides in human cortical bone and the dentine of teeth, Nature 164:625–26.

SCHUBERT, M., and HAMERMAN, D. 1956. Metachromasia: Chemical theory and histochemical use, J. Histochem. Cytochem. 4:159–89.

SEIFTER, S., FRANZBLAU, C., HARPER, E., and CALLOP, P. M. 1965. Special aspects of the primary structure of collagen. *In:* S. FITTON JACKSON *et al.* (eds.), Structure and function of connective tissue. London: Butterworth.

UDENFRIEND, S. 1966. Formation of hydroxyproline in collagen, Science 152:1335–40.

VEIS, A. 1964. The macromolecular chemistry of gelatin. New York: Academic Press, Inc.

WASSERMANN, F. 1963. The ground substance of connective tissue in a foreshortened historical perspective. *In:* W. BARGMAN (ed.), Aus der Werkstatt der Anatomen, 177–92. Stuttgart: Georg Thieme Verlag.

WISLOCKI, G. B., BUNTING, H., and DEMPSEY, E. W. 1947. Metachromasia in mammalian tissues and its relationship to mucopolysaccharides, Am. J. Anat. 81:1–37.

WOODS, J. F., and NICHOLS, G., JR. 1965. Collagenolytic activity in rat bone cells. Characteristics and intracellular location, J. Cell Biol. 26: 747–57.

CHAPTER V

CRYSTAL STRUCTURE AND CHEMICAL COMPOSITION OF BONE MINERAL

ARMSTRONG, W. D., and SINGER, L. 1965. Composition and constitution of the mineral phase of bone, Clin. Orthop. 38:179–90.

BACHRA, B. N. 1966. Calcification: A problem in molecular biology. *In:* P. M. JAMES, K. E. KÖNIG, and H. R. HELD (eds.), Adv. in fluorine research and dental caries prevention, 4:95–101.

BJERRUM, N. 1959. Calcium orthophosphates, Harwell, Berkshire: Atomic Energy Research Establishment, United Kingdom.

BOGERT, L. J., and HASTINGS, A. B. 1931. The calcium salts of bone, J. Biol. Chem. 94:473–81.

BROWN, W. E. 1962. Octacalcium phosphate and hydroxyapatite, Nature 196:1048–50.

———. 1966. Crystal growth of bone mineral, Clin. Orthop. 44:205–20.

BROWN, W. E., SMITH, J. P., LEHR, J. R., and FRAZIER, A. W. 1962. Crystallographic and chemical relations between octacalcium phosphate and hydroxyapatite, Nature 196:1050–54.

CARLSTRÖM, D. 1955. X-ray crystallographic studies on apatites and calcified structures, Acta Radiol. *Suppl.* 121:1–59.

CARTIER, P., and PICARD, J. 1955. La minéralisation du cartilage *in vitro*, Bull. Soc. Chim. Biol. 37:485–94.

DALLEMAGNE, M. J. 1952. Some recent facts about the properties of tricalcium phosphate and the composition of the bone salt, Trans. Macy Conf. on Metabolic Interrelations 4:154–68.

EANES, E. D., GILLESSEN, I. H., and POSNER, A. S. 1965. Intermediate states in the precipitation of hydroxyapatite, Nature 208:365–67.

EANES, E. D., and POSNER, A. S. 1965. Kinetics and mechanism of conversion of noncrystalline calcium phosphate to crystalline hydroxyapatite, Trans. N.Y. Acad. Sci. 28:233–41.

EDELMAN, L. S., JAMES, A. H., BADEN, H., and MOORE, F. D. 1954. Electrolyte composition of bone and the penetration of radiosodium and deuterium oxide into dog and human bone, J. Clin. Invest. 33:122–31.

EISENBERGER, S., LEHRMAN, M., and TURNER, W. D. 1940. The basic calcium phosphates and related systems: Some theoretical and practical aspects, Chem. Rev. 26:257–96.

ENGSTRÖM, A. 1960. The structure of bone: An excursion into molecular biology, Clin. Orthop. 17:34–37.

FERNÁNDEZ-MORÁN, H., and ENGSTRÖM, A. 1957. Electron microscopy and X-ray diffraction of bone, Biochim. Biophys. Acta 23:260–64.

MCCONNELL, D. 1965. Crystal chemistry of hydroxyapatite. Its relation to bone mineral, Arch. Oral Biol. 10:421–31.

MACGREGOR, J. E., and BROWN, W. E. 1965. Blood-bone equilibrium in calcium homeostasis, Nature 205:359–61.

MCLEAN, F. C., and BUDY, A. M. 1964. Radiation, isotopes, and bone. New York: Academic Press, Inc.

MELLORS, R. C. 1964. Electron probe microanalysis, Lab. Invest. 13:183–95.

MOLNAR, Z. 1960. Additional observations on bone crystal dimensions, Clin. Orthop. 17:38–42.

NEUMAN, W. F., and MULRYAN, B. J. 1967. Synthetic hydroxyapatite crystals. III. The carbonate system, Calcified Tissue Res. 1:94–104.

NEUMAN, W. F., and NEUMAN, M. W. 1958. The chemical dynamics of bone mineral. Chicago: The University of Chicago Press.

POSNER, A. S., HARPER, R. A., and MULLER, S. A. 1965. Age changes in the crystal chemistry of bone apatite, Ann. N.Y. Acad. Sci. 131:421–31.

POSNER, A. S., and PERLOFF, A. 1957. Apatites deficient in divalent cations, J. Res. Natl. Bureau Standards 58:279–86.

QUINAUX, N., and RICHELLE, L. J. 1967. X-ray diffraction and infra-red analysis of bone specific gravity fractions in the growing rat, Israel J. Med. Sci. 3:677–90.

RICHELLE, L. J., and ONKELINX, C. 1968. Recent advances in the physical biology of bone and other hard tissues. *In:* C. COMAR and F. BRONNER (eds.), Mineral metabolism, An advanced treatise. New York: Academic Press, Inc. (in press).

SOBEL, A. E., and HANOK, A. 1948. Calcification of teeth. I. Composition in relation to blood and diet, J. Biol. Chem. 176:1103–22.

STRANDH, J., BENGSTON, A., and JORULF, H. 1965. The rate of uptake of calcium and phosphorus in microscopic bone structures, J. Bone Jt. Surg. 47-A:146–54.

TERMINE, J. D. 1966. Amorphous calcium phosphate: The second mineral of bone. Thesis, Cornell University.

URIST, M. R., and DOWELL, T. A. 1967. The newly deposited mineral in cartilage and bone matrix, Clin. Orthop. 50:291–308.

WEBER, J. C., and EANES, D. 1967. Electronmicroscopic study of non-crystalline calcium phosphate, Arch. Biochem. Biophys. 120:723–24.

WINAND, L. 1960. Etude physico-chimique des phosphates de calcium de structure apatitique. Thesis, University of Liège.

WINAND, L., and DALLEMAGNE, M. J. 1962. Hydrogen bonding in the calcium phosphates, Nature 193:369–70.

CHAPTER VI

DYNAMICS OF BONE MINERAL

BACHRA, B. N., SOBEL, A. E., and STANFORD, J. W. 1959. Calcification. XXIV. Mineralization of collagen and other fibers, Arch. Biochem. Biophys. 84:79–95.

BORLE, A. B., NICHOLS, N., and NICHOLS, G., JR. 1960. Metabolic studies of bone *in vitro*. I. Normal bone, J. Biol. Chem. 235:1206–10.

FLEISCH, H., and NEUMAN, W. F. 1961. Mechanisms of calcification: Role of collagen, polyphosphates, and phosphatase, Am. J. Physiol. 200: 1296–1300.

GLIMCHER, M. J. 1959. Molecular biology of mineralized tissues with particular reference to bone, Rev. Mod. Physics 31:359–93.

GLIMCHER, M. J., FRANÇOIS, C., and KRANE, S. M. 1965. Possible role of phosphate in the calcification of collagen and enamel proteins. *In:* S. FITTON JACKSON *et al.* (eds.), Structure and function of connective and skeletal tissue, pp. 342–47. London: Butterworth.

GLIMCHER, M. J., HODGE, A. J., and SCHMITT, F. O. 1957. Macromolecular aggregation states in relation to mineralization: The collagen-hydroxyapatite system as studied *in vitro*, Proc. Nat. Acad. Sci. 43:860–67.

GLIMCHER, M. J., and KRANE, S. M. 1962. Studies of the interactions of collagen and phosphate. I. The nature of inorganic orthophosphate binding. *In:* F. C. MCLEAN, P. LACROIX, and A. M. BUDY (eds.), Radioisotopes and bone. Philadelphia: F. A. Davis Company.

GLIMCHER, M. J., and KRANE, S. M. 1964. The incorporation of radioactive inorganic phosphate by collagen fibrils *in vitro*, Biochem. J. 31: 195–202.

HOWLAND, J. 1923. The etiology and pathogenesis of rickets, Harvey Lect., Ser. XVIII, pp. 189–216.

HOWLAND, J., and KRAMER, B. 1921. Calcium and phosphorus in the serum in relation to rickets, Am. J. Dis. Child. 22:105–19.

IRVING, J. 1963. The sudanophilic material at sites of calcification, Arch. Oral Biol. 8:735–43.

IRVING, J. T., SCHIBLER, D., and FLEISCH, H. 1966. Effect of condensed phosphates on vitamin D–induced aortic calcification in rats, Proc. Soc. Exptl. Biol. (N.Y.) 122:852–56.

LEVINSKAS, C. J. 1953. Solubility studies of synthetic hydroxylapatite (the lattice of bone mineral). Rochester, N.Y.: Univ. of Rochester Reports, No. 273.

LOGAN, M. A., and TAYLOR, H. L. 1937. Solubility of bone salt, J. Biol. Chem. 119:293–307.

MACGREGOR, J., and NORDIN, B. E. C. 1960. Equilibration studies with human bone powder, J. Biol. Chem. 235:1215–18.

MCLEAN, F. C. 1960. Phosphorus metabolism. *In:* K. RODAHL, J. T. NICHOLSON, and E. M. BROWN (eds.), Bone as a tissue. New York: McGraw-Hill Book Co., Inc.

MCLEAN, F. C., LIPTON, M. A., BLOOM, W., and BARRON, E. S. G. 1946. Biological factors in calcification in bone, Tr. Conf. Metab. Aspects of Convalescence 14:9–19, Figs. 1–4. New York: Josiah Macy, Jr. Foundation.

MARSHALL, J. H., ROWLAND, R. E., and JOWSEY, J. 1959. Microscopic metabolism of calcium in bone. V. The paradox of diffuse activity and long-term exchange, Radiat. Res. 10:258–70.

MILLER, Z. B., WALDMAN, J., and MCLEAN, F. C. 1952*a*. The effect of dyes on the calcification of hypertrophic rachitic cartilage *in vitro*, J. Exptl. Med. 95:497–508.

———. 1952*b*. Rapidity of calcification *in vitro*, Proc. Soc. Exptl. Biol. (N.Y.) 79:606–7.

MOSS, M. J., and URIST, M. R. 1964. Experimental cutaneous calcinosis A.M.A. Arch. Path. 78:127–34.

NEUMAN, W. F. 1950. Trans. Second Conf. on Metab. Interrelations, p. 187. New York: Josiah Macy, Jr. Foundation.

NEUMAN, W. F., and NEUMAN, M. W. 1958. The chemical dynamics of bone mineral. Chicago: The University of Chicago Press.

ROWLAND, R. E., and MARSHALL, J. H. 1959. Radium in human bone: The dose in microscopic volumes of bone, Radiat. Res. 11:299–313.

SELYE, H. 1962. Calciphylaxis. Chicago: The University of Chicago Press.

SHIPLEY, P. G., KRAMER, B., and HOWLAND, J. 1925. Calcification of rachitic bones *in vitro*, Am. J. Dis. Child. 30:37–39.

SOBEL, A. E., BURGER, M., and NOBEL, S. 1960. Mechanisms of nuclei formation in mineralizing tissues, Clin. Orthop. 17:103–23.

SOLOMONS, C. C., and NEUMAN, W. F. 1960. On the mechanisms of calcification: The remineralization of dentin, J. Biol. Chem. 235:2502–26.

SPEER, D., and URIST, M. R. 1965. Intracellular calcification of muscle, Clin. Orthop. 39:213–31.

TAVES, D. R. 1965. Mechanisms of calcification, Clin. Orthop. 42:207–20.

TEREPKA, A. R., DOWSE, C. M., and NEUMAN, W. F., 1960. Unifying concepts of parathyroid hormone action, USAEC Report UR-577, pp. 1–28, Rochester, N.Y.: Univ. Rochester Atomic Energy Project.

URIST, M. R. 1964. Recent advances in the physiology of calcification, J. Bone Jt. Surg. 46-A:889–900.

———. 1966. Origins of ideas about the local mechanism of calcification, Clin. Orthop. 44:13–39.

———. 1967. Effects of calcium ion upon the structure and calcifiability of tendon, Clin. Orthop. (in press).

URIST, M. R., and ADAMS, J. M., JR. 1966. The effect of blocking reagents on the calcifiability of tendon, A.M.A. Arch. Path. 81:325–42.

URIST, M. R., MOSS, M., and ADAMS, J. M., JR. 1964. Calcification of tendon: A triphasic local mechanism, A.M.A. Arch. Path. 77:594–608.

VAN DE PUTTE, K. A., and URIST, M. R. 1965. Experimental mineralization of collagen sponge and decalcified bone, Clin. Orthop. 40:48–56.

WALDMAN, J. 1948. Calcification of hypertrophic epiphyseal cartilage *in vitro* following inactivation of phosphatase and other enzymes, Proc. Soc. Exptl. Biol. (N.Y.) 69:262–63.

WALTON, A. G. 1965. Nucleation of crystals from solution, Science 148: 601–7.

WEIDMANN, S. M. 1963. Calcification of skeletal tissues, Internat. Rev. Connect. Tis. Res. 1:339–77.

CHAPTER VII

ENZYME SYSTEMS AND METABOLIC PATHWAYS IN BONE AND CARTILAGE

ALBAUM, H. G., HIRSCHFELD, A., and SOBEL, A. E. 1952. Calcification. VIII. Glycolytic enzymes and phosphorylated intermediates in preosseous cartilage, Proc. Soc. Exptl. Biol. (N.Y.) 79:682–86.

CARTIER, P. 1952. Mécanisme enzymatique de l'ossification, Exposés Ann. Biochim. Méd. 14:73–86.

CARTIER, P., and PICARD, J. 1955*a*. La minéralisation du cartilage ossifiable. I. La minéralisation du cartilage *in vitro*, Bull. Soc. Chim. Biol. 37:485–94.

———. 1955*b*. La minéralisation du cartilage ossifiable. III. Le mécanisme de la réaction ATPasique du cartilage, Bull. Soc. Chim. Biol. 37:1159–68.

DUVE, C. DE. 1963. The lysosome concept. *In:* A. V. S. DE REUCK and M. P. CAMERON (eds.), Lysosomes, p. 1. London: Churchill.

DZIEWIATKOWSKI, D. D. 1966. Role of proteinpolysaccharides in calcification, Birth Defects Original Article Series 2:31–34.

FLEISCH, H. 1964. Role of nucleation and inhibition in calcification, Clin. Orthop. 32:170–80.

FLEISCH, H., and NEUMAN, W. F. 1960. On the role of phosphatase in the nucleation of calcium phosphate by collagen, J. Am. Chem. Soc. 82: 3783–84.

GUTMAN, A. B. 1951. Current theories of bone salt formation, with special reference to enzyme mechanisms in endochondral ossification, Bull. Hosp. Jt. Dis. 12:74–86.

GUTMAN, A. B., and GUTMAN, E. B. 1941. A phosphorylase in calcifying cartilage, Proc. Soc. Exptl. Biol. (N.Y.) 48:687–91.

GUTMAN, A. B., and YU, T. F. 1950. A concept of the role of enzymes in endochondral ossification. *In:* Metabolic interrelations. Transactions of the second conference, pp. 167–90. New York: Josiah Macy, Jr. Foundation.

HARRIS, H. A. 1932. Glycogen in cartilage, Nature 130:996–97.

KRANE, S. M., and GLIMCHER, M. J. 1962. Studies of the interactions of collagen and phosphate. II. Nucleotidase activity and binding of nucleotide phosphorus. *In:* F. C. MCLEAN, P. LACROIX, and A. M. BUDY (eds.), Radioisotopes and bone. Philadelphia: F. A. Davis Company.

KUHLMAN, R. E. 1965. Phosphatases in epiphyseal cartilage. Their possible role in tissue synthesis, J. Bone Jt. Surg. 47-A:545–50.

MOOG, F. 1946. The physiological significance of the phosphomonoesterases, Biol. Rev. 21:41–59.

PERKINS, H. R., and WALKER, P. G. 1958. The occurrence of pyrophosphate in bone, J. Bone Jt. Surg. 40-B:333–39.

PICARD, J. 1955. Relations entre la minéralisation du cartilage ossifiable et son métabolisme chez l'embryon de mouton et le rat. Thesis, Faculté de Médecine, Hôpital des Enfants Malades, Paris.

PRITCHARD, J. J. 1952. A cytological and histochemical study of bone and cartilage formation in the rat, J. Anat. 86:259–77.

ROBISON, R. 1923. The possible significance of hexosephosphoric esters in ossification, Biochem. J. 17:286–93.

———. 1932. The significance of phosphoric esters in metabolism. New York: New York University Press.

ROBISON, R. 1936. Chemistry and metabolism of compounds of phosphorus, Ann. Rev. Biochem. 5:181–204.

ROBISON, R., MACLEOD, M., and ROSENHEIM, A. H. 1930. The possible significance of hexosephosphoric esters in ossification. IX. Calcification *in vitro*, Biochem. J. 24:1927–41.

ROBISON, R., and ROSENHEIM, A. H. 1934. Calcification of hypertrophic cartilage *in vitro*, Biochem. J. 23:684–98.

VAN REEN, R. 1965. The influence of parathyroid extract on bone metabolism and the levels of nicotinamide nucleotides. *In:* P. J. GAILLARD, R. V. TALMAGE, and A. M. BUDY (eds.), The parathyroid glands, pp. 211–20. Chicago: The University of Chicago Press.

ZAMBOTTI, V. 1957. The biochemistry of preosseous cartilage and of ossification, Sc. Med. Ital. 5:614–43.

CHAPTER VIII

RESORPTION OF BONE

ARNOLD, J. S., and JEE, W. S. S. 1957. Bone growth and osteoclastic activity as indicated by radioautographic distribution of plutonium, Am. J. Anat. 101:367–418.

BÉLANGER, L. 1965. Osteolysis: An outlook on its mechanism and causation. *In:* P. J. GAILLARD, R. V. TALMAGE, and A. M. BUDY (eds.), The parathyroid glands, pp. 137–43. Chicago: The University of Chicago Press.

BHASKAR, S. N., MOHAMMED, C. I., and WEINMANN, J. P. 1956. A morphological and histochemical study of osteoclasts, J. Bone Jt. Surg. 38-A:1335–45.

CAMERON, D. A., and ROBINSON, R. A. 1958. The presence of crystals in the cytoplasm of large cells adjacent to sites of bone absorption, J. Bone Jt. Surg. 48-A:414–18.

GAILLARD, P. J. 1961. Parathyroid and bone in tissue culture. *In:* R. O. GREEP and R. V. TALMAGE (eds.), The parathyroids. Springfield, Ill.: Charles C Thomas.

GOLDHABER, P. 1960. Behavior of bone in tissue culture. *In:* R. F. SOGNNAES (ed.), Calcification in biological systems, pp. 349–72. Washington, D.C.: Am. Assoc. Adv. Science.

HANCOX, N. M., and BOOTHROYD, B. 1961. Motion picture and electron microscope studies on the embryonic avian osteoclast, J. Biophys. and Biochem. Cytol. 11:651–61.

JOWSEY, J., ROWLAND, R. E., MARSHALL, J. H., and MCLEAN, F. C. 1958. The effect of parathyroidectomy on haversian remodeling of bone, Endocrinol. 63:903–8.

KÖLLIKER, A. 1873. Die normale Resorption des Knochengewebes und ihre Bedeutung für die Entstehung der typischen Knochenformen. Leipzig: F. C. W. Vogel.

KROON, D. B. 1954. The bone-destroying function of the osteoclasts (Koelliker's "brush border"), Acta Anat. 21:1-18.

LINDQUIST, B., BUDY, A. M., MCLEAN, F. C., and HOWARD, J. L. 1960. Skeletal metabolism in estrogen-treated rats studied by means of Ca^{45}, Endocrinol. 66:100–111.

MCLEAN, F. C. 1954. Biochemical and biomechanical aspects of the resorption of bone, J. Periodontol. 25:176–82.

MCLEAN, F. C., and BLOOM, W. 1941. Calcification and ossification. Mobilization of bone salt by parathyroid extract, Arch. Path. 32:315–33.

PECK, W. A., and DIRKSEN, T. R. 1966. The metabolism of bone tissue *in vitro*, Clin. Orthop. 48:243–65.

POMMER, G. 1924. Bemerkungen zu den Lehren von Knochengeschwund, Arch. Mikr. Anat. 102:324–36.

SCOTT, R. L., and PEASE, D. C. 1956. Electron microscopy of the epiphyseal apparatus, Anat. Rec. 126:465–95.

SLEDGE, C. B. 1966*a*. Lysosomes and cartilage resorption in organ culture. *In:* H. FLEISCH, H. J. J. BLACKWOOD, and M. OWEN (eds.), Third European symposium on calcified tissues, pp. 52–55. Heidelberg: Springer-Verlag.

———. 1966*b*. Some morphologic and experimental aspects of limb development, Clin. Orthop. 44:241–64.

TONNA, E. A. 1960. Osteoclasts and the aging skeleton: A cytological, cytochemical, and autoradiographic study, Anat. Rec. 137:251–70.

VAES, G. 1967. La résorption osseuse et l'hormone parathyroïdienne. Brussels: A. de Visscher, Éditeur.

WALKER, D. C., LAPIERE, C. M., and GROSS, J. 1964. A collagenolytic factor in rat bone promoted by parathyroid extract, Biochem. Biophys. Res. Commun. 15:397–402.

CHAPTER IX

REGULATORY PROCESSES AND BONE. A. BONE MATRIX

ASLING, C. W., and EVANS, H. M. 1956. Anterior pituitary regulation of skeletal development. *In:* G. H. BOURNE (ed.), The biochemistry and physiology of bone, pp. 671–704. New York: Academic Press, Inc.

BARNICOT, N. A. 1950. The local action of vitamin A on bone, J. Anat. 84: 374–87.

BAUER, G. C. H., CARLSSON, A., and LINDQUIST, B. 1955. Evaluation of accretion, resorption, and exchange reactions in the skeleton, Kungl. Fysiogr. Sällskap. Lund Förhandl. 25:1–16.

BLOOM, W., BLOOM, M. A., and MCLEAN, F. C. 1941. Calcification and ossification. Medullary bone changes in the reproductive cycle of female pigeons, Anat. Rec. 81:443–75.

BLOOM, M. A., DOMM, L. C., NALBANDOV, A. V., and BLOOM, W. 1958. Medullary bone of laying chickens, Am. J. Anat. 102:411–53.

BLOOM, M. A., MCLEAN, F. C., and BLOOM, W. 1942. Calcification and ossification. The formation of medullary bone in male and castrate pigeons under the influence of sex hormones, Anat. Rec. 83:99–120.

BUDY, A. M. 1960. Skeletal distribution of estrone-16-C^{14}, Clin. Orthop. 17:176–85.

BUDY, A. M., URIST, M. R., and MCLEAN, F. C. 1952. The effect of estrogens on the growth apparatus of the bones of immature rats, Am. J. Path. 28:1143–67.

DINGLE, J. T., and WEBB, M. 1965–66. Mucopolysaccharide metabolism in tissue culture, *In:* E. N. WILLMER (ed.), Cells and tissues in culture, pp. 353–96. New York: Academic Press, Inc.

FELL, H. B. 1964*a*. The role of organ cultures in the study of vitamins and hormones, Vit. and Horm. 22:81–127.

———. 1964*b*. Some factors in the regulation of cell physiology in skeletal tissues. *In:* H. M. FROST (ed.), Bone biodynamics, pp. 189–207. Boston: Little, Brown and Co.

HENNEMAN, P. H., FORBES, A. P., MOLDAWER, M., DEMPSEY, E. F., and CARROLL, E. L. 1960. Effects of human growth hormone in man, J. Clin. Invest. 39:1223–38.

HORSTMANN, P. 1949. Dwarfism: A clinical investigation with special reference to the significance of endocrine factors, Acta Endocrinol. 3, *Suppl. 5,* 1–175.

HULTH, A. and OLERUD, S. 1963. The effect of cortisone on growing bone in the rat, Brit. J. Exptl. Path. 44:491–96.

KYES, P. and POTTER, T. S. 1934. Physiological marrow ossification in female pigeons, Anat. Rec. 60:377–79.

LINDQUIST, B., BUDY, A. M., MCLEAN, F. C., and HOWARD, J. L. 1960. Skeletal metabolism in estrogen-treated rats studied by means of Ca^{45}, Endocrinol. 66:100–111.

MCINDOE, W. M. 1959. A lipophosphoprotein complex in hen plasma associated with yolk production, Biochem. J. 72:153–59.

ROSENBLOOM, A. L. 1966. Growth hormone replacement therapy. J.A.M.A. 198:364–68.

SCHEIDE, O. A., and URIST, M. R. 1959. Proteins and calcium in egg yolk, Exptl. Cell. Res. 17:84–94.

SIMMONS, D. J. 1966. Collagen formation and endochondral ossification in estrogen treated mice, Proc. Soc. Exptl. Biol. (N.Y.) 121:1165–68.

TAPP, E. 1966. The effects of hormones on bone in growing rats, J. Bone Jt. Surg. 48-B:526–31.

URIST, M. R. 1959. The effects of calcium deprivation upon the blood, adrenal cortex, ovary, and skeleton in domestic fowl, Recent Prog. Hormone Res. 15:455–81.

URIST, M. R., BUDY, A. M., and MCLEAN, F. C. 1948. Species differences in the reaction of the mammalian skeleton to estrogens, Proc. Soc. Exptl. Biol. (N.Y.) 68:324–6.

———. 1950. Endosteal-bone formation in estrogen treated mice, J. Bone Jt. Surg. 32-A:143–62.

URIST, M. R., SCHEIDE, O. A., and MCLEAN, F. C. 1958. The partition and binding of calcium in the serum of the laying hen and of the estrogenized rooster, Endocrinol. 63:570–85.

CHAPTER X

REGULATORY PROCESSES AND BONE. B. VITAMIN D–PARATHYROID COMPLEX

ALBRIGHT, F., and REIFENSTEIN, E. C., JR. 1948. The parathyroid glands and metabolic bone disease; Selected studies. Baltimore: Williams & Wilkins Co.

AUBERT, J-P., and BRONNER, F. 1965. A symbolic model for the regulation by bone metabolism of the blood calcium level in the rat, Biophys. J. 5:349–58.

BARNICOT, N. A. 1948. The local action of the parathyroid and other tissues on bone in intracerebral grafts, J. Anat. 82:233–48.

BLOOM, W., NALBANDOV, A. V., and BLOOM, M. A. 1960. Parathyroid enlargement in laying hens on a calcium-deficient diet, Clin. Orthop. 17:206–9.

COPP, D. H., CAMERON, E. C., CHENEY, B. A., DAVIDSON, A. G. F., and HENZE, E. G. 1962. Evidence for calcitonin—A new hormone from the parathyroid that lowers blood calcium, Endocrinol. 70:638–49.

COPP, D. H., COCKCROFT, D. W., and KUSH, Y. 1967. Ultimobranchial origin of calcitonin. Hypocalcemic effect of extracts from chicken glands, Canad. J. Physiol. Pharmacol. (in press).

DELUCA, H. F., and SALLIS, J. D. 1965. Parathyroid hormone: Its subcellular actions and its relationship to vitamin D. *In:* P. J. GAILLARD, R. V. TALMAGE, and A. M. BUDY (eds.), The parathyroid glands, pp. 181–96. Chicago: The University of Chicago Press.

FREEMAN, S., and BREEN, M. 1960. The influence of alterations in parathyroid function on the distribution of plasma calcium, Clin. Orthop. 17:186–94.

HASTINGS, A. B., and HUGGINS, C. B. 1933. Experimental hypocalcemia, Proc. Soc. Exptl. Biol. (N.Y.) 30:458–59.

HELLER, M., MCLEAN, F. C., and BLOOM, W. 1950. Cellular transformations in mammalian bones induced by parathyroid extract, Am. J. Anat. 87:315–48.

HIRSCH, P. F., GAUTHIER, G. F., and MUNSON, P. L. 1963. Thyroid hypocalcemic principle and recurrent laryngeal nerve injury as factors affecting the response to parathyroidectomy in rats, Endocrinol. 73:244–52.

JOWSEY, J., ROWLAND, R. E., MARSHALL, J. H., and MCLEAN, F. C. 1958. The effect of parathyroidectomy on haversian remodeling of bone, Endocrinol. 63:903–8.

LOUW, G. N., SUTTON, W. W., and KENNY, A. D. 1967. Action of thyrocalcitonin in the teleost fish *Ictalurus melas*, Nature 215:888–89.

MCLEAN, F. C. 1937. The parathyroid hormone and bone, Clin. Orthop. 9:46–60.

MELICK, R. A., AURBACH, G. D., and POTTS, J. T., JR. 1965. Distribution and half-life of ^{131}I-labeled parathyroid hormone in the rat, Endocrinol. 77:198–202.

NEUMAN, W. F. 1965. The influence of parathyroid hormone on the cellular exchange and transport of phosphate. *In:* P. J. GAILLARD, R. V. TALMAGE, and A. M. BUDY (eds.), The parathyroid glands, pp. 175–80. Chicago: The University of Chicago Press.

PATT, H. M., and LUCKHARDT, A. B. 1942. Relationship of a low blood calcium to parathyroid secretion, Endocrinology 31:384–92.

POTTS, J. T., JR., and AURBACH, G. D. 1965. The chemistry of parathyroid hormone. *In:* P. J. GAILLARD, R. V. TALMAGE, and A. M. BUDY (eds.), The parathyroid glands, pp. 53–67. Chicago: The University of Chicago Press.

POTTS, J. T., JR., REISFELD, R. F., HIRSCH, P. F., COOPER, C. W., WASTHED, A. B., and MUNSON, P. L. 1967. Current status of the purification of thyrocalcitonin, Proc. European Sympos. on Calcified Tissues, Vol. 5 (in press).

RASMUSSEN, H. 1961. Parathyroid hormone, nature and mechanism of action, Am. J. Med. 30:112–38.

TALMAGE, R. V., DOTY, S. B., COOPER, C. W., YATES, C., and NEUENSCHWANGER, J. 1965. Cytological and biochemical changes resulting from fluctuations in endogenous parathyroid hormone levels. *In:* P. J. GAILLARD, R. V. TALMAGE, and A. M. BUDY (eds.), The parathyroid glands, pp. 107–24. Chicago: The University of Chicago Press.

TEREPKA, A. R., DOWSE, C. M., and NEUMAN, W. F. 1960. Unifying concepts of parathyroid hormone action, US-AEC (UR-577).

WOODS, K. R., and ARMSTRONG, W. D. 1956. Action of parathyroid extract on stable bone mineral using radiocalcium as tracer, Proc. Soc. Exptl. Biol. (N.Y.) 91:255–58.

CHAPTER XI

MINERAL METABOLISM

BAUER, G. C. H. 1954. Metabolism of bone sodium in rats investigated with Na^{22}, Acta Physiol. Scand. 31:334–50.

BAUER, G. C. H., CARLSSON, A., and LINDQUIST, B. 1955. Evaluation of accretion, resorption, and exchange reactions in the skeleton, Kungl. Fysiogr. Sällskap. Lund Förhandl. 25:1–16.

———. 1961. Metabolism and homeostatic function of bone. *In:* C. L. COMAR and F. BRONNER (eds.), Mineral metabolism, An advanced treatise 1:608–76. New York: Academic Press, Inc.

BERGSTROM, W. H., and WALLACE, W. M. 1954. Bone as a sodium and potassium reservoir, J. Clin. Invest. 33:867–73.

BERNARD, C. 1878. Leçons sur les phénomènes de la vie communs aux animaux et aux végétaux, Vol. 1, p. 113. Paris: Ballière et Fils.

BJERRUM, N. 1958. Calciumorthophosphate. I. Die festen Calciumorthophosphate. II. Komplexbildung in Lösungen von Calcium- und Phosphate-Ionen, Mat. Fys. Medd. Dan. Vid. Selsk. 31, no. 7,:1–79. *See translation as follows:*

BJERRUM, N. 1959. Calcium orthophosphates, Harwell, Berkshire: Atomic Energy Research Establishment, United Kingdom.

BORLE, A. B., NICHOLS, N., and NICHOLS, G., JR. 1960*a*. Metabolic studies of bone *in vitro*. I. Normal bone, J. Biol. Chem. 235:1206–10.

———. 1960*b*. Metabolic studies of bone *in vitro*. II. The metabolic patterns of accretion and resorption, J. Biol. Chem. 235:1211–14.

CARTTAR, M. S., MCLEAN, F. C., and URIST, M. R. 1950. The effect of the calcium and phosphorus of the diet upon the formation and structure of bone, Am. J. Path. 26:307–31.

CHIEWITZ, O., and HEVESY, G. 1935. Radioactive indicators in the study of phosphorus metabolism in rats, Nature 136:754–55.

DICKENS, F. 1941. The citric acid content of animal tissues, with reference to its occurrence in bone and tumour, Biochem. J. 35:1011–23.

DIXON, T. F., and PERKINS, H. R. 1956. Citric acid and bone. *In:* G. H. BOURNE (ed.), The biochemistry and physiology of bone, pp. 309–24. New York: Academic Press, Inc.

DUCKWORTH, J., and HILL, R. 1953. The storage of elements in the skeleton, Nutrition Abstr. Rev. 23:1–17.

EICHELBERGER, L. 1960. Hyaline cartilage: the histochemical characteristics of the extracellular and intracellular compartments, Clin. Orthop. 17:77–91.

FANCONI, A., and ROSE, G. A. 1958. The ionised, complexed, and protein-bound fractions of calcium in plasma, Quart. J. Med. 27:463–94.

Food and Nutrition Board. 6th ed. 1964. Recommended dietary allowances. National Academy of Sciences—National Research Council, Publication 1146.

FOURMAN, P. 1960. Calcium metabolism and the bone. Springfield, Ill.: Charles C Thomas.

HASTINGS, A. B., MCLEAN, F. C., EICHELBERGER, L., HALL, J. L., and DACOSTA, E. 1934. The ionization of calcium, magnesium, and strontium citrates, J. Biol. Chem. 107:351–70.

HEANEY, R. P. 1963. Evaluation and interpretation of calcium-kinetic data in man, Clin. Orthop. 31:153–83.

HEANEY, R. P., and WHEDON, G. D. 1958. Radiocalcium studies of bone formation rate in human metabolic disease, J. Clin. Endocrinol. 17: 1105–23.

HODGE, H. C., NEUMAN, M. W., and BLANCHET, H. J., JR. 1960. Studies of the oral toxicity of strontium chloride in rats, Clin. Orthop. 17:265–68.

HODGE, H. C., and SMITH, F. A. 1965. J. H. SIMONS (ed.), Fluorine chemistry. New York: Academic Press, Inc.

HOWARD, J. E. 1957. Calcium metabolism, bone and calcium homeostasis. A review of certain current concepts, J. Clin. Endocrinol. 17:1105–23.

IRVING, J. T. 1957. Calcium metabolism. London: Methuen & Co., Ltd.

JOHNSON, L. C. 1964. Morphologic analysis in pathology: The kinetics of disease and general biology of bone. *In:* H. M. FROST (ed.), Bone biodynamics, pp. 543–654. Boston: Little, Brown and Company.

LLOYD, H. M., and ROSE, G. A. 1958. Ionised, proteinbound, and complexed calcium in the plasma in primary hyperparathyroidism, Lancet 2:1258–61.

LLOYD, H. M., ROSE, G. A., and SMEENK, D. 1962. The ability of plasma proteins to bind calcium in normal subjects, in patients with primary hyperparathyroidism both pre- and post-operatively, and in other hypercalcemic conditions, Clin. Sci. 22:353–62.

MCLEAN, F. C. 1942*a*. Activated sterols in the treatment of parathyroid insufficiency. *In:* Glandular physiology and therapy, Chap. XXVII, pp. 461–93. Chicago: A.M.A.

———. 1942*b*. The economy of phosphorus in the animal organism. *In:* E. A. EVANS, JR. (ed.), The biological action of the vitamins, pp. 185–201. Chicago: The University of Chicago Press.

McLean, F. C., Barnes, B. O., and Hastings, A. B. 1935. The relation of the parathyroid hormone to the state of calcium in the blood, Am. J. Physiol. 113:141–49.

McLean, F. C., and Hastings, A. B. 1934. A biological method for the estimation of calcium ion concentration, J. Biol. Chem. 107:337–50.

———. 1935*a*. Clinical estimation and significance of calcium ion concentrations in the blood, Am. J. Med. Sci. 189:601–12.

———. 1935*b*. The state of calcium in the fluids of the body. I. The conditions affecting the ionization of calcium, J. Biol. Chem. 108:285–322.

McLean, F. C., and Hinrichs, M. A. 1938. The formation and behavior of colloidal calcium phosphate in the blood, Am. J. Physiol. 121:580–88.

Malm, O. J. 1958. Calcium requirement and adaptation in adult man, Scandinav. J. Clin. Lab. Invest., *Suppl.* 10:1–290.

Marshall, J. H. 1964. Theory of alkaline earth metabolism. The power function makes possible a simple but comprehensive model of skeletal systems, J. Theoret. Biol. 6:386–412.

Nicolaysen, R. 1960. The calcium requirement of man as related to diseases of the skeleton, Clin. Orthop. 17:226–34.

Norris, W. P., and Kisieleski, W. 1948. Comparative metabolism of radium, strontium and calcium, Cold Spring Harbor Symp. Quant. Biol. 13:164–72.

Norris, W. P., Tyler, S. A., and Brues, A. M. 1958. Retention of radioactive bone-seekers, Science 128:456–62.

Perkins, H. R., and Walker, P. G. 1958. The occurrence of pyrophosphate in bone, J. Bone Jt. Surg. 40-B:333–39.

Prasad, A. S., and Flink, E. B. 1958. The base binding property of the serum proteins with respect to calcium, J. Lab. Clin. Med. 51:345–50.

Rose, G. A. 1957. Determination of the ionised and ultrafilterable calcium of normal human plasma, Clin. Chim. Acta 2:227–36.

Sherman, H. C. 1947. Calcium and phosphorus in foods and nutrition. New York: Columbia University Press.

Sognnaes, R. F. 1965. Fluoride protection of bones and teeth, Science 150:989–93.

Thomas, R. O., Litovitz, T. A., Rubin, M. I., and Geschickter, C. F. 1952. Dynamics of calcium metabolism. Time distribution of intravenously administered radiocalcium, Am. J. Physiol. 169:568–75.

Vincent, J. 1959. Distribution of sodium in compact bone, as revealed by autoradiography of neutron-activated sections, Nature 184:1332.

———. 1960. Autoradiographies au Na^{22} de l'os compact du Cercopithèque, Bull. Acad. Roy. Méd. Belg. 25:283–95.

CHAPTER XII

Radiation, Isotopes, and Bone

Amprino, R. 1952. Rapportin fra processi di ricostruzione e distribuzione dei minerali nella ossa. II. Richerche con metodo autoradiografico. Ztschr. Zellforsch. Mikr. Anat. 37:240–73.

Aub, J. A., Evans, R. D., Hempelmann, L. H., and Martland, H. S. 1952. The late effects of internally-deposited radioactive materials in man, Medicine 31:221–329.

Bauer, G. C. H., Carlsson, A., and Lindquist, B. 1961. Metabolism and homeostatic function of bone. *In:* C. L. Comar and F. Bronner (eds.), Mineral metabolism 1:608–76. New York: Academic Press, Inc.

Bauer, G. C. H., and Ray, R. D. 1958. Kinetics of strontium metabolism in man, J. Bone Jt. Surg. 40-A:171–86.

Bauer, G. C. H. and Scoccianti, P. 1961. Uptake of Sr-85 in non-malignant vertebral lesions in man, Acta Orthop. Scand. 31:90–102.

Bauer, G. C. H., and Wendeberg, B. 1959. External counting of Ca-47 and Sr-85 in studies of localized skeletal lesions in man, J. Bone Jt. Surg. 41-B:558–80.

Bloom, W. (ed.). 1948. Histopathology of irradiation from external and internal sources. New York: McGraw-Hill Book Co., Inc.

Boyd, J., Neuman, W. F., and Hodge, H. C. 1959. On the mechanism of skeletal fixation of strontium. Part II, Arch. Biochem. Biophys. 80: 105–13.

Brues, A. M. 1955. Radiation as a carcinogenic agent, Radiat. Res. 3: 272–80.

Caldecott, R. S., and Snyder, L. A. (eds.). 1960. A symposium on radioisotopes in the biosphere. Minneapolis: University of Minnesota.

Chiewitz, O., and Hevesy, G. 1935. Radioactive indicators in the study of phosphorus metabolism in rats, Nature 136:754–55.

Comar, C. L. 1955. Radioisotopes in biology and agriculture. Principles and practice. New York: McGraw-Hill Book Co., Inc.

Comar, C. L., and Wassermann, R. H. 1960. Radiation absorption and methods of elimination: Differential behavior of substances in metabolic pathways. *In:* R. S. Caldecott and L. A. Snyder (eds.), A symposium on radioisotopes in the biosphere, pp. 526–40. Minneapolis: University of Minnesota.

Corey, K. R., Kenny, P., Greenberg, E., and Laughlin, J. S. 1962. Detection of bone metastases in scanning studies with calcium-47 and strontium-85, J. Nucl. Med. 3:454–71.

DUDLEY, H. C., MARKOWITZ, H. A., and MITCHELL, T. G. 1956. Studies of the localization of radioactive gallium (Ga^{72}) in bone lesions, J. Bone Jt. Surg. 38-A:627–37.

DUNHAM, C. L. 1958. Fallout from nuclear weapons tests, Adv. Biol. Med. Physics 6:175–201.

ENGSTRÖM, A., BJÖRNERSTEDT, R., CLEMEDSON, C.-J., and NELSON, A. 1958. Bone and radiostrontium. Stockholm: Almquist & Wiksell.

FINKEL, M. P., BERGSTRAND, P. J., and BISKIS, B. O. 1960. The consequences of the continuous ingestion of Sr^{90} by mice, Radiology 74:458–67.

GRAN, F. C. 1960. Studies on calcium and strontium-90 metabolism in rats, Acta Physiol. Scand. 48 (*Suppl.* 167):1–109.

HASTERLIK, R. J. 1960. Radiation neoplasia, Proc. Inst. Med. Chicago 23:37–46.

International Atomic Energy Agency. 1960. Radiation damage in bone. Vienna.

JOWSEY, J., SISSONS, H. A., and VAUGHAN, J. 1956. The site of deposition of Y^{91} in the bones of rabbits and dogs, J. Nucl. Energy 2:168–76.

LOONEY, W. B. 1958. Effects of radium in man, Science 127:630–33.

MACDONALD, N. S. 1960. The radioisotope osteogram—kinetic studies of skeletal disorders in humans, Clin. Orthop. 17:154–66.

MARINELLI, L. D. 1958. Radioactivity and the human skeleton, Am. J. Roentgenol. 80:729–39.

MARSHALL, J. H., ROWLAND, R. E., and JOWSEY, J. 1959. Microscopic metabolism of calcium in bone. IV. Ca^{45} deposition and growth rate in canine osteons, Radiat. Res. 10:243–57.

MARSHALL, J. H., WHITE, V. K., and COHEN, J. 1929. Microscopic metabolism in bone. I. Three-dimensional deposition of Ca^{45} in canine osteons, Radiat. Res. 10:197–212.

MULRY, W. G., and DUDLEY, H. C. 1951. Studies of radiogallium in bone tumors, J. Lab. Clin. Med. 37:239–52.

NORRIS, W. P., TYLER, S. A., and BRUES, A. M. 1958. Retention of radioactive bone-seekers, Science 128:456–62.

PONLOT, R. 1959. Le radiocalcium dans l'ètude des os. Brussels: Arscia.

ROSENTHAL, M. W. 1960. Radioisotope absorption and methods of elimination: Factors influencing elimination from the body. *In:* R. S. CALDECOTT and L. A. SNYDER (eds.), A symposium on radioisotopes in the biosphere, pp. 541–63. Minneapolis: University of Minnesota.

ROWLAND, R. E. 1960. The deposition and the removal of radium in bone by a long-term exchange process, Clin. Orthop. 17:146–53.

ROWLAND, R. E., JOWSEY, J., and MARSHALL, J. H. 1959. Microscopic metabolism of calcium in bone. III. Microradiographic measurements of mineral density, Radiat. Res. 10:234–42.

ROWLAND, R. E., MARSHALL, J. H., and JOWSEY, J. 1959. Radium in human bone: The microscopic appearance, Radiat. Res. 10:323–34.

SCHACHTER, D., and ROSEN, S. M. 1959. Active transport of Ca^{45} by the small intestine and its dependence on vitamin D, Am. J. Physiol. 196: 357–62.

STROMINGER, D., HOLLANDER, J. M., and SEABORG, G. T. 1958. Table of isotopes, Rev. Mod. Physics 30:585–904.

VINCENT, J. 1955. Recherches sur la constitution de l'os adulte. Brussels: Arscia.

WENDEBERG, B. 1961. Mineral metabolism of fractures of the tibia in man studied with external counting of Sr-85, Acta Orthop. Scand., *Suppl.* 52:1–79.

CHAPTER XIII

POSTFETAL OSTEOGENESIS

BILLINGHAM, R. E. 1959. Reactions of grafts against their hosts, Science 130:947–53.

———. 1966. Tissue transplantation: Scope and prospect, Science 153: 266–70.

BLOOM, W. 1937. Cellular differentiation and tissue culture, Physiol. Rev. 17:589–617.

BONFIGLIO, M., JETER, W. S., and SMITH, C. L. 1955. The immune concept: Its relation to bone transplantation, Ann. N. Y. Acad. Sci. 59:417–32.

BRIDGES, J. B. 1959. Experimental heterotopic ossification, Internat. Rev. Cytol. 8:253–78.

BRIDGES, J. B., and PRITCHARD, J. J. 1958. Bone and cartilage induction in the rabbit, J. Anat. 92:28–38.

BÜRING, K., and URIST, M. R. 1967. Transfilter bone induction, Clin. Orthop. (in press).

BURNET, F. M. 1961*a*. Immunological recognition of self, Science 133:307–11.

———. 1961*b*. The mechanism of immunity, Scient. Am. 204:58–67.

BURWELL, G. 1964. Biological mechanisms in foreign bone transplantation. *In:* J. M. P. CLARK (ed.), Modern trends in orthopedics. Washington, D.C.: Butterworth.

CHASE, S. W., and HERNDON, C. H. 1955. The fate of autogenous and homogenous bone grafts. A historical review, J. Bone Jt. Surg. 37-A: 809–41.

COHEN, J., and LACROIX, P. 1955. Bone and cartilage formation by periosteum. Assay of experimental autogenous grafts, J. Bone Jt. Surg. 37-A:717–30.

Cohen, J., Maletskos, C. J., Marshall, J. H., and Williams, J. B. 1957. Radioactive calcium tracer studies in bone grafts, J. Bone Jt. Surg. 39-A:361–77.

Curtiss, P. H., Jr., Powell, A. E., and Herndon, C. H. 1959. Immunological factors in homogenous bone transplantation. III. The inability of homogenous rabbit bone to induce circulation antibodies in rabbits, J. Bone Jt. Surg. 41-A:1482–88.

D'Anis, A. 1957. Étude de l'ossification dans les greffes de moelle osseuse, Acta Med. Belg., *Suppl.* 3:1–120.

Duthie, R. B. 1958. A histochemical study of transplanted skeletal tissue during tissue culture "*in vivo*," Brit. J. Plast. Surg. 11:1–30.

Enneking, W. F. 1957. Histological investigation of bone transplants in immunologically prepared animals, J. Bone Jt. Surg. 39-A:597–615.

Enneking, W. F., and Gratch, A. 1959. The effect of total body irradiation on bone transplants in parabiosed animals, J. Bone Jt. Surg. 41-A:463–75.

Fell, H. B. 1953. Recent advances in organ culture, Sc. Prog. 162:212–31.

Hammack, B. L., and Enneking, W. F. 1960. Comparative vascularization of autogenous and homogenous bone transplants, J. Bone Jt. Surg. 42-A:811–17.

Heinen, J. H., Jr., Dabbs, G. H., and Mason, H. A. 1949. Experimental production of ectopic cartilage and bone in muscles of rabbits, J. Bone Jt. Surg. 31-A:765–75.

Heslop, B. F., Zeiss, I. M., and Nisbet, N. W. 1960. Studies on transference of bone. I. A comparison of autologous and homologous bone implants with reference to osteocyte survival, osteogenesis, and host reaction, Brit. J. Exptl. Path. 41:269–87.

Holmstrand, K. 1957. Biophysical investigations of bone transplants and bone implants, Acta Orthop. Scand., *Suppl.* 26:1–66.

Johnson, F. R., and McMinn, R. M. H. 1956. Transitional epithelium and osteogenesis, J. Anat. 90:106–16.

Johnson, L. C. 1960. Mineralization of turkey leg tendon. I. Histology and histochemistry of mineralization. *In:* R. F. Sognnaes (ed.), Calcification in biological systems, pp. 117–28. Washington, D.C.: Am. Assoc. Adv. Science.

Lash, J., Holtzer, S., and Holtzer, H. 1957. An experimental analysis of the development of the spinal column. VI. Aspects of cartilage induction, Exptl. Cell. Res. 13:292–303.

Likins, R. C., Piez, K. A., and Kunde, M. L. 1960. Mineralization of turkey leg tendon. III. Chemical nature of the protein and mineral phases. *In:* R. F. Sognnaes (ed.), Calcification in biological systems, pp. 143–50. Washington, D.C.: Am. Assoc. Adv. Science.

Longmire, W. P., Jr., Cannon, J. A., and Weber, R. A. 1954. General surgical problems of tissue transplantation. *In:* G. E. Westerholme,

M. P. Cameron, and J. Etherington (eds.), Preservation and transplantation of normal tissues, pp. 23–40. Boston: Little, Brown and Co.

Medawar, P. B. 1957. The immunology of transplantation, Harvey Lect., Ser. LII, 144–76.

———. 1959*a*. Reaction to homologous tissue antigens in relation to hypersensitivity. *In:* H. S. Lawrence (ed.), Cellular and humoral aspects of the hypersensitive state, pp. 504–34. New York: Hoeber Med. Division, Harper and Row.

———. 1959*b*. Zoologic laws of transplantation. *In:* L. A. Peer (ed.), Transplantation of tissues, II, 41–69. Baltimore: Williams & Wilkins.

———. 1961. Immunological tolerance, Science 133:303–6.

Nisbet, N. W., Heslop, B. F., and Zeiss, I. M. 1960. Studies on transference of bone. III. Manifestations of immunological tolerance to implants of homologous cortical bone in rats, Brit. J. Exptl. Path. 41: 443–51.

Nylen, M. U., Scott, D. B., and Mosley, V. M. 1960. Mineralization of turkey tendon. II. Collagen-mineral relations revealed by electron and X-ray microscopy. *In:* R. F. Sognnaes (ed.), Calcification in biological systems, pp. 129–42. Washington, D.C.: Am. Assoc. Adv. Science.

Selle, R., and Urist, M. R. 1961. Calcium deposits and new bone formation in muscle in rabbits, J. Surg. Res. 1:132–41.

Smith, D. M., Zeman, W., Johnson, C. C., Jr., and Deiss, W. P. 1966. Progressive myositis ossificans, Metabolism 15:521–28.

Russell, P. S., and Monaco, A. P. 1965. The biology of tissue transplantation. Boston: Little, Brown and Co.

Urist, M. R. 1953. Physiologic basis of bone-graft surgery, with special reference to the theory of induction, Clin. Orthop. 1:207–16.

———. 1965. Bone: Formation by autoinduction, Science 150:893–99.

Urist, M. R., MacDonald, N. S., and Jowsey, J. 1958. The function of the donor tissue in experimental operations with radioactive bone grafts, Ann. Surg. 147:129–45.

Urist, M. R., and McLean, F. C. 1952. Osteogenetic potency and new-bone formation by induction in transplants to the anterior chamber of the eye, J. Bone Jt. Surg. 34-A:443–70.

Urist, M. R., Wallace, T. H., and Adams, T. 1965. The function of the fibrocartilaginous fracture callus, J. Bone Jt. Surg. 47-B:304–18.

Van de Putte, K. A., and Urist, M. R. 1965. Osteogenesis in the interior of intramuscular implants of decalcified bone matrix, Clin. Orthop. 43:257–70.

Weiss, P. 1949. Differential growth. *In:* A. K. Parpart (ed.), The chemistry and physiology of growth, pp. 135–86. Princeton: Princeton University Press.

———. 1950. Perspectives in the field of morphogenesis, Quart. Rev. Biol. 25:177–98.

Zaccalini, P. S., and Urist, M. R. 1964. Traumatic periosteal proliferations in rabbits. The enigma of myositis ossificans traumatica, J. Trauma 43:344–57.

CHAPTER XIV

Healing of Fractures

Banks, H. H. 1965. The healing of intra-articular fractures, Clin. Orthop. 40:17–29.

Bauer, G. C. H. 1960. Epidemiology of fractures in aged persons. A preliminary investigation in fracture etiology, Clin. Orthop. 17:219–25.

Cooley, L. M., and Barker, A. N. 1955. The effects of transplantation and X-irradiation on the repair of fractured bones, Am. J. Anat. 102: 167–81.

Duthie, R. B., and Barker, A. N. 1955. An autoradiographic study of mucopolysaccharide and phosphate complexes in bone growth and repair, J. Bone Jt. Surg. 37-B:304–23.

Lacroix, P. 1953. Sur la réparation des fractures. Les mécanismes locaux, Compt. Rend. Soc. Internat. Chir., 15 Congr., pp. 553–63.

MacDonald, N. S., Lorick, P. C., and Petriello, L. I. 1957. Healing bone fractures and simultaneous administration of radioisotopes of sulfur, calcium, and yttrium, Am. J. Physiol. 191:185–88.

Nilsonne, U. 1959. Biophysical investigations of the mineral phase in healing fractures, Acta Orthop. Scand., *Suppl.* 37:1–81.

Ollier, L. 1867. Traité expérimental et clinique de la régénération des os et de la production artificielle du tissu osseux, 2 vols. Paris: Victor Masson et Fils.

Paget, J. 1860. The repair of fractures, *In:* Lectures on surgical pathology delivered at the Royal College of Surgeons of England, pp. 160–73. 2d Am. ed. Philadelphia: Lindsay & Blakiston.

Phemister, D. B. 1951. Biologic principles in the healing of fractures and their bearing on treatment, Ann. Surg. 133:433–46.

Pritchard, J. J., and Ruzicka, A. J. 1950. Comparison of fracture repair in the frog, lizard and rat, J. Anat. 84:236–61.

Stinchfield, F. E., Sankaran, H., and Samilson, R. 1956. The effect of anticoagulant therapy on bone repair, J. Bone. Jt. Surg. 38-A:270–82.

Urist, M. R., and Johnson, R. W., Jr. 1943. Calcification and ossification. IV. The healing of fractures in man under clinical conditions, J. Bone Jt. Surg. 25-A:375–426.

URIST, M. R., and McLEAN, F. C. 1941*a*. Calcification and ossification. I. Calcification in the callus in healing fractures in normal rats, J. Bone Jt. Surg. 23-A:1–16.

———. 1941*b*. Calcification and ossification. II. Control of calcification in the fracture callus in rachitic rats, J. Bone Jt. Surg. 23-A:283–310.

———. 1950. Bone repair in rats with multiple fractures, Am. J. Surg. 80:685–95.

———. 1953. The local physiology of bone repair with particular reference to the process of new bone formation by induction, Am. J. Surg. 80:444–49.

URIST, M. R., MAZET, R. JR., and McLEAN, F. C. 1954. The pathogenesis and treatment of delayed union and non-union, J. Bone Jt. Surg. 36-A:931–67.

CHAPTER XV

PATHOLOGIC PHYSIOLOGY OF BONE

ALBERS-SCHÖNBERG, H. E. 1907. Eine bisher nicht beschriebene Allgemeinerkrankung des Skeletts in Röntgenbild, Fortschr. a. d. Geb. d. Röntgenstr. 11:261–63.

ARNOLD, J. S. 1960. Quantitation of mineralization of bone as an organ and tissue in osteoporosis, Clin. Orthop. 17:167–75.

BARTTER, F. C. 1960. Hypophosphatasia. *In:* J. B. STANBURY, J. B. WYNGAARDEN, and D. S. FREDRICKSON (eds.), The metabolic basis of inherited disease, pp. 1367–78. New York: McGraw-Hill Co., Inc.

BASSETT, S. H., FIGUEROA, W. G., TUTTLE, S. G., and JORDAN, T. 1960. Metabolic studies in Cushing's syndrome. The effect of steroid withdrawal, androgen, and vitamin D on calcium, phosphorus and nitrogen balance, Clin. Orthop. 17:304–32.

BERGLUND, G., and LINDQUIST, B. 1960. Osteopenia in adolescence, Clin. Orthop. 17:259–64.

BERNSTEIN, D. S., SADOWSKY, N., HEGSTED, D. M., GURI, C. D., and STARE, F. J. 1966. Prevalence of osteoporosis in high and low fluoride areas, J.A.M.A. 198:499–504.

CALDWELL, R. A., and COLLINS, D. H. 1961. Assessment of vertebral osteoporosis by radiographic and chemical methods post-mortem, J. Bone Jt. Surg. 43-B:346–61.

DORFMAN, A., and LORINCZ, A. E. 1957. Occurrence of urinary acid mucopolysaccharides in the Hurler syndrome, Proc. Nat. Acad. Sci. 43:443–46.

DOW, E. C., and STANBURY, J. B. 1960. Strontium and calcium metabolism in metabolic bone diseases, J. Clin. Invest. 39:885–903.

Engfeldt, B. 1958. Recent observations of bone structure, J. Bone Jt. Surg. 40-A:698–706.

Engfeldt, B., and Zwetterström, R. 1956. Osteodysmetamorphosis foetalis. *In:* G. E. Wolstenholme and C. M. O'Connor (eds.), Ciba Foundation symposium on bone structure and metabolism, pp. 258–71. Boston: Little, Brown and Co.

Engfeldt, B., Zwetterström, R., and Winberg, J. 1956. Primary vitamin D resistant rickets. III. Biophysical studies of skeletal tissue, J. Bone Jt. Surg. 38-A:1323–34.

Erdheim, J. 1907. Ueber Epithelkörperbefunde bei Osteomalacie, Sitzber. Akad. Wiss. Wien, math.-naturw. Kl. 116, III:311–70.

———. 1914. Rachitis und Epithelkörperchen, Denkschr. Akad. Wiss. Wien, math.-naturw. Kl. 90:363–683.

Fanconi, G. 1955. Variations in sensitivity to vitamin D: From vitamin D resistant rickets, vitamin D avitaminotic rickets and hypervitaminosis D to idiopathic hypercalcemia. *In:* G. E. W. Wolstenholme and C. M. O'Connor (eds.), Ciba Foundation symposium on bone structure and metabolism, pp. 187–205. Boston: Little, Brown and Co.

Fawcett, D. W. 1942. The amedullary bones of the Florida manatee (Trichechus latirostris), Am. J. Anat. 71:271–309.

Fraser, D. 1957. Hypophosphatasia, Am. J. Med. 22:730–46.

Freeman, S., and McLean, F. C. 1941. Experimental rickets. Blood and tissue changes in puppies receiving a diet very low in phosphorus, with and without vitamin D, Arch. Path. 32:387–408.

Granstrom, K. O., and Hed, R. 1966. Idiopathic hypoparathyroidism with cataract and spontaneous hypocalcemic hypercalciuria, Acta Med. Scand. 178:417–21.

Harrison, H. E. 1957. The varieties of rickets and osteomalacia associated with hypophosphatemia, Clin. Orthop. 9:61–74.

Hinkel, C. L. 1957. Developmental affections of the skeleton characterized by osteosclerosis, Clin. Orthop. 9:85–106.

Hooft, C., and Vermassen, A. 1960. De Toni-Debré-Fanconi syndrome in nephrotic children, Ann. Paediat. 194:193–216.

Howard, J. E. 1961. The clinical picture of hyperparathyroidism. *In:* R. O. Greep and R. V. Talmage (eds.), The parathyroids, pp. 460–66. Springfield, Ill.: Charles C Thomas.

Hsia, D. Y. 1960. Inborn errors of metabolism. Chicago: The Year Book Publishers, Inc.

Jowsey, J. 1960. Age changes in human bone, Clin. Orthop. 17:210–18.

Leaf, A. 1960. The syndrome of osteomalacia, renal glycosuria, aminoaciduria, and hyperphosphaturia (the Fanconi syndrome). *In:* J. B.

STANBURY, J. B. WYNGAARDEN, and D. S. FREDRICKSON (eds.), The metabolic basis of inherited disease, pp. 1222–45. New York: McGraw-Hill Book Co., Inc.

LEONE, N. C., SHIMKIN, M. B., ARNOLD, F. A., STEVENSON, C. A., ZIMMERMAN, E. R., GEISER, P. B., and LUBERMAN, J. E. 1954. Medical aspects of excessive fluoride in a water supply, Public Health Reports 69:925–36.

MANDL, F. 1925. Therapeutischer Versuch bei Ostitis fibrosa generalisata mittels Extirpation eines Epithelkörperchentumors. Wien. Klin. Wschr. 38:1343–44.

MAXWELL, J. P., and MILES, L. M. 1925. Osteomalacia in China, J. Obst. Gynec. Brit. Empire 32:433–73.

MELTZER, W., LYON, I., MENSEN, E. D., and RAY, R. D. 1960. Radioisotope studies of generalized skeletal disorders. Vitamin D–resistant rickets, Clin. Orthop. 17:269–87.

MEYER, K., GRUMBACH, M. W., LINKER, A., and HOFFMAN, P. 1958. Excretion of sulfated mucopolysaccharides in gargoylism (Hurler's syndrome), Proc. Soc. Exptl. Biol. (N.Y.) 97:275–79.

MILCH, R. A. 1960. Studies of alcaptonuria: Inheritance of 47 cases in eight highly interrelated Dominican kindreds, Am. J. Human Genet. 12:76–85.

MOON, N. F., and URIST, M. R. 1962. Gerontal and gerontoid osteoporosis, Clin. Orthop. 23:269–82.

IX INTERNAT. CONGR. PAEDIAT. 1959. Symposium on bone metabolism, Helvet. Paediat. Acta 14:433–646.

NORDIN, B. E. C. 1960. Osteomalacia, osteoporosis, and calcium deficiency, Clin. Orthop. 17:235–58.

———. 1966. International patterns of osteoporosis, Clin. Orthop. 45: 17–30.

REIFENSTEIN, E. C., JR. 1957*a*. Anabolic steroid therapy for the protein depletion and osteoporosis induced corticoid hormones, Clin. Orthop. 9:75–84.

———. 1957*b*. Definitions, terminology and classification of metabolic bone disorders, Clin. Orthop. 9:30–45.

———. 1957*c*. The relationships of steroid hormones to the development and the management of osteoporosis in aging people, Clin. Orthop. 10: 206–53.

RICH, C., ENSINCK, J., and IVANOVICH, P. 1964. The effects of sodium fluoride on calcium metabolism of subjects with metabolic bone disease, J. Clin. Invest. 43:545–56.

ROSE, G. A. 1964. The study of osteoporosis and osteomalacia, Postgrad. Med. J. 40:158–63.

SAVILLE, P. D., NASSIM, R., STEVENSON, F. H., MULLIGAN, L., and CAREY, M. 1955. The Fanconi syndrome. Metabolic studies on treatment, J. Bone Jt. Surg. 37-B:529–39.

SMITH, R. W., and RIZEK, J. 1966. Epidemiologic studies of osteoporosis in women of Puerto Rico and southeastern Michigan with special reference to age, race, national origin, and other related findings, Clin. Orthop. 45:31–48.

SNAPPER, I. 1957. Bone diseases in medical practice. New York: Grune & Stratton.

SOLOMON, G. F., DICKERSON, W. J., and EISENBERG, E. 1960. Psychologic and osteometabolic responses to sex hormones in elderly osteoporotic women, Geriatrics 15:46–60.

STORSTEEN, K. A., and JANES, J. M., 1954. Arteriography and vascular studies in Paget's disease of bone, J.A.M.A. 154:472–74.

TROTTER, M., BROMAN, G. E., and PETERSON, R. R. 1960. Density of bones of white and Negro skeletons, J. Bone Jt. Surg. 42-A:50–58.

URIST, M. R. 1960. Observations bearing on the problem of osteoporosis. *In:* K. RODAHL, J. J. NICHOLSON, and E. M. BROWN (eds.), Bone as a tissue. New York: McGraw-Hill Book Co.

———. 1964. Accelerated aging and premature death of bone cells in osteoporosis. *In:* O. H. PEARSON and G. F. JOPLIN (eds.), Dynamic studies of metabolic bone disease. Oxford: Blackwell Sci. Publ.

URIST, M. R., and DEUTSCH, N. M. 1960*a*. Effects of cortisone upon blood, adrenal cortex, gonads, and the development of osteoporosis in birds, Endocrinol. 66:805–18.

———. 1960*b*. Influence of ACTH upon avian species and osteoporosis, Proc. Soc. Exptl. Biol. (N.Y.) 104:35–39.

URIST, M. R., MACDONALD, N. S., MOSS, M. J., and SKOOG, W. A. 1963. Rarefying disease of bone. *In:* R. SOGNNAES (ed.), Mechanisms of hard tissue destruction. Washington, D.C.: Am. Assoc. Adv. Sci.

URIST, M. R., and VINCENT, P. J. 1961. The excretion of various fractions of the 17-ketosteroids in the urine of women with postmenopausal or senile osteoporosis, Clin. Orthop. 19:245–52.

URIST, M. R., ZACCALINI, P. S., MACDONALD, N. S., and SKOOG, W. A. 1962. New approaches to the problem of osteoporosis, J. Bone Jt. Surg. 44-B:464–84.

VILLANUEVA, B. S., RAMSER, J. R., FROST, H. M., ARNSTEIN, A. R., FRAME, B., and SMITH, R . W. 1966. Tetracycline-based quantitative measurements of the tissue and cell dynamics in 10 cases of osteoporosis, Clin. Orthop. 46:203–17.

VINCENT, P. J., and URIST, M. R. 1961. The appearance of osteoporosis in ambulatory institutionalized males, Clin. Orthop. 19:245–52.

WHEDON, G. D. 1959. Effects of high calcium intakes on bones, blood, and soft tissue; relationship of calcium intake to balance in osteoporosis, Fed. Proc. 18:1112–18.

WILLIAMS, T. F., WINTERS, R. W., and BURNETT, C. H. 1960. Familial hypophosphatemia and vitamin D–resistant rickets, *In:* J. B. STANBURY, J. B. WYNGAARDEN, and D. S. FREDRICKSON (eds.), The metabolic basis of inherited disease, pp. 177–221. New York: McGraw-Hill Book Co., Inc.

CHAPTER XVI

EVOLUTION OF BONE

CARLSTRÖM, D. 1963. A crystallographic study of vertebrate otoliths, Biol. Bull. 125:441–63.

DENISON, R. H. 1963. The early history of vertebrate calcified skeleton, Clin. Orthop. 31:141–52.

GORDON, M. S., SCHMIDT-NIELSON, K., and KELLY, H. M. 1961. Osmotic regulation in the crab-eating frog (Rana cancrivora), J. Exptl. Biol. 38: 659–78.

LUND, R. 1966. Intermuscular bones in *Pholidophorus bechei* from the lower Ilias of England, Science 152:348–49.

ROBERTSON, J. D. 1954. The chemical composition of the blood of some aquatic chordates, including members of the Tunicata, Cyclostomata, and Osteichthyes, J. Exptl. Biol. 31:424–42.

ROMER, A. S. 1946. The early evolution of fishes, Quart. Rev. Biol. 21: 33–69.

SMITH, H. W. 1936. The retention and physiological role of urea in the Elasmobranchii, Biol. Rev. 11:49–62.

TARLO, B. J., and TARLO, L. B. H. 1965. The origin of teeth, Discovery 26 (September):1–7.

URIST, M. R. 1961. Calcium and phosphorus in the blood and skeleton of of the Elasmobranchii, Endocrinology 69:778–801.

———. 1962*a*. The bone-body fluid continuum, Perspect. Biol. Med. 6: 75–115.

———. 1962*b*. Calcium and other ions in the blood and skeleton of the Nicaraguan fresh water shark, Science 137:984–86.

———. 1963. The regulation of calcium and other ions in the serums of hagfish and lampreys, Ann. N.Y. Acad. Sci. 109:294–311.

———. 1964*a*. Further observations bearing on the bone-body fluid continuum. *In:* H. M. FROST (ed.), Bone biodynamics, pp. 151–78. Boston: Little, Brown and Co.

———. 1964*b*. The origin of bone, Discovery 25:13–19.

———. 1964*c*. Accelerated aging and premature death of bone cells in osteoporosis. *In:* G. H. Pearson and G. F. Joplin (eds.), Dynamic studies of metabolic bone disease, pp. 127–60. Oxford: Blackwell Sci. Pub.

———. 1966*a*. Humoral factors in prolonged inactivity, Ann. N.Y. Acad. Sci. (in press).

———. 1966*b*. Calcium and electrolyte control mechanisms in lower vertebrates, including some data obtained from the ratfish (*Hydrolagus colliei*). *In:* R. T. Smith, R. A. Good, and P. A. Miescher (eds.), Phylogenic approach to immunity. Gainesville: University of Florida Press.

———. 1966*c*. Comparative biochemistry of the blood of fishes. *In:* J. R. Olive (ed.), Current investigations dealing with biology of Elasmobranch dishes, Washington, D.C.: Am. Inst. of Biol. Sciences.

Urist, M. R., MacDonald, N. S., Moss, M. J., and Skoog, W. A. 1963. Rarefying disease of the skeleton: Observations dealing with aged and dead bone in patients with osteoporosis. *In:* R. F. Sognnaes (ed.), Mechanisms of hard tissue destruction, pp. 385–446. Washington, D.C.: Am. Assoc. Adv. Science.

Urist, M. R., and van de Putte, K. A. 1967. Comparative biochemistry of the blood of fishes. *In:* P. W. Gilbert, R. F. Mathewson, and D. P. Rall (eds.), Sharks, skates, and rays, pp. 271–85. Baltimore, Md.: The Johns Hopkins Press.

Index

Index